To

Dr. J. W. Christoffersen

from

Robert H. Harafson Jr. M.D.

MEDICINA CLASSICA

MEDICAL ECONOMY
DURING THE
MIDDLE AGES

MEDICAL ECONOMY

DURING THE

MIDDLE AGES

A Contribution To The History of European Morals
From The Time of The Roman Empire To The
Close of The Fourteenth Century

By

GEORGE F. FORT

[1883]

With an Introduction By

MORRIS H. SAFFRON, M.D., PH.D.

AUGUSTUS M. KELLEY · PUBLISHERS
NEW YORK 1970

First Published 1883
(London: B. Quaritch)
(New York: J. W. Bouton)

Reprinted 1970 By
AUGUSTUS M. KELLEY, PUBLISHERS
NEW YORK, NEW YORK 10001

SBN 678 03758 2
Library of Congress Catalogue Card Number
71-95625

Printed in the United States of America

Notes on George Franklin Fort (1843-1909) and Medical Economy in The Middle Ages

A good many years ago and after a lengthy search, I was finally able to acquire a copy of the present book. When a cursory examination indicated that both the publisher and the printer were American the thought occurred to me that possibly the author might also prove to be a native of this country. Turning to my trusted Allibone I found my man quickly (or so I then thought) in one of the supplementary volumes:

> Fort, George Franklin, M.D., b. 1809, at Pemberton, N. J. graduated at the medical department of the University of Pennsylvania in 1830; held various political offices in New Jersey, where he was elected governor, serving from 1850 to 1854 and was afterward a judge of the court of errors and appeals, The Early History of Freemasonry, as connected with the Ancient Norse Guilds and the Oriental and Mediaeval Building Fraternities, Phila., 1875, cr 8vo.

Now here was a rare specimen indeed, a typical Renaissance humanist in arid nineteenth century New Jersey, a man whose interests embraced not only medicine and law, but politics and scholarship as well. Certainly such a phenomenon deserved further attention, and at the earliest opportunity I continued my search in the library of the New Jersey Historical Society. Here I immediately ran into a problem: Appleton's *Cyclopedia of American Biography* gave Fort's date of death as 1872, but it seemed highly improbable that *Medical Economy* which bore the copyright date 1883 should have been published posthumously, eleven years after the author's death. I began to suspect a comedy of errors in the offing, a confusion of namesakes and dates. Nor was I mistaken. Further investigation revealed the true identity of our Fort as the nephew and namesake of the governor, and his junior by thirty-four years.

Having once settled the fact that the reference books were definitely in error in attributing *The Early History* (and the other writings as well) to the governor, I became increasingly curious about the personality of the younger man. Why did the nephew make no effort to point out these errors for subsequent editions of the reference works? Was he accessory to a hoax meant to enhance either the reputation of a revered relative or his own writings, or was his reticence merely a supreme example of self-effacement and lack of vanity? There is reason to believe that our author was amused at the confusion and chose deliberately to let the errors go uncorrected as evidence of complete indifference to public acclaim.

George Franklin Fort, the son of an itinerant Methodist preacher, John Fort, and his wife Elizabeth Emley, was born in the parsonage at Absecon, Atlantic County, on November 20, 1843. The family claimed descent from the Norman "Le Fort", captain of the bodyguard of William the Conqueror at Hastings, and it may well have been this romantic connection which first inspired George's lifelong involvement with the history and culture of the middle ages. The New Jersey Forts are said to have settled in the vicinity of Pemberton, Burlington County in 1695, and through the centuries numerous members of the family gained prominence in the political and professional life of the state. Thus at the time of our author's death in 1909 a cousin, John Franklin Fort, was serving as governor.

Having completed with unusual brilliance the classical courses offered at several public schools and the Pennington Seminary, George was sent at his uncle's expense on a *wanderjahr* to Europe. Here he quickly acquired fluency in French, Spanish and German. His brother states (and there is no reason to doubt him) that George audited certain law lectures at Heidelberg, and there developed a serious interest in Anglo-Saxon and other Germanic dialects. Several other visits to Europe were to follow, and the young student is said to have walked over large sections of the continent, often visiting obscure sites of romantic interest.

There is an appealing picture to be conjured up of this provincial youth from America, wandering leisurely through the old world, absorbing with his truly remarkable memory a mélange of long-forgotten dialects, and historical lore. Family tradition credits George with a knowledge of no less than seventeen languages. Brother John informs us "If no glossary was available he would dig out certain roots from dictionaries and in a short time would construct a grammar and glossary, and soon be reading the language as readily as English". Of the remarkable range of Fort's linguistic attainments there can be no doubt, but McDaniell rightly notes "the curious blend of Germanic idiom" which affected adversely his English style.

Apparently George was a true medievalist in a day when such studies were practically unknown in this country, and would undoubtedly have preferred spending his years in the cloisters of academe. However the exigencies of life prevailed and young Fort returned home to "read" law in the office of Abraham Browning of Camden, at that time attorney-general of New Jersey. In 1866 he passed the bar and three years later at the age of 26 became a counselor-at-law. But the prosaic practice of law could not hold indefinitely a mind already captivated by the most obscure details of medieval history and legend. During his visits to the various cathedrals of Europe Fort had developed a keen interest in the wandering fraternity of master-builders who were responsible for the construction of these marvels, and this in turn led him to a study of the origins of freemasonry. Having founded with a brother and friends at Camden a lodge of the Masonic order, he soon inaugurated a series of lectures on the origins of freemasonry, and these were so well received by large audiences that he was urged to publish the results of his research. *The Early History and Antiquities of Freemasonry* which appeared in 1875 was immediately recognized as authoritative, and "one of the most remarkable books that has ever been written concerning Freemasonry". The 11th editon of the Encycolepdia Britannica referred to the book as "instructive in throwing light on certain phases of Middle Age Life". In fact Fort's work is based solidly on adherence to the written records, and in it he made a serious effort to relegate to oblivion many fanciful tales which had gathered around the origin of freemasonry. After describing the debased state of the arts during the Dark Ages Fort carefully traced the early revival in architecture which took place in Lombard northern Italy through the mingling of Byzantine and Germanic artistic strains. He may have been the first to emphasize the role of the Comacini masters as the indermediate link between ancient and medieval builders; certainly this theory was later adopted and elaborated by Leader Scott and W. Ravenscroft. The publication of his first major work brought Fort into correspondence with scholars from all parts of the world; much additional data was later incorporated in two related works: *A Critical Inquiry into the Condition of the Conventual Builders and their Relation to the Secular Guilds of the Middle Ages* (1884) and *A Historical Treatise on Early Builders' Marks* (1885).

We turn now to the present book which provides the primary reason for our interest in Fort's biography. The circumstances leading to the actual writing of *Medical Economy* are not without interest. In 1866 the Medical Society of New Jersey, the oldest in the United States, was celebrating its first centennial. So little was then known of medieval medicine that a prominent physician was quoted as saying "that medicine had no history beyond Galen and Hippocrates". When Fort objected to this preposterous statement he was challenged by a committee "to write a history of the ancient cult". Either the task took much longer than he had anticipated or the work was frequently set aside in favor of the books mentioned earlier. At any rate is was not before seventeen years had elapsed that *Medical Economy* finally came off the press. When the book did appear "some of the critics thought he should literally translate the authorities, as but few could read the original; this he always refrained from doing as he claimed the quotation was the authority". Indeed the impartial reader will undoubtedly be impressed by the evidence of wide reading which is apparent on every page. Fort was never content to depend on secondary sources, but, whenever possible went directly to the original authority. Some of these texts were undoubtedly available at the splendid library of the Pennsylvania Hospital in Philadelphia, but his brother states that he had his own "extensive library in foreign languages", and on one trip to Europe he spent most of his time pouring over books at the British Museum, the Bodleian and the Vatican.

Of Fort's personal life we know something from the memoirs already quoted of a younger brother, John H. Fort, who was the publisher of several newspapers in South Jersey, and a local historian. George had married on March 2, 1869 Hattie R. Bird of Camden, with his father the Reverend John Fort officiating. Apparently there were no children of this union, nor is his wife listed as a survivor at George's death. There is good reason to believe that our author's health had always been precarious and this may account for a gradual withdrawal from society. "He was a modest and retiring man and any attempt to draw him out into a discussion was fruitless". However his range of interests was enormous, including not only "archaic research and antiquities . . . but science, belles-lettres, literature, mathematics, astronomy and ancient history". When compelled to speak "his erudition was apparent at once, and in a few minutes extemporaneously a magnificent oration was delivered upon any subject." John likened his brother to a "prophet speaking", and even allowing for the exaggerated reverence of a surviving younger brother we can readily understand how this withdrawn scholar, with his seemingly encyclopedic grasp of even the most recondite subject, must have aroused in his listeners a very real sense of awe. But as time went on the "chronic asthma" which is listed as the cause of death must have imposed more and more restrictions on his activities. He gave up law completely, and undertook various editorial assignments, writing for his brother's newspapers, for a Masonic paper, *The Keystone*, and finally for *American Notes and Queries, a* Philadelphia publication which appeared between 1886 and 1892, and which Fort edited during its last two years. For this periodical Fort wrote numerous articles and brief comments on the most esoteric subjects, usually, but not always in response to questions submitted by correspondents, indeed it is here that we can best gauge the enormous range of Fort's reading and erudition. Probably the best essay is again on his favorite subject of the master-builders of the middle ages, a few of whom he could now identify by name. Other sketches run the gamut from early Norse legal customs and literature to contemporary writers of the Iberian peninsula; from obscure 11th century poetry to Rosicrucians and the plays of Ibsen. He deplored as inadequate and misleading recent translations from French to Spanish and from Arabic to Portuguese. That Fort was a typical nineteenth century liberal of the same stamp as Henry C. Lea is obvious from a strongly anti-clerical tone which repeats itself throughout his writings. At one point he praises Galdos for an "aimiable and ennobling presentation of the persecuted Jewish race". It seems unfortunate that A. E. Bear and brother John did not (at least to my knowledge) carry out their expressed intention of collecting "from periodicals and newspapers his fugitive pieces".

In the remaining years of his life Fort became practically a recluse. Poor health combined with a compulsive urge to complete the projected (but never published) work on *Norse Mythology* caused him to shun society. In 1959 I spoke to Mrs. William F. Fort of Atlantic City, widow of George's nephew. She told me that he paid frequent and lengthy visits to their home in search of relief from his asthmatic attacks; and it was there that on March 30, 1909 he breathed his last.

As McDaniell points out George Fort was the first medical historiographer in this country who was not himself a physician. Aside from this distinction he was undoubtedly the only scholar in America then capable of undertaking so difficult and unusual an assignment as a history of medieval medicine. *Medical Economy* was published in a small edition, probably at the author's own expense. Certainly the book received little attention, although *The New York Medical Journal* gave it a pleasant but superficial review. Strangely enough the Surgeon-General's offprint of 1912 listing *Texts Illustrating the History of Medicine* does not mention this work, and this would seem to indicate that Garrison did not then know of its existence, although it was later included in the *Garrison and Morton.* Riesman quoted from Fort on at least five occasions and Cecelia Mettler also mentions the book. Nevertheless, it is safe to say that this source-book of medieval life and culture has yet to attain the recognition which its high standards of scholarship fully justify. Let us admit at once that Fort is not easy to read. His deliberate use of semi-obsolete words, his involved phraseology and sentence structure and a general tendecy to pomposity and redundancy are real impediments; nor are his data and interpretations always beyond reproach. Yet I know of no American or English writer on medieval medicine who brings to us a closer sense of familiarity with the original sources and texts. Futhermore, although medicine is the ostensible theme of *Medical Economy* Fort's vast knowledge flows over to illuminate many subjects only distantly related to the medical profession. Now that this book will become available to a wider public, I feel certain that it will at last receive the appreciation long overdue a neglected monument of early American scholarship.

MORRIS H. SAFFRON, M.D. Ph.D.

Rutgers Medical School
September, 1969

REFERENCES

1. Appleton's Cyclopedia, New York, 1887 Vol II,p. 507; entry remains unchanged in the edition of 1889.
2. Mackey, Albert G. *Encyclopedia of Freemasonry,* Revised and enlarged by Robert I. Clegg, with a Supplemental Volume by H. L. Hayward, Chicago, 1946 Vol. I, p. 363, Vol. III, pp. 1230-1.
3. Encyclopedia Britannica, 11th ed. "Freemasonry".
4. Fort, John Henry, *The Builder,* a Journal for the Masonic Student, Anamosa, Iowa, Vol. 4, 1918, pp. 171-2.
5. Street, Oliver Day, The Masonic Writings of George Franklin Fort, *The Builder,* Vol. 4, 1918, pp. 210-13.
6. Bear, A. E. *Miscellanea Latomorum,* London, Vol. 3 (New Series), 1916 pp. 12-14.
7. *New York Medical Journal,* Vol. 38, 1883, p. 237.
8. Riesman, David, The Story of Medicine in the Middle Ages, New York, 1936.
9. Mc Daniell, W. B. 2nd. *Bulletin of the History of Medicine.* Baltimore, 1959 Vol. 23, pp. 431-2. The author credits the present writer with first noting that Fort was an American and not the physician-governor of the same name.
10. *Camden Post-Telegram,* Tuesday, March 30, 1909.

MEDICAL ECONOMY

DURING THE

MIDDLE AGES:

A CONTRIBUTION TO THE HISTORY OF EUROPEAN MORALS, FROM THE TIME OF THE ROMAN EMPIRE TO THE CLOSE OF THE FOURTEENTH CENTURY.

BY

GEORGE F. FORT,

AUTHOR OF THE

"EARLY HISTORY AND ANTIQUITIES OF FREEMASONRY."

NEW YORK:

J. W. BOUTON, 706 BROADWAY.

LONDON:

B. QUARITCH, 15 PICCADILLY.

1883.

INQUIRER P. & P. CO.,
PRINTERS,
LANCASTER, PA.

PREFACE.

IN its general purpose the object of the treatise now published under the preceding title may be stated to be an historical inquiry into the practical effect upon social life throughout the period traversed, of that singular credence which involved preternatural agencies. Perhaps no portion of society of the Middle Ages reveals greater susceptibility to these curious influences than that appertaining to the preservation and restoration of bodily vigor.

It is especially the tendency of this disquisition to elucidate, so far as was deemed commensurate with the design of the work, the more significant relationship existing—as understood in the period designated—between supernal or angelic puissance and the human or physical constitution. Conclusions reached and indications drawn within the limits of the subject thus marked, will, it is believed, be found fully substantiated by reference to marginal annotations.

The labor required to collect, investigate, and suitably arrange indispensable material, will doubtless suggest itself to the reader. This toil was largely increased on account of the author's profession—to the bar—oftentimes necessitating his vigilant attention elsewhere; although the greater part of the authorities quoted, constituting an essential portion of his private collection, to some extent modified the more onerous perplexities of the task. In addition to these, through the courtesy of the officials of the British Museum, the writer was enabled to pursue his researches among the accumulations in that institution.

The scope of the work includes the narration of medical art under the Roman Emperors to Galen's time, and the modifying influences of the Alexandrine Schools in producing a regular system of magic cures. The progress of this interesting phenomenon, as a moralistic episode of the Middle Ages, concurrent with ancient medical text-books in the cloisters, and the gradual development of the science, aided by Arabic erudition in the Italian Universities, together with alchemy and astrology, are also subjected to careful scrutiny. Among other features of this history are treatises on the curative power of gems, incantations, etc., an elaboration of the condition and attempts to reform abandoned women at the several epochs, and curious facts touching the status of physicians of both sexes.

In the several appendices subjoined will be found original and ancient records used in the preparation of the text, and reproduced in full for more extended use. A complete analytical and subjective index concludes the work, in order to facilitate its utility.

GEORGE F. FORT.

CONTENTS.

CHAPTER VIII.

PAGE.

CHAPTER IX.

CHAPTER X.

CHAPTER XI.

CHAPTER XII.

CHAPTER XIII.

CHAPTER XIV.

CHAPTER XV.

CHAPTER XVI.

CHAPTER XVII.

CHAPTER XVIII.

CHAPTER XIX.

APPENDICES.

HISTORY

OF

MEDICAL ECONOMY

DURING THE

MIDDLE AGES.

CHAPTER I.

Conquest of Greece by Rome attracts Grecian Artists to the Metropolis—Arrival of Medical Men—Their Depraved Character—Romans Imitate the Hellenistic Medical Art—Its Use Claimed by Priesthood—Curative force of Number 3—Cato's Hatred of Greek Medicine—Inhuman Surgery of Archagathus—Immunities to Physicians in the Julian Age—Aesclepiades Celebrated Founder of a School of Medicine—Royal Rescript Favors the Professors of this Art—Thessalus and his Troop of Ambulatory Artificers—Hospitals—Celsus' Encyclopedia of Medicine—Professors of this Art Charged with Unscrupulous Deportment—Imperial Ordinance Published to Correct this—Compensation how to be Paid—The Free System—Rescript Reaffirmed in the year 321—The Archiatri.

BY the conquest of Greece through the invincible armies of Lucullus and Pompey, the capital of the Roman government remained without serious rival in the development of those arts which were to embellish the great metropolis. An immediate result of the subjugation of the Greek provinces, was the steady and ceaseless tide of artistic labor towards Rome, where the attraction of enlarged emoluments for their skill quickly drew these adventurers.[1] Mingled with the troops

[1] Cicero attests the inroads of Grecian learning, and admits its superiority. Tuscul., I. 1. Horace, Epistolæ, II. 1, likewise avows it in the following metrical formula:

" Graecia capta ferum victorem cepit, et artes
Intulit agresti Latio : sic horridus ille
Defluxit numerus Saturninus ; et gravi virus
Munditiæ pepulere," etc. V. 156.

of rhetoricians, philosophers[2] and poets, the first to present themselves in the universal concurrence, were numerous medical men.[3] Although the increasing luxury and consequent diminishing forces of the Romans necessitated more frequent recourse to the secrets of curative or preservative art subsequent to the Augustan era, it would appear that, as early as the time of Cato, foreign physicians were domiciled in the Latin emporium, plying their craft and obtaining enormous compensation for professional services.[4] The earliest of these stranger empirics in chronological gradation were Etruscans, whose skill in fine arts and science largely aided in aggrandizing and embellishing the ancient Roman metropolis.[5] However welcome may have been these ancient Etruscans, the subsequent arrival in Rome of adventurous Greek physicians, excited the anger and contempt of the illustrious Censor.[6]

The vigilant and political scrutiny of Cato had, prior to the total extinction of Grecian nationality beneath the ponderous pressure of victorious Latin arms, realized the possible domination of Hellenistic art on the people of Rome.[7] It may indeed be accredited that the specific charges urged by the distinguished patrician against Greek medical adventurers, were

[2] Rhetoricians, by an ancient decree of the Roman Senate, were liable to forcible expulsion from the city. Sueton. De claris Rhetoribus, cap. 1, seq., and Aulius Gellius, Noctes Atticæ, Lib. XV., c. 2. Touching the statue to Musa, Sueton. Vita Augusti, cap. 59.

[3] Dio Cassius, apud fin. Hadriani Historiæ, Lib. LXIX., cap. 22.

[4] Gaupp, De Professoribus et Medicis eorumque Privilegiis in jure Romano, p. 26.

[5] Tiraboschi, Storia della Letteratura Italiana, Tom. 1, p. 32. Egyptians also, at a later period, practiced medical art at Rome. "Adveneruntque ex Ægypto talium vitiorum medici, hanc solam operam afferentes, magna sua prædia." Plinii, Historiæ Naturalis, Lib. XXVI., cap. 3.

[6] Plinii, Historiæ Naturalis, Lib. XXIX., c. 6–7.

[7] Plutarch, Vita Catonis Major, c. 23, reproduces Cato's letter to his son on this subject. "Quid Athenis exquisitum habeam, et quod bonum sit illorum literas inspicere, non perdiscere, vincam. Nequissimum et indocile genus illorum: et hoc puta vatem dississe: Quandocunque ista gens suas literas dabit, omnia corrumpit." Plinii, op. cit., Lib. XXIX., cap. 7.

grounded in justice, and in exact accord with the unequivocally vile conduct of these surgical charlatans, who prostituted the dignity of a divine art to debased purposes of extorting gain from credulous and suffering patrons.[8] So long, indeed, as the cohesive principle remained intact and unshattered in those patriarchial elements with which the older families of Rome were constituted, the use and application of medicine passed under the immediate direction of the Pater-familias.[9]

The Latins appear to have had, in the more remote adoptation of medical practice, a comparative immunity from hierarchical intervention, within whose sacerdotal seclusion was absorbed and jealously maintained the custody of medicine and other arts.[10] At Rome, where exclusive practice of medicine was not claimed by the priesthood, Cato,[11] with other families, was especially zealous in the use and administration of this domestic medication, and on this subject drew up a short treatise, still extant.

Among sovereign remedies which he recommends as infallible, is the colewort or brassica. He held the Number Three in highest veneration, similar to the Phythagoreans, and hesitated not to commit to writing a magic formula by the aid of which luxations and fractures were readily cured.[12] This household system of medicine undoubtedly subserved an excellent and salutary purpose so long as the healthy vigor and robust

---

[8] Gaupp, De Professor. et Medic., p. 26. The statue to Æsculapius, described by Callistratus, Descriptiones, cap. 10, typified the sacred origin of medicine.

[9] Plinii, op. cit., Lib. XXIX., cap. 8.

[10] Salverte, Sciences Occultes, pp. 330–345, and Matter, Ecole D'Alexandrie, Tom. II., p. 19.

[11] De Re Rustica, cc. 2, 39 and 70. He appears to have possessed a receipt-book of curatives especially adapted to slaves and cattle. Cato advises the use of a certain preparation by which gourmands might indulge in excessive drinking without inebriety. Ib., cap. 156.

[12] "Et luxatum si quod est, bis die aqua calida foveto, brassicam tritam apponito, cito sanum feciet." De Re Rustica, cap. 157. Women were urged to freely use this specific: "Et si mulier eo lotio locos fovebit, nunquam ii virosi fieunt," etc. For advice to use magic words over luxations, vide Ib. cap. 160.

vitality of the Latins were left unimpaired by the luxurious influences which gradually crept into the metropolis upon the footsteps of invincible legions and victorious heroes, and preserved a probable existence down to the Julian age.

The earliest Greek medical operators, who as surgeons sought the Roman capital, where their services were gradually became indispensible, deduced their origin from the most degraded of the conquered populace—such for example as attended on the public and private baths, servants in the gymnasiums of the diverse municipalities of Greece, or assistants in the Hellenistic pharmacies.[13] Frequently these adventurers arriving from their country as slaves and bondmen, and quickly assuming at Rome the title and condition of freedmen, opened booths on the public streets and offered their wares for sale—medicaments prepared by themselves.[14] In these places the indolent and unoccupied assembled, for the purpose of whiling away the time, as in modern cafés and in quest of the news of the day.[15] Consequently the practitioners of medicine at Rome presented no unusual attraction for the gracious respect of the citizens; and as the healing art remained in the hands of freedmen, it was regarded indeed as a vile and degraded traffic, suitable only for the servile condition of slaves.

Greed of gold, unscrupulous of the means by which their thirst for gain might be satisfied, and totally depraved, these practitioners of a craft originally sanctioned under the attributes of divinity, soon acquired the uncompromising hatred of the Roman patricians, and among these M. Porticus Cato, the famed Censor.[16] So profound, indeed, was his con-

[13] "Sed quod ad medicinam attinet, eadem olim potissimum a servis libertisque exercitam esse satis constat." Gaupp, De Professor. et Medicis, etc., p. 16, and Buddeus, Critica Sacra, p. 22.

[14] Friedlander, Geschichte der Heilkunde, p. 137.

[15] Lessing, Geschichte der Medezin, Th. 1, p. 73; and Hirschel, Geschichte der Medezin, p. 72.

[16] Plutarchus, Vita Catonis Major, cap. 22, and Plinii, Histor. Naturalis, Lib. XXIX., cap. 6.

tempt for Grecian physicians, and Hellenistic art and science, that he wrote to his son, then sojourning at Athens, to avoid a searching study of those arts and letters, which, although desirable as an agreeable pastime, were utterly unworthy serious attempt of acquisition. Moreover, that the wily Greek would surely impress the Latin mind with corrupting influences; and as a transcendant instrument of debasement should be cited their physicians, who, as urged the indignant Roman, had sworn by mutual oaths to exterminate all barbarians by the potential means of medicine—and yet they require enormous fees from those whom they attend, in order the more readily to captivate the confidence of those selected as victims.[17] He concludes by emphatically interdicting his son the society of medical men.

Notwithstanding the hate of Cato seems exaggerated and ridiculous, it is but just to avow that the Greek physicians who came to Rome in his day and later were, as hitherto mentioned, men of intriguing character, and having the single object in view to acquire affluence, were not over scrupulous as to the means by which such fortune should be obtained.[18]

At least this is the portraiture sketched out by Galen.[19] From whatever causes were developed Roman hatred, it appears to have extended back as far as the second century prior to the Christian era, to the time of Archagathus, a Peloponnesian surgeon who came to the city of Rome in order to exercise his vocation. From the Senate he received the right of citizenship, Jus Quiritum, and a medical booth purchased for him with public funds. He subsequently lost the respect of the patricians and fell into contempt on account of the cruel

---

[17] "Tum etiam magis si medicos suos hunc mittet. Jurarent inter se barbaros necare omnes medicina. Et hoc ipsum mercede faciunt, ut fides iis sit, et facile disperdant. Nos quoque dictitant barbaros, et spurcius nos, quam alios opicos, appelatione fœdant. Interdixi tibi de medicis." Plinii, op. cit., Lib. XXIX., c. 7, and Plutarch, op. cit., cap. 23.

[18] Plinii Histor. Natural., Lib. XXIX., cap. 8.

[19] Galeni De Libris propriis, cc. 1 and 2.

nature of his surgical operations, which, as in more ancient times, consisted in cauterizing and incisions.[20]

On Archagathus was bestowed the dishonorable nomenclature of Vulnarius et Carnifex, as a just appellation for his reckless and indifferent cruelty.[21] Towards the age of Julius Cæsar, Greek physicians began to acquire greater privileges, induced, perhaps primarily, by the increasing interest and zeal for Grecian arts and letters, which swept into the capital like a rising flood, and gave a decided character to its ornamentation. One of the foreign surgeons who appears to have fully merited the considerate immunities extended to medical men at this period, Æsclepiades of Bithynia, succeeded in grounding his curative system upon a philosophic or scientific basis.[22]

Although this celebrated physician was not entirely exempt from the debasing tendencies which inspired the conduct, so reprehensible, of his associates, and caused them to have recourse to a nefarious charlatanism and shameful trickery, yet he was honored with the amity of the illustrious orators, Crassus and Cicero.[23] This generous friendship may have arisen from the graces of intellectual culture, the undisguised talents, and attractive personality of Æsclepiades. He came to Rome skilled in the highest exercise of elocutionary art, and in the pronouncing of philosophical discourses was already distinguished: more conversant with the fluency of rhetoric and precision of grammar, it had been his well-defined intention to open a series of public readings on dialectics.

After some years of flourishing success as teacher of elocu-

---

20 "Medicina cum ferro et poculo occurrit," Tertullian, Contra Gnosticos, cap. 1.

21 Plinii, op. cit., Lib. XXIX., cap. 6, and Gaupp, De Professor. et Medicis, p. 27.

22 "Mutata et quam postea Æsclepiades invenerat." Plinii Histor. Naturalis, Lib. XXIX., cap. 5. The deplorable state of medicine in Rome in Æsclepiades' day may be gathered from his professional treatises. Fragmenta, p. 37.

23 Cicero, De Oratore, II., c. 1.

tion,[24] then in high repute in Rome,[25] he abandoned the career of letters and devoted himself assiduously to the practice of medicine. The successful resurrection of an apparent cadaver excited popular interest, and advanced him to the apex of professional glory.[26] The medical economy of Æsclepiades involved largely the use of wine as a medicament and frequent baths of cold water as a sanitary element.[27] During the government of the Roman commonwealth by the Senate, in early ages, the practitioners of medicine possessed, as a body, no legal status, neither were they distinguished as artisans of curative craft from the more ignorant operative; but entirely abandoned to their own conscience and skill, to advance the art without the inducement of municipal recognition. The enlightened policy of Julius Cæsar elevated the character of the surgeons and physicians of the metropolis by conceding to them the franchises of citizenship.[28] By such judicious concessions, this valuable profession was at once made honorable in the eyes of the people, and henceforth stood forth as an avocation which had obtained the honors of specific illustration at the hands of the celebrated warrior and statesman.

Of the scholars of Æsclepiades, whose scientific abilities and skill aided in elevating the dignity of the curative art, Antoninus Musa was without question the most commendable, inasmuch as his successful treatment of the future Emperor Augustus, by means of cold lotions and saturated wraps, saved him from a dangerous illness.[29] Marcus Artorus, also a medical disciple of Æsclepiades, at the battle of Philippi cer-

---

[24] On the pharmaceutical writings of Æsclepiades, Fragmenta, p. 4.

[25] Quintill. De Orat., Instit., Lib. I., c. 1.

[26] Like skill attributed to Rhazes in 998, Leo Afric. De Med. et Philosoph., cap. 27.

[27] Fragmenta, p. 120, seq.

[28] Suetonius, Vita Julii Cæsar., cap. 42. Reserved from expulsion by Augustus, Ib., Vita Augusti, cc. 42 and 84.

[29] Plinii Natur. Histor., Lib. XXIX., c. 5, Livii Histor. Rom., Lib. CXXV., c. 2, and Sueton. Vita Augusti, c. 81. For this successful result a bronze statue of Musa was erected to commemorate imperial gratitude, Ib. cap. 19.

tainly contributed to the kind recognition which the profession ultimately obtained from this emperor, by saving his sovereign's life.[30]

Of all the prerogatives with which the devotees of medical science had been previously endowed, none equalled the grateful immunities of Augustus after his preservation by Musa. By a rescript promulgated by the imperial authorities, all surgeons were declared thenceforth forever free from public impositions of every description and enfranchised of all taxes, while at the court of the emperor a highly salaried surgeon was regularly engaged.[31] Such arrangements unquestionably largely aided in permanently establishing the social dignity of members of this avocation, and contributed to the development of medical science. Since the time of Julius Cæsar, great numbers of Greek surgeons were domiciled in Rome; about which period the names of several army surgeons of this nationality appear.

For example, Glyken is mentioned as a field-officer in that capacity to consul Pansa; while under the four first emperors, Cassius, who applied opium as a medicinal alleviant,[32] Calpentranus, Arruntius, Albutius, Reubrius, Q. Stertinus, and Charkles,[33] were selected as royal physicians. Themison of Laodicea, a scholar of the Æsclepidean system, and enjoying the friendship of Cicero,[34] prepared, it is stated, the earliest encyclopædia of chronic maladies.

[30] Lessing, Geschichte der Medezin, Th. I., p. 79.

[31] Gaupp, De Professoribus et Medicis eorumque Privilegiis in Jure Romano, pp. 50 and 52. Notwithstanding the acknowledged elevation of medicine through the favors accorded its professors by early emperors, frequent mention is made of manumitted and enslaved male and female physicians during the first and second century. Sueton. Vita Caligulæ, c. 81, and Ib. in Vita Nero, cap. 2.

[32] Lessing, Geschichte der Medezin, Th. I., p. 80.

[33] Plinii Historiæ Naturalis, Lib. XXIX., cap. 5, and Suetonius, Vita Tiberii, cap. 79. This physician discovered the symptoms of the emperor's sudden death by feeling his pulse, on leaving a banquet: existimans tentatas ab eo venas, Ib.

[34] Also his surgeon, Cicero De Oratore, I. c. 14. Themison was highly lauded by Thessalus. Galeni, De Methodo Medendi, Lib. I., cap. 2. Vide Plinii, op. cit., cap. 5.

Although in a measure successful in the treatment of diseases, this surgeon was severely satirized by Juvenal,[35] who accuses him of great slaughter in the experiments incident to the application of a new theory.[36] Such of the disciples of Themison as Scribonius Largus and Vectius Valens the surgeon of Claudius, who drew up treatises on subjects cognate with medicine, sought the popular remedies of peasants and huntsmen, whose superstitious notions they readily engrafted upon the body of their system. For instance, the liver of a dead athlete was a sovereign talisman against epilepsy.[37] Scribonius made the earliest known direct application of electricity to cure bodily infirmities, although the continuance of science within the close custody of the hierarchy in more ancient times, doubtless electrical forces were well understood and skilfully adapted to maintain the vulgar belief in the extraordinary potency of the sacerdoty.[38]

It was at this period in the first century that Nero, to distinguish his personal surgeon, Andromachus of Crete, the inventor of the Theriac,[39] from other medical men, elevated him to the dignity of Archiater, or Superpositus Medicorum.[40]

---

[35] Satira, Lib. X., v. 221.

[36] By a law of the German Empire, A. D. 1532, physicians experimenting with the lives of their patients are to be treated as highway robbers and broken on the wheel. Carciani, Leg. Barb, cap. 134; Tom. I., p. 543.

[37] "Item ex jecinore gladiatoris particulam aliquam datam consumat." Scribonii Largi Composit. Medic., cap. II., § 17. Ad comitialem Morbum. He adds, however, Ib., § 18: "Remedies of this kind are outside of medicine—extra medicinam—but are known to have been very successful." One of his maxims was that men were easier cured than women; boys, than girls; especially post complexum et devirginationem, Ib., p. 26. On Valens, vide Plinii, op. cit., c. 5.

[38] Salverte, Sciences Occultes, p. 98, and Goujet, Origin des Arts et Metiers, Tom. III., p. 104.

[39] Lessing, Geschichte der Medezin, Th. I., p. 84.

[40] Gothofredus, Comment in Cod. Theodos., Tom. V., pp. 52 and 55 seq. for the minute details concerning the character and significance of this dignity. Gaupp, De Professor. et Medic. in Jure Romano, p. 38, states that the name of Archiater is not met with in the Digestæ. Vide Du Cange, Med. et Infimi Latinit. sub v. Archiatria.

Notwithstanding the interest manifested by Augustus and his immediate successors to the imperial throne, in aggrandizing the social rank of physicians and surgeons, and although in numerous instances this watchful zeal was duly appreciated by those who used the enfranchisement thus granted, to advance more swiftly toward an affluent independence with reasonable scruples, there were, unfortunately, other devotees to the curative art who boldly abused the privileges of their condition.

Of these, Thessalus of Tralles at Rome[41] was indeed a typical example. Originally sprung from a servile source, by his sagacity, prudence, and impenetrable hypocrisy he attained to a wide-spread celebrity. In attendance upon his patients, he assumed the rôle of servant rather than physician. The economy of his medical art seems to have consisted mainly in permitting the diseased and infirm to act entirely to suit individual impulse and to force away other surgeons, of whose approaches he asserted himself to be a guard of undiminishing watchfulness. Living constantly among and accompanied by the vilest of the populace, such as cobblers, weavers, tailors, and equally degraded artisans, who idolized him,[42] he publicly and impudently taught a physician need know nothing of medicine; and that the entire body of this art could be readily acquired in six months.[43]

In his attendance upon the sick and infirm, Thessalus was invariably escorted by a troop of ambulatory artificers whom he denominated his disciples, similar to the ancient Pythagoreans. The noise and tumult which necessarily arose whenever this empiric appeared may be readly imagined,—a cus-

[41] On the fatal antagonism of his system to that of Galen, vide De Methodo Medendi, Lib. IV., c. 4.

[42] Friedlander, Geschichte der Heilkunde, p. 140, and Reynouard, Histoire de la Médecine, Tom. I., p. 401.

[43] Lessing, Geschichte der Medezin, Th. I., p. 84. Galen seems to have entertained a sincere respect for the medical acquirements of Thessalus' son, who lived on familiar terms with Archaeles, king of Macedonia, Com. in Hippoc. De Natura Hominis, Proem., Tom. XIX., p. 12.

tom which the pungent pen of a Roman satirist has made ridiculous.[44] To such extent indeed was the pompous insolence of Thessalus carried that he wrote a letter to Nero, boldly asserting that before him no physician had ever invented anything useful to the preservation of health or the cure of maladies, and that he alone had discovered the veritable, the indisputable accessory to such cases.[45] As an able diagnostician, Soranus under the emperors Trajan and Hadrian, accurately delineated the essential differences of diseases, and wrote a work on chronic maladies. But the most illustrious surgical skill emanating from the methodical system of Themison and the second century, may be justly claimed for Cælius Aurelianus, a Numidian, among whose merits the censure has been joined that his treatise on acute and chronic diseases[46] is a Latin version of Soranus. In this shape the writings of Soranus passed into the hands of the mediæval monks and were largely used by them in conjunction, as we shall hereafter observe, with Hippocrates and Galen, and the practical administration of medicine.[47]

To this epoch should be assigned the creation of the Valetudiarium and Veterinarium,[48] in order the more fittingly to treat infirm and disabled soldiers and their horses. Frequent notice is made of surgeons recruited for the Roman legions under the distinctive nomenclature of medici legionum and medici cohortum. Soranus, surnamed the younger, in order to distinguish him from the renowned physician of the first century, also a follower of the school of Themison, prepared

---

[44] Martial, Epigram, V. v. 9.

[45] Galeni, De Methodo Medendi, Lib. I., c. 2: Thessalus charges; "Hippocrates, inquit, noxia præcepta tradidit." Ib.

[46] Still extant under the title: Acutis Morbis et Chronicis Libri Octo. The methodical system pursued and described in Lib. V., De Morbis Chronicis.

[47] Richerius, Historiar. Lib. IV., cap. 50, in the middle of the tenth century, avows his acquaintance with the writings of Soranus.

[48] Celsus, De Medicina, praef., and Vegitius, De Re Militar. 2, 10; 3, 2, and Columella, De Re Rustica, cc. 7, 5, 14.

an elaborate work on obstetrical treatment—a branch of surgery anciently intrusted to female care,[49] and in the Roman Empire regulated by proper legislation.[50] Soranus the younger is known as the oldest historian of the curative art.[51]

Moschion, apparently his disciple, distinguished himself as author of the first treatise on midwifery, entitled De Mulierum Passionibus Liber.[52] He especially cautioned in such cases against an antiquated custom of severing the umbilical cord with a wooden or glass fragment, but in the place of these directed the use of a sharp blade.[53] Roman zeal for the cultivation of a taste for natural history and the kindred science of medicine, unattached to the inflexible demands of a system, influenced two illustrious citizens of the Empire to acquire the mastery of the entire range of contemporary sciences, and although subject to the curious superstitions of the age, to become profoundly skilled in a knowledge of the curative art. Of these, Aulus Cornelius Celsus, in the time of Augustus, carefully collated an enormous encyclopædia, of which the sections treating of medicine are yet extant, in eight books.[54]

In this work we possess a magnificent specimen of the intellectual industry and scientific research of an enthusiastic scholar; written in a vigorous but somewhat inelegant style, whose classical frame is at times so varied by unusual words as to render his meaning obscure, he has, notwithstanding, collected the wisdom of preceding ages and aggregated in exact adjustment the productions of learning of Hippocrates and

---

[49] Goujet, Orig. des Arts et Metiers, Tom. I., p. 216.

[50] XII. Tabul. Leg., c. V., § 4.

[51] Fabricius, Biblioth. Græca, Tom. XI., p. 714.

[52] Friedlander, Geschichte der Heilkunde, p. 144.

[53] Lessing, Geschichte der Medezin, Th. I., p. 87.

[54] This work, entitled De Medicina Libri Octo, appears to have been much used in the Middle Ages. MSS. copies of the tenth century are still in existence. Choulant, Prodromus Novæ Edit. Celsi, p. 2, asserts that Celsus' writings have suffered neglect on account of their unusual Latinity, which caused them to be left: "doctoque pulvere."

Æsclepiades, Archagathus,[55] and Israelitish[56] and Arabic[57] physicians.

The character of this encyclopædia may justly open a question touching the practical skill of its compiler, but the results of his labors embody the substantial elements of a science, and fully illustrate the epoch which produced the medical digest. A few of the operations described by Celsus may be reproduced. One of these, the cure of stammering by cutting the lingual ligament, although carefully portrayed,[58] was certainly known at the time of Cicero.[59]

An additional and not less instructive phase of Latin society is exhibited by the encyclopædist in a description of the means by which an artificial growth of the preputium may be produced, and further the so-called process of infibulation.[60] The other celebrated scholar, Cajus Plinius Secundus, of Como, on a more enlarged scale indeed than Celsus, and with almost superhuman forces, mastered the entire range of natural science and arts, and reduced them into encyclopædiac form. The thirty-seven books of Natural History present a marvelous repertoire of manifold wisdom, in the midst of which the vast culture and sagacious reflection of the illustrious author are the chief embellishment.

In its broadest signification Pliny was less a friend than an inactive enemy to physicians and surgeons, yet he aggregated, with the most scrupulous care and vigilant search into diversified sources and by the most untiring industry, such natural productions, endowed with medicinal properties, as should elicit the profoundest attention of coeval medical men.

Conforming to the elaborate development of social sensuousness, the principal object of the curative art seems to have

---

[55] Celsi, De Medicina, Lib. V., c. 19, § 27.

[56] Ibid, Lib. V., c. 19, § 11, and c. 22, § 4.

[57] Ibid, Lib. V., c. 18, § 16.

[58] Ibid, Lib. VII., c. 12, § 4.

[59] De Divinat. II., c. 46.

[60] Celsi, op. cit., Lib. VIII., c. 25, § 3.

been the invention of unusual remedies, strangely compounded, while the medical adviser assumed the attitude of a professional empiric.

Out of this system grew unnumbered receipt-books prepared for practical use, the value of which was attested by actual experiment. None of these collections attained the celebrity enjoyed by the comprehensive work on herbal medicaments of Dioscorides, a native of Anazarabia, in the reign of Nero. This compilation maintained its repute with undiminished vitality through the Middle Ages[61] to modern times.[62]

Among vegetable remedies known and recommended by Dioscorides, were ginger, pepper, aloes, sugar or saccharine matter, etc. In addition to these he suggests the free use of elm bark against pustular maladies. Rules were established by him for the prompt detection of adulterated medicaments, while his intimacy with metallic remedies, whose preparation evidently required an apparatus of fine implements, presupposes a knowledge of chemical action.[63] Influenced by the illogical credulity of his age, Dioscorides professed absolute faith in the curative property of dove's milk for opthalmic disorders, quartain fever and hysteria.

Under the beneficent rule of Trajan a slight progress was made towards a more exact understanding of the anatomical construction of the human body. Rufus of Ephesus wrote a treatise on anatomy which reproduces with accuracy the general condition of this science at that period.[64]

He used almost exclusively the labors of Herophile and

---

[61] Photii, Bibliotheca, p. 156, asserts that it was known positively to be in existence in the ninth century. In the year 1198 reference is made by the annalist of an English convent, to the presentation of a copy of Dioscorides De Virtutibus Herbarum; Swaphami, Coenobii Burg. Histor. sub an. cit. Dioscorides was also military surgeon under Claudius, Præfat. ad Dioscorid., p. 11.

[62] Lessing, Geschichte der Medezin, Th. I., p. 92.

[63] Lessing, Geschichte der Medezin, Th. I., p. 92.

[64] Celsus, De Medicina, Præf., p. 19, states the absolute necessity of dissecting *cadavera*, but declares vivisection as "crudele et supervacuum"—cruel and useless.

Eudemus, and sometimes dissected apes, in the pursuit of personal information.[65] The incessant struggle of more advanced physicians and theorists to give the economy of medicine a homogeneous form animated by the quickening principle of a spiritual essence, originated a sect of devotees, the founder of whom, Athenæus of Cilicia, a renowned Roman surgeon, in the year 68, declared that the dynamic force of the soul or pneuma was the indispensable element of medical art.[66] No new principles seem to have existed among the practitioners of this school; but, on the contrary, refuge was had to the expansive teachings of more ancient philosophers and sophists, whose fundamental theories were intimately interwoven with the pneuma or soul-power. According to their sophistical expounder, the eventualities of a healthy or infirm existence were without variance derived from the movable and fleeting essence designated, to which, as especially subject to its influences, Athenæus added the four elements, not in their material types, but in the dynamical qualities, which he classified as forces.[67]

Since indeed these material essences were so finely spiritualized, it became in the highest degree perplexing to know by what approaches a transition to the application of medical knowledge could be made practicable, consequently a Lacedemonian, Agathines, in the year 90, opened a new school of medicine, which while accepting the dynamic force of the pneuma or soul, boldly selected the choicest theories and best usages from other sects. From this systematic adaptation of alien schools arose the name of Eclecticism.[68]

To this system properly belonged Archigenes, the Syrian,

---

[65] Lessing, op. cit., Th. I., p. 89.

[66] Friedlander, Geschichte der Heilkunde, p. 143.

[67] Freidlander, Geschichte der Heilkunde, p. 143. Vide Osterhausen, Dissertatio exhibit. Sectæ Pneumaticorum Medicor. Histor. passim and Galen, Opera., Tom. VII., p. 57.

[68] Friedlander, op. cit., p. 144, and Lessing, Geschichte der Medezin, Th. I., p. 94.

a most distinguished and enlightened professor of this avocation about the year 100. His eminent abilities and cultured skill enabled him to practice the healing art at will throughout its entire scope, especially in its strictest pathological branches. Little is known of him beyond the gracious commendation of Galen,[69] although it is claimed that he was elevated to the archiatria by Hadrian as a just recognition of transcendent talents.[70] Touching his erudition and quarrelsome nature the attestation of writers is unanimous, while the just commendation is as freely awarded of brilliancy and subtilty of genius, especially in the accuracy of his distinction between diverse physical pain and the careful analysis of pulse and fevers.[71] Such of these diagnoses as portray the variations of pain, traced to its origin or seat, have escaped the dissipating effect of intermediate ages, and with slight modification are adopted as authority in the present day.[72] Not less valuable were the services of this scholastic in the department of surgery. His descriptions of the solution of the members and limbs of the human frame are portrayed by the hand of a skilled master.

As a sanitary precaution against poisoned wounds, he applied the simplest specifics, and is claimed to have been the first[73] who solved mineral waters into their chemical analyses, such for instance as soda, alum, sulphur, iron, copper, etc.[74] A pustular malady, in its general characteristics exhibiting a close identity with the variole, was sketched out so early as the beginning of the second century by Herodotus, a disciple of Agathinus. From this description his writings have often-

---

69 Galeni De Composit. Medic., Lib. II., c. 1.

70 Hieronym. Mercurialis, De Arte Gymnast, Lib. VII., c. 8.

71 Galen, De Composit. Medic., Lib. II., c. 1.

72 "Und ist mit einigen modificationen in die heutige zeichenlehre übergangen," Lessing, Geschichte der Medezin, Th. I., p. 94.

73 Lessing, op. cit., Th. I., p. 95.

74 Galeni Medicamenta ad Sugillationes, Tom. XII., p. 808. Ibid. Tom. XIII., p. 167.

times furnished possible argumentation to those advocating the high antiquity of the dread disease alluded to.[75]

Of all the medical writers and practitioners of the first century, Aretæus of Cappadocia was pre-eminently supreme in the remarkable exemption from that dwarfed spirit and narrowed intellectual culture which preferred the binding authority of theorists or zealous sectarians to the substantial advantages of extended experience guided by the salutary promptings of a healthy and robust reason. His eight books on the examination and treatment of chronic diseases[76] are indeed an example, marked for its rarity, especially in those remote times, of freedom from the servile guidance of schools, and above all noticeable for their tenacious fidelity to the systematic procedure urged by Hippocrates. Aretæus may claim the appellation of eclectic in its most elevated conception. As an anatomist, from whatever authorities he procured his knowledge of this science, he was unequivocally far in advance of the medical men of his day.

It would seem[77] that such information as he possessed touching the mysterious construction of the human body was obtained by personal dissection, whether of animals by comparative anatomy or otherwise, does not appear.[78] At all events, as a rare concession of illustrious worth, Aretæus has received the distinction to be declared equal to Hippocrates in the fidelity of describing maladies, and to his successor, Galen, in the exquisite discrimination of his judgment of diseases.[79]

---

[75] Lessing, op. cit., p. 95.

[76] The work of Aretæus, De Re Pharmaceutica, is lost, Kuhn Vita Aretæi, p. XIII., § 4. The exact age of this celebrated writer has been made the subject of dispute over a period of time not earlier than Julius Cæsar, nor later than Galen. He evidently belonged to a country open to Roman traffic, as he recommends for maladies Findanum, Falernum, and Signium wines, ib. p. 8.

[77] Lessing, Geschichte der Medezin, Th. I., p. 97.

[78] Anatomy of human *cadavera* in Celsus' day strongly probable, De Medicina. Prœm., p. 19.

[79] Friedlander, Geschichte der Heilkunde, p. 147.

Towards the middle of the second century, Iasistrohist Cassius, proceeding in the line of disciples of the renowned Agathinus, prepared a treatise which he denominated, "Eighty-four questions: Natural and Medicinal,"[80] in which the Aristotelian problems are closely imitated, but furnished a singular paucity of original notions germane to medicine. This work conveys a most disadvantageous idea of the condition of the curative art in his time. For instance, to the query, as one of a series for popular use, why a person sneezes twice consecutively, he responds: "For the reason that there are two nostrils."[81]

Up to the time of Galen trifling alterations had occurred in the ethics of the medical profession which increased popular esteem, or rendered physicians objects of general favor. Even the illustrious Galen himself distinctly charged[82] that in the favoring obscurity of a great metropolis it was easy for a citizen, and particularly a stranger, to conceal his name, his fortune, and his conduct; that a man was only judged by the splendor of his private life and the glitter of public display. If arrogant, he was assured of becoming the centre of zealous favor, and in case the debased deportment or the vileness of his origin were discovered, he could with perfect safety change his habitation to another quarter of the imperial city and renew his extravagances until misfortune again compelled him to migrate.

Such portraiture of the facilities with which impudent adventurers found access to favor corresponds with the scathing rebuke administered to the citizens of Rome by Ammianus Marcellinus,[83] for their eagerness to welcome strangers of recent arrival, make them the object of personal interest some-

---

[80] De Animalibus Medicinæ Questiones et Problemata, quæ hactenus non videre, 84 Questiones.

[81] "Sternutatio raro simul causa in promptu est; nunquam bina sint narium foramina," Iasistr. Cass. De Animalib, Quest. qu. 37, p. 28.

[82] Galeni De Libris Propriis, cc. 1 and 2.

[83] Gesta Roman. Lib. XIV., c. 6.

what ostentatiously for a period, and then abandon them to the perplexities of an adventurous career. In the midst of troops of adventurers who displayed their nefarious skill in the metropolis of the empire, when, as Galen judiciously observes,[84] it would be impossible to deceive in a provincial town, naturally enough the sanitary condition of the Roman capitol suffered by being abandoned to the first medical charlatan, who volunteered to cure impossible maladies, or sought to prolong these ills in order to extort pecuniary compensation. For a prolonged period it was impracticable to distinguish between the knavish empiric who prostituted the slight knowledge of surgery and medicine obtained in the bathing establishments or barber shops, to trafficking in the credulity of the sick and infirm, from the earnest and dignified professor who identified his practice with the system of Æsculapius or Hippocrates, or enlarged upon the experience of Æsclepiades.

No examinations, no legal proofs that the practitioner was possessed of suitable qualifications in the art of healing; in a word, absolute insecurity for the valetudinarian under the disorganized state of medical practice, maintained its supremacy until the time of Antoninus Pius.[85] Notwithstanding the apparent necessity for such legislative interference, almost a century and a half from the age of Julius Cæsar elapsed before the sick and infirm were protected by imperial edicts. As hitherto stated, in the earlier days of the Roman Empire, the judicious sagacity of Augustus, by direct intervention, advanced the science of medicine and its professors from the low degradation to which they had descended to a dazzling and abrupt transition of royal favorites.[86]

Especially was this difference publicly marked between the comparative abject servility of earlier surgeons, and the titled

---

[84] Galeni, op. cit., cc. 1 and 2.

[85] On the mendacity and avaricious charges of the Roman medicists in Hadrian's age, vide Dio Cassius, Histor., Lib. LXIX., cap. 22.

[86] Gaupp, De Professorib. et Medicis in Jure Romano, pp. 38, 76. Slight illustration of early medical writers, Cuvier, Hist. des Sciences Naturelles, Tom. I., p. 366 seq.

honor bestowed upon Andromachus of the Archiatria Palatina.[87] This dignity, with which the imperial surgeons were honored—Archiatri Sacri Palatii[88]—involved the franchises of guildic community whose aggregate number and positions were, as other regal arrangements of the court, liable, under changing emperors, to sensible modifications.

In the fourth century the title and rank distinction of the Perfectissimi Dignitatis conveyed to these ennobled personages valuable immunities, sometimes of a descendable nature inherited by their posterity.[89] Added to this was the illustration of the Comitava or Comitis dignitas, sacri palatii, equivalent to the honorary position of Count, divided into three classes or grades, of which the Comitava Primi Ordinis, usually addressed as praesul spectabilis, was the personal medical adviser of the emperors, although the whole were indifferently styled comites archiatrorum, or archiatri sacri palatii.[90]

It is doubtless beyond controversy[91] that this honorable distinction accorded Andromachus as physician to Nero was not borne by Galen under the philosophic emperor Marcus Aurelius, although conferred by Pagan rulers. To the epoch of Christian emperors must be assigned the first serious attempt at medical organization. Accompanying this dignity were invaluable prerogatives and profitable immunities, exemptions from public assessments and burthensome duties, such for example as acceptance of guardianship.[92] At a later date the comes archiatrorum was placed on equal footing with the Vicar and Dukes of the Empire. The rapid increase of surgeons ultimately necessitated their subjection to a supreme head whose

[87] Gaupp, op. cit., p. 41 seq.

[88] Gothofred, Cod. Theodos., Tom. V., pp. 27–48, and Ibid, Tom. II., p. 106, seq.

[89] Gaupp, De Professor, et Medic, p. 76, § 7.

[90] Gothofred, op. cit., Tom. V., p. 52 seqq. Dujardin et Peyrille, Hist. de la Chirurgie, Tom. II., p. 715.

[91] Reynouard, Hist. de la Médicine, Tom. I., p. 403.

[92] This exemption of tutelage was caused by Hadrian, Gaupp, op. cit., p. 79; XIII. Codex Theodos. Tit. III., Lex 1.

dignity was designated as Archiatrus popularis, whose official duty was identical with that of physician salaried by the state.

These medical professors were invariably selected by favor or influence of a provincial governor for candidature to such citizens and landed proprietors as exercised electoral rights.[93] In addition to this, a confirmation by the college of older archiatri populares was imperative, of whom according to a rescript of the emperor, Valentinian, in the year 364, and of Valens, in the year 370 respectively, at least seven affirmative votes were necessary to ratify such choice.[94]

However, in order that such immunities might not excite the disaffection of other civilians of the empire, entire freedom from assessments was not conceded to the whole body of surgeons, but restricted alone to the Archiatria.[95] For the purpose of establishing the lawful privileges of this profession on a basis of correlative duties and substantial enfranchisement, the Emperor, Antoninus Pius, about the middle of the second century, issued an edict in the nature of a medicinal ordinance,[96] which prescribed that cities of the smallest number of inhabitants should be entitled to have and maintain five physicians absolutely freed of all and every kind of public service—intermediate towns and villages were privileged to possess seven,[97] while the largest metropolitan cities obtained an enlargement of privileged surgeons to the number of ten,[98] within the municipal limits of the great capital of the empire, each of the fourteen regiones or departments was allowed a

---

93 Codex Justinian. Tit. 52, Lex 9.

94 XIII. Cod. Theodos., Tit. 3, Lex 9.

95 "Archiatri omnes et ex-Archiatri, ab universis muneribus," Cod. Theodos. cit. Lex 2. Gaupp, De Prof. et Medic. p. 50, for additional information on this subject.

96 X Codex Justinianus, Tit. 52.

97 Under Alexander Severus there were seven of these highly privileged personages, Lampred, Vit. Alex. Severi, c. 42. This number was reaffirmed by the Valentinian rescript of the year 370, Cod. Theod., cit. Lex 9.

98 Codex Justin, cit. Tit. 52.

medical attendant whose salary was fixed by law.[99] The Vestals and Gymnasia also were permitted a surgeon regularly employed at public expense.[100]

Compensation for professional skill under these venerable edicts consisted chiefly in kind—annonaria commoda,[101] or natural productions, sometimes in money, or its current equivalent, usually styled salara, as distinguished from the honorarium or fees, which more accurately applied to the law than to medicine.[102] Upon the principle of receiving state or government patronage, the members of the medical profession thus salaried, were likewise obliged to perform certain functions partaking eminently of a public service. Consequently it was their official duty to render attendance to the impoverished without compensation,[103]—a system of absolute necessity arising from the disinclination of the affluent and aristocratic Roman to subject himself to the hazard of infection, which was carefully avoided on the return of the messenger to sick friends, by compelling the servant to bathe himself before presenting the result of his inquiry.[104]

In the case of wealthy sufferers the departmental physician was allowed to demand his honoraria or fees. To these emoluments arising from their official position, municipal surgeons added the substantial benefits of the dignified Archiatria, by an exemption from such imposts as military obligations, quartering, forced loans, etc.[105] In matters requiring ju-

[99] XIII. Codex Theodos., Tit. 3, Lex 8. Lampridius, Vita Alex. Severi, c. 42, mentions a salaried physician of that emperor's reign. Vide Gaupp, De Profess. et Medic., p. 52. On public salaries, Codex Theodos., cit. Tit. IV., Lex 1.

[100] Codex Theodos., cit., Lex 8.

[101] Ibid.

[102] The facility with which the young lawyers secured the confidence of their clients to advise them into expensive litigation, where the client became poor and the lawyer rich, is noted by Am. Marcellinus, Gesta Rom., Lib. XXX., c. 4.

[103] Codex Theodos., cit. Lex 8.

[104] Ammian. Marcellinus, op. cit., Lib. XIV., c. 6.

[105] "Eosdem ad militiam minime comprehendi placeat: sed nec hospites militares recipiant." Ibid., Lex 10.

dicial inquiry, these privileged officials were favored with a speedier disposition of their causes before the tribunals where they were called,—a prerogative of the highest value under the complicated and tedious proceedings which the Roman barristers were skilled in prolonging in exact proportion as the gilded honoraria of the clientièle failed to stimulate his judicious hesitancy.[106] Antoninus Pius enacted that these public surgeons should be exempt from summary process, and interdicted the issuance of a warrant against them to bring their body before the courts.

This rescript was reaffirmed by Constantine in the year 321, under a most exemplary fine and the penalty of being flayed alive.[107] The deduction from the Antonine ordinances and their succeeding reproduction, that the archiatri in some way were associated with a perfunctionary duty of inquiring into the qualifications of medical students prior to their admission to the profession, seems to come within the intention of these several edicts.

Upon what plan such examination was conducted, or tuition in the art given, if at all, is in the highest degree uncertain, and involved in great obscurity.[108] It is indeed improbable that these disciples, the future devotees of a vacillating science, possessed the appliances of regularly organized institutions of learning, but rather followed the instruction of a selected teacher, and aggregated themselves to hear the accumulated wisdom of personal experience, joined perhaps to the frail and timid outlines of a scientific system. From the careful legislation promulgated during several centuries, having direct reference to the ability of medical professors, it is equally clear that no surgeon or physician was permitted to teach the prin-

---

[106] Ammianus Marcellinus, Gesta Rom., Lib. XXX., c. 4.

[107] XIII. Codex Theodos., Tit. III., Lex I.

[108] This much may be gathered from the rescript of 364, Codex cit., Lex V., which decrees: "Quisque docere vult, non repente nec temere prosiliat ad hoc munus," etc.

ciples of his art without consent of the surgical commune,[109] and to a certain extent the ranks of the avocation were recruited only from such as passed triumphantly a prescribed examination.[110]

Violation of this regulation caused a forfeiture of two thousand drachms. In this arrangement making it mandatory for the collegiate members to impart medicinal knowledge to students, nothing further can be gleaned from the law which directs it, than a puzzled inquirer applying to a public official for mental assistance which strict legislation compelled him to give. The scholars in the law schools of the empire were far more carefully tutored.[111]

Government subsidy was freely employed in maintaining these institutions and filling professorial positions with the most cultured talent which the vast extension of imperial authority could procure.[112] By the policy of the Antonine enactment, midwives, wound-dressers, and dentists were also placed under the vigilant scrutiny of the college of surgeons.[113] Notwithstanding this medical constitution, infrequent fragments reward research into the civil law, which would warrant the assumption that a regular governmental organization existed for the propagation of this science. Towards the commencement of the third century an edict was promulgated which rendered medical practitioners responsible for the pathological treatment of their patients,[114] and forbid for such

---

[109] "Sed judicio ordinis probatus decretum curialium mereatur, optimorum conspirante consensu." XIII. Cod. Theodos. Tit. III., Lex 5.

[110] Cod. Justinian. Tit. 52.

[111] Law students were required to give their first years to the study of Greek letters, Heineccius, Juris Civilis Romani, Tom. I., cap. 154.

[112] Berytus was the most distinguished law school of the empire, Eunapius, Vit. Sophistor. v. Proehaersius, p. 490, and was exempted from the edict closing these schools, Heineccius, op. cit., Tom. I., cap. 387.

[113] Cod. Just. cit., Lib. 52.

[114] A similar custom of more ancient date, Goujet, Origin des Arts et Métiers, Tom. II., p. 229. Physicians punished if their patients were not cured according to Egyptian rules, Gothofred, Com. in Cod. Theod., Tom. V., p. 35.

purpose the application of magic.[115] Permission, however, restoring certain remedies of a magical nature was subsequently decreed by Constantine the Great, in the year 321.[116] In order to hold in subjection a tendency so rapidly increasing at this epoch, to apply supernatural curatives, a law was passed adjudging the delinquent to the death penalty.[117]

At a comparatively early period of the Roman government, legislative ordinances compelled the presence of selected midwives in all cases demanding a judicial investigation.[118] To these statutes other laws were added for the preservation of human life against the prevailing crime of infanticide and exposure of new-born children.[119] Idiots, or such as were mentally unsound according to the economy of the Twelve Tables,[120] passed to the custody of relatives, who subsequently were required to secure for them their privileges, possessions and official dignities.

A wife's insanity or imbecility of three years, or a five year's idiocy of a husband entitled the aggrieved party to a separation in case no inculpation by way of recrimination was made.[121] One of the most singular and, in its moral influences on the Roman society, destructive customs, traceable to the deteriorating presence of Greek refugees in the imperial metropolis, was the universal extension of the emasculation of

115 Am. Marcellinus, Gesta Romanor. Lib. XVI., c. 4.

116 IX. Codex Theodos., Tit. XVI., De Maleficiis, Lex 3.

117 Spartianus, Vita Caracallæ, sub. fin.

118 Consult Gothofred, ut sup., p. 35, col. 5, for the status under the law of the earlier and later Roman midwives.

119 V. Codex Theodos., Tit. VII., De Expositis, Lex 2; and IX. Cod. Theod., Tit. XIV., De Sicariis, Lex 1. On the prevalence of this crime Juvenal, Satira VI., says: "Quae steriles facit atque homines in ventre necandos." Also, Tertullian, ad Nationes, Lib. I., c. 15.

120 Leg. XII. Tabul., Lex 5.

121 Another cause of divorce, added by Constantine in the year 331, was the accusation and proof of a wife being Medicamentariae, evidently a medical sorceress, III. Cod. Theod., Tit. XVI., Lex 1.

infants to qualify them for a terrible servitude.[122] The mortality of this deformity may be conjectured when it is stated that only one of thirty survived the mutilation. Severe laws were promulgated by the emperors in order to totally extinguish this inhuman practice.

Impartial justice should record as a commendation of Domitian that one of his earliest imperial acts was a decree interdicting this crime.[123] The penalties inflicted for violating these ordinances were emasculation by way of retaliation, banishment, and confiscation of the offender's personal possessions. In the time of Justinian extraordinary efforts were made to crush out beneath the ponderous influences of statutory edicts the widely indulged criminality of Paiderastia.[124] None of the habits surviving the wreck of Grecian nationality seem to have been more promptly imported into Rome, with the increasing afflux of adventuresome spirits, than this social immorality.

It can not be presumed that the earlier Roman emperors struggled to successfully impede its progress and check the frightful demoralization following in its advance. Christian rulers doubtless vindicated personal dignity in erecting a legal barrier against it, and sought to make such interdict vital by subjecting the guilty to castration. Under the Roman law, poisoning was regarded as more heinous crime than forcible homicide, and notwithstanding the frequent occasions which compelled judicial investigation into the unlawful use of poisons, the means of testing their presence was totally divested of accurate detection.[125] In general, toxicology was divided into

[122] As late as the year 949 merchants from France sought the Grecian empire, and bought eunuchs of youthful age and sold them in Spain at lucrative prices. Liutprand, Antapodos. Lib. VI., c. 6.

[123] "Vetent in ejus contumeliam, ne quis in postremum intra fines Romani imperii castraretur." Xiphil. in Domitian, p. 255. Philostratus Vita Apol. Tyan., Lib. VI., c. 42.

[124] Lecky, History of European Morals to Charlemagne, Vol. II., p. 311, may be advantageously consulted.

[125] The example of Mithridates certainly influenced many of the citizens of declining Rome to inquire into this science. Fabricius, Biblioth. Græca, Tom. XIII., p. 344.

two branches by legislation, the bonum venenum, et malum, noxious, and the innocuous or beneficial poison.[126] It may be added here, as connected with the subject, that toward the conclusion of the third century the first indications present themselves of the existence of a class of citizens to whose vigilant care was confided the preparation of medicaments ordered by attendant physicians.[127] Prior to this epoch, for several centuries it had been the most usual method for medical practitioners to compound their own medications and administer them to their suffering patients.[128]

Regular pharmacists were entirely unknown, excepting perhaps the Herbarii, who disposed of their commodities at trifling prices in the public markets or along the highways. There was indeed a class of medicinal compounders whose operations were mainly limited to the preparation of such remedies as experience or current rumor suggested to be most suitable for popular merchandise, and offered their wares upon benches or stalls, in booths denominated apothecæ, directly for public sale.[129]

For this reason they were classified as medici sellurlarii, but the market vendors of medicaments by outcry were known as medici circumforanei, or circulatores. Physicians themselves, in preparing proper remedies for their sick, usually purchased pharmaceutical supplies from these medicinal merchants. At the period under notice, the functions of the apothecary began to assimilate with the duties of a modern druggist, although comparison between the obscure predecessors of the present pharmacists would be manifestly unjust. Prior to this epoch, medical men were accustomed to the assistance of their disciples, or servants, in suitably compounding prescribed re-

---

126 In this sense it is used by Lucan, Pharsalia, Lib. VIII., v. 690 seq., sic:

"Putris ab alto
Humor, et infuso facies solidata veneno est."

127 Oribasius, in tres Euporiston Libros, ad Eunapium Præfatio.

128 Dujardin et Peyrille, Histoire de la Chirurgie, Tom. II., p. 61; and Galen, De Compos. Medicam., Lib. VI., c. 1.

129 Dujard. et Peyrille, op. cit., p. 60 seq.

ceipts,[130] or perhaps in the emergencies continually arising in the career of practitioners, such remedies doubtless were constantly ready for physicians, surgeons, and others.[131] Medicaments thus compounded for the immediate necessities as simple curatives, and sold publicly in the booths skirting the streets of Rome or Athens, were not, in the technical signification, chemical compositions, although a knowledge of this science was extant at this period.[132]

---

130 "L'état ni les fonctions de l'apothicaire n'existoient point alors; chaque medécin préparait lui-même, ou faisoit préparer par ses disciples et ses serviteurs," Dujardin et Peyrille, Histoire de la Chirurgie, Tom. II., p. 60 seq.

131 Ibid, p. 60.

132 Goujet, Origin des Arts et Métiers, Tom. III., p. 104.

CHAPTER II.

Galen: His Beneficial Influence on Medicine—Its Deplorable State Prior to his Time—Arrests a Complete Downfall—Degeneration of the Empire at this Epoch—Galen, a Native of Pergamos, in the second Century—First Studies Philosophy—Is Directed by a Dream to Devote Himself to Medicine—Goes to Alexandria for Anatomical Instruction—Is Domiciled at Rome—Excites Envy of the Professors There—Leaves this City on Account of their Indignities—No Complete Method before his day—Galen Conversant with Mosaic Doctrines—Revered with Honors almost Divine.

IMMEDIATELY preceding the era of Galen, medical science had succumbed to the deplorable influences of contentions and zealous sects. While empiricism and speculation sought to mutually crush each other in order that the dogmatic and triumphant rival might pass onward upon an unimpeded plane of success, the more correct principles of the curative art gradually decline before its own expounders. Galen's advent arrested the complete downfall of medicine as a scientific method of cure, and maintained through his authoritative exposition, the outlines at least of treating maladies for centuries upon the basis of a reasoning philosophy. At this epoch the Roman empire had extended its domination by invincible armies from the outlets of the Rhine to the deserts of Africa, from the pillars of Hercules, the ancient Ultima Thule, to the Caspian Sea and the Persian Gulf. All the glittering splendor of this mighty exterior was impotent to arrest the disintegrating effects of internal decay, and the quickening principles of dissolution which had so insidiously crept in behind the burnished chariot wheels of Julius Cæsar.

Barbarism permanently domiciled by the side of a corrupting Grecian civilization, mournfully predicted and justly forecast by the inflexible Censor of Republican Rome,[1] mutually

[1] Livii Histor. Naturalis, Lib. XXIX., cap. 7.

strained the social fabric by their perverted humanity,[2] which dissipated the martial essence of the colossal government. The reigns of Trojan and the Antoninii, indeed, stand out in marked distinction to the remorseless tyranny of their predecessors, but succeeding rulers wasted the beneficent influences by imperial excesses.

Rude and insolent pomp, inordinate vanity of an unhealthy social existence, swelled the immorality of the affluent Roman into unnatural indulgences and abandoned the popular impulses to the vilest criminalities. Within the narrowed limits of royal authority no barrier was elevated to resist the ceaseless shocks which weakened the moralistic cohesion of society —everywhere apathetic indifference to the restrictive forces of religious principle and a palpable inertness against elevating the mind to the inspiration of sublime virtue. Naturally enough, the social debasement of the great metropolis radiated through the smaller cities, and finally corrupted the villages and hamlets of the empire, where vigilant prætors gathered up budgets of gossip and news of suspected citizens for the imperial ear.[3] The immediate result of this deplorable degradation manifested itself in dwarfed art[4] and a lamentable decay of medical science.

Although the ponderous weight of unnatural vices and startling immoralities weakened the nervous energies of the citizens of declining Rome, there were bold and brilliant men of great culture who scourged the terrible excesses of their

---

[2] The Historiæ Augustæ Scriptores Sex., and the fragmentary writings of Ammianus Marcellinus draw a picture of the awful depravity of the third and fourth centuries, only equalled by the brutal ferocity of the Roman soldiery. The following military chant attests this inhumanity: "Mille, mille, mille, mille, mille, mille decollavimus; Unus homo mille, mille, mille, mille, mille, decollavimus; Mille, mille, mille, vivat, qui mille, mille occidit; Tantum vini habet nemo, quantum fudit sauguinis." Vopisci, Vita Div. Aureliani, cap. 6.

[3] Plinii Epistolæ ad Trajan. Lib. X., Epp. 30, 40–42.

[4] The superstitious ferocity of Tiberius in summarily executing a skilled artificer, is sagely commented on by Pancirolus, Rerum Memorabil. sive Deperdit., Tom. I., p. 126 seq.

degraded contemporaries and cauterized their infamies with bitter satire, or laid bare the moral depravity of the Latin race, in glorifying the virtues of the illustrious heroes of antiquity. Such mirrored reflections were reproduced under the burning stylus of Plutarch; painted in the brilliant hues of impressive truth by Suetonius in his "Lives of the Cæsars"—while Cornelius Tacitus unveiled the sombre and hideous corruption which disintegrated the fast waning vitality of civil life and appealed to the dispassionate severity of the tribunal of the universe.

Poetry, incapable of original inspiration, found nourishment in the calamitous debasement of the age, and nerved the hand of Juvenal, Petronius, and Lucan, with the unsparing scourge of satire. Philosophy, which under the earlier Romans[5] and the later emperors, had never found subjects of independent and scholastic research, shackled with dilettantism, was associated with trickery and superstitious usages.[6] While the devotees of Aristippus and Epicurus practiced their sensuous teachings in the most ordinary details of life, or sought the abandonment of a bold skepticism, the merited exercises of the Stoa found infrequent but illustrious advocates in Seneca and the emperor Marcus Antoninus, who struggled with unavailing example to oppose the debasing tendencies of the period.[7]

Other causes were co-operating to modify and perhaps precipitate a dissolution of heathen philosophy, and newer elements were actively engaged in supplanting the Paganistic doctrines by the subrogation of a youthful and vigorous rival,

---

[5] Cato, in the exercise of censorial functions, ordered Grecian philosophers domiciled at Rome to return to their own country. Gaupp, De Professor. in Jure Romano, p. 22 seq.

[6] Rhetoricians appear to have shared the fortunes of their confreres, the philosophers, and were ordered into exile, Suetonius, De Claris Rhetoribus, Lib. I., cap. 1.

[7] Julius Capitolinus, Vita M. Anton. Philosoph., cap. 1, awards him the panegyric of being the most enlightened ruler, on account of his philosophy and purity of morals: "Sanctitate vitæ omnibus principibus antecellit."

whose successful industry rejuvenated society, infused it with purity, but corrupted medical economy. Prior to the consummation of those events which crowned Christianity, after the edict of Milan, as the religion of the Roman Empire, for a century a spiritless eclecticism, which deteriorated with the general decline of science, had revealed itself among the professors of medicine and threatened at length to destroy the unstable vitality of scientific development.

At this critical epoch in the second century, Claudius Galen temporarily arrested the hastening decay of medical science. Of all the sectarians of curative dogmatism he was the most fertile, the most dexterous and puissant, and in the universality of professional scope the most extensive. Born in the city of Pergamos, in Asia Minor, towards the close of the first portion of the second century, he began his useful existence amid the cultured surroundings of a municipality long celebrated for its temple dedicated to Æsculapius,[8] the colossal dimensions of a carefully selected library and its school of medicine.[9] His father, Nikon, an architect of renown, under the reign of Hadrian, with parental devotion, largely aided by the accomplishment of a polished mind, had been his earliest preceptor.

Upon attaining to his fifteenth year he was placed under the tutelage of the academician Gajus, and other equally illustrious philosophers of Pergamos. Here, where the scholastic exercises of the Peripaticians were carefully taught, Galen was enabled to fully gratify a predilection for Aristotle, Theophrastus, and Plato,[10] and thorough culture in dialectic declamation. Within two years, the youthful student under his Pergamic instructors obtained an extraordinary celebrity, and at a time when abundantly equipped for disputation with the profoundly learned of his native city in grammar, history, phil-

8 Philostratus, Vita Apollon. Tyan, Lib. IV., c. 11, § 1.

9 Matter, École d'Alexandrie, Tom. I., p. 214.

10 Vide Galeni De Hippocrat. et Platon. Placitiis, Lib. V., c. 3, where his profound acquaintanceship with the Platonic dogma of the soul-principle reveals itself.

ϙsophy, and mathematical science, through the express intervention or advice of pagan divinities,[11] he instantly abandoned the agreeable pastime of polite and instructive arts, and devoted himself to the study of medicine.

He recounts with charming complaisance that this divine admonition having been twice given to him by Apollo,[12] he was unable longer to resist such impressive manifestation of supernal direction. His numerous and sagacious writings doubtless better justify the medical vocation of Galen than these mystical reminiscences. In his seventeenth year he received the first tuition in anatomical science and therapeutics from Satyrus Stratonickus, and the empiric Æschion.[13] Four years later proceeding to Smyrna for the purpose of attending the instruction of Pelops in dissection, thence to Corinth to listen to the Numescarius, and finally to Alexandria, where he devoted himself exclusively to anatomy, and, as it appears, to vivisection, at the instance of Boethius,[14] of such subjects as were procurable, where he sojourned for an extended period to complete his studies.

On returning to Pergamus in his twenty-eighth year, he was specifically intrusted by the Pagan pontiff with the surgical care of such athletes as were wounded in the gladiatorial combats, and in the application of his professional skill readily manifested marvelous knowledge of surgery and its cognate science.[15] Three years subsequent to his departure from the Alexandria scholastic institutions, he domiciled himself permanently in Rome,[16] where he became quickly and intimately

---

[11] Galeni, Prænot. ad Posthum, cap. 2; and Ibid, De Methodo Medendi, Lib. IX., cap. 4.

[12] Galeni, De Prænot, ad Posthum, cap. 2, and Ibid, De Method. Medendi, cap. 4.

[13] Inflexibility to principle seems to have characterized the empirics. One refused to attend a sectio operation as against reason, Richter, De Veter. Empiricor. ingenitate, p. 8.

[14] Galeni, De Anatomicis Administrationibus, Lib. I., cap. 1.

[15] Ibid., De Composit. Medicam., Lib. III., c. 2.

[16] Ibid., De Libriis Propriis, cc. 1 and 2.

associated with the most erudite scholars of the empire, and advanced to close companionship with the metropolitan surgeons.[17]

At this epoch of Galen's life, it is evident that the dialectic culture of his earliest youth exercised a ponderous influence in deciding the nature of that devotion to the details of medicine which afterward rendered him famous. Soon after arriving in the imperial capital, Galen seems to have assumed an undisputed superiority over the most distinguished medical professors there, and to whom he apparently abandoned the practical drudgery of the avocation, and illustrated his own scientific acquisitions by the fascinating method of public readings.[18] But his rapid success and the widely extending fame of his professional dexterity in anatomy and ophthalmy,[19] his unseasonable tumid boasting, his undisguised and contemptuous indifference for his professional confrères, which he wholly declined to conceal, his natural irascibility, provoked exasperating enmities and made his sojourn at Rome so extremely hazardous that he left the city and returned to Pergamus.[20]

His route homeward to the distant city of Asia Minor was diversified by erratic voyages on foot in the interest of medical science, through Thrace and Macedonia, in search of such medicamental herbs as grew in these localities.[21] Notwithstanding the undisputed irritability of Galen's temperament, a turgid haughtiness, frequently inseparable from recognized ability, which, in the great Pergamic scientist's career, were evidently the direct outgrowth of unstinted adulation to a distinguished personage of thirty-three years, the portraiture which he has

---

[17] Ibid.

[18] Ibid.

[19] Professional consultations were forwarded to him from Iberia, Celtica, Thrace, and Asia. Galeni, Lib. IV., c. 2, Kühn, Tom. VII., p. 454; and Hieron. Mercurial. De Arte Gymnas., Lib. VI., c. 10., p. 374.

[20] Galeni, Prænotat. ad Epigenem, Kühn, Tom. VIII.

[21] Ibid., De Simplic. Medic., Lib. IX., c. 1.

traced of the medical gentlemen of the Roman capital would seem to be a life-like resemblance, reproduced in the vivid coloring of veracity.

With imbittered hatred, he lays them under the sweeping charge of ignoble jealousy, accuses them of stupid ignorance, inculpates them as thieves[22] and poisoners, and finishes his burning censoriousness by declaring that, having finally unmasked such villains, he will thenceforth place himself beyond the reach of their vindictive snares and accursed malevolence, by abandoning the great and populous metropolis, where no one is considered as respectable only in proportion to ostentatious splendor, and where shameless charlatanism usurped the confidence of a frivolous and perverse people; and would thenceforth inhabit a humble village, where each citizen is intimately known to the other, whose birth, education, fortune, and morals, are matters upon which public judgment is rarely at fault.[23] After an absence from Rome of about a year, Galen was ordered to return by the enlightened emperor, Marcus Aurelius, and was appointed surgeon to Commodus,[24] during the time that Aurelius was actively engaged in his campaign against the Germans. He also enjoyed the confidence of the succeeding emperor, Septimus Severus.

In the year 169, Galen left the imperial city, as is stated, on account of the pestilence raging there, and returned to Pergamus.[25] The time of his death is uncertain, but it is presumed that he died about the age of seventy, or in the opening year

---

[22] Legislation as early as Antoninus Pius, and reaffirmed by later emperors, was compelled to add the force of rescripts to restrict physicians to liberal compensation under their oath, Juramentum Hippocrates, which the law of the fourth century repealed, Gothofred, Com. in Cod. Theodos., Tom. V., p. 37.

[23] Galen. De Libriis Propriis, c. 2; and Ibid., Prænot. ad Epigenem, Kühn, Tom. VIII.

[24] Ibid., De Libriis Propriis, c. 2. Kühn, Vita Galeni, p. 29, states that in this emperor's day the Temple of Peace was destroyed by fire, in which conflagration many manuscript copies of Galen's writings perished. Galeni, De Antidotis, Lib. I., c. 13.

[25] Galeni, De Libriis Propriis, cc. 1 and 2.

of the third century, while revisiting his native city. From the voluminous aggregation of his treatises saved from loss, it would seem that a large part of the later years of his life was devoted to the preparation of medical compositions, and given to the public or professors as readings or lectures. A dream, sent by Æsculapius prevented Galen from accompanying Marcus Aurelius in his expedition against the Teutonic races. An enthusiastic monk has confidently asserted that this illustrious surgeon finished his life while on a pilgrimage to the Holy Land.[26]

Among the manifold writings of Galen on the subject of medicine and its associate branches, the influence of the liberal education of early youth appears to have survived the less attractive investigation into a deteriorated science, inasmuch as nearly a hundred and twenty-five treatises have perished, elaborating philosophical, grammatical, geometrical, and juristic subjects.[27]

In the scientific treatment of his medical essays, he most unequivocally asserts that he is totally disconnected with and unattached to any of the numerous sects which divided the profession of his day. On the contrary, he boldly charged almost abject servitude upon those who arrogated to themselves the title of Hippocratians, Praxaguereans, or Herophilians. Full adhesion to this inculpation would be perhaps unjust, especially when he claimed to hold the exact equilibrium between diverse doctrines, and should be accepted as the pardonable autocracy of a voluminous writer, or the trivial artifice of a rhetorician who uses a figurative phrase in order to surprise an auditor into admitting his claim to independence and impartiality. His predilection for Hippocrates is so visible that he comments and explains the venerable father of

[26] Reynouard, Histoire de la Medécine, Tom. I., p. 322. The utter absurdity of this partisan claim may be seen by comparing Galen's own notions touching Christianity; De Differentia Pulsuum, Lib. II., cc. 3 and 4.

[27] Some of these on Galen's own testimony, Fabricius, Bibliotheca Græca, Tom. II., p. 435. Excellent resumé of Galen's life in Fabricius, op. cit., Tom. V., pp. 378–390.

medicine, and while amplifying these different propositions he refutes the objections made against the Hippocratian method, in order to render its triumph easy and complete.

In the exegetical treatises by Galen, he holds up Thessalus to merited scorn on account of his malediction of Hippocrates.[28] He distinctly states, however, with the satisfactory consciousness of his great authority, that before him no one had furnished a complete method for the treatment of maladies. While avowing that his ancient predecessor had indicated the plan by which the adaptation of medicine as a scientific cure of disorders might be rendered systematic and rational, he maintained that Hippocrates had failed to pursue the course described; that a vicious order in the treatment of infirmities was adopted by the illustrious physician of Cos, which compelled him to omit certain important indications, while his obscurity, the usual style of the ancients, arose from a desire for excessive precision. In a word, Hippocrates had barely sketched the outlines, and formally opened the way to scientific cure of disease; the enlargement of this system to practical use, and the establishment of medicine as a science,[29] Galen attributed to himself.

Without doubt anatomical knowledge of that epoch was largely increased by the Pergamic scientist, who followed this valuable branch of medicine with assiduity—a study much neglected by the dominant schools, and suffered to decline into desuetude. Utilizing the studious results of his predecessors, he obtained such practical information from dissecting cadavera, animals, and especially apes, or by vivisection,[30] as the circumscribed permission to anatomize the human body of the period would permit.[31] Marinus, in the first century, and the

[28] Galeni, De Methodo Medendi, Lib. I., cap. 2.

[29] Galeni, De Methodo Medendi, Lib. IX., cap. 8.

[30] Celsus, De Medicina, Lib. I., Prœm., p. 19.

[31] It is possible that anatomy may have developed from the Egyptian embalming, the professors of which, after preparing the cadaver, were usually driven away by survivors with stones and curses, Goujet. Origin des Arts et Metiers, Tom. I., p. 222. Alexandria derived especial permission from the Ptolemies to dissect human cadavera, Plinii Histor. Naturalis, Lib. XIX., c. 26.

Ephesian Rufus under Trajan, appear to have obtained distinction in anatomy through their writings prior to the time of Galen.[32]

The Galenic system of medicine, thus established by the practical skill of its founder upon the most accessible materials which intelligent zeal could use, was so servilely followed throughout the Middle Ages in a deteriorated adaptation, and conjoined with the assumed potency of external but divinized influences, that a fleeting outline of the same is indispensable. According to this methodical treatment of medicine, there were in man three principles or actuating impulses: spirit, humors, and solids.[33] Inasmuch as he accepted the dynamical forces of the soul, or pneuma, with Hippocrates, he also admitted the four primordial qualities of heat, cold, dryness, and humidity, which, in their individual or united action, sufficiently influenced the transformation of the human system.[34]

In close harmony with the theories of the Peripatician essences, he avows three original powers; natural force located in the liver, vital force in the brain, and sensual force in the heart,[35] which were vitalized in their respective habitations by a concealed pneuma or soul.[36] These natural essences, which directly supervise the action of production, nutrition, and growth, in their turn are controlled by four, the attractive, differential, preservative, and exclusive powers, and collectively act under the domination of a circulating spirit, which moves through the arteries, and have their central organism in the liver, where the veins originate, blood is prepared, and nutriment distributed to the entire body. In the pathological method of Galen's treatment, the aggregation of entities, either

---

[32] Friedlander, Geschichte der Heilkunde, p. 151.

[33] Kühn, Vita Galeni, p. 56, seq.

[34] Galeni, De Hippocrat. et Platonis Placitiis, Lib. I.. cap. 1.

[35] Ibid., Lib. V., cap. 3. Philo. Judæus, Leg., Lib. II., c. 110; Tom. I., p. 57 seq., accords the liver as the seat of cupidity.

[36] Galeni, De Hip. et Plato. Placit:, Lib. V., cc. 1, 2 and 3.

imaginary or in the abstract, may be found—to which are attributed acts and powers incident to realistic beings.[37]

From the character of Galen's distribution of the sanguinary fluids throughout the veins, it is a rational conclusion to assume his practical acquaintanceship with the circulation of the blood, to whose knowledge the utility of venal valves was alone essential to complete the universality of his anatomical learning.[38] In the psychological or pneumatic essence of Galen, is to be found the earliest serious effort of a cultivated and scholastic mind to delineate with tolerable accuracy the exact correlation so palpably existing between the secret impulses of the soul and their demonstrable effect on the physical system of man. So far indeed as this explanation of a close but independent unity is visible in Galen's demonstration, it was evidently the development of his profound knowledge of Platonic philosophy; but unfortunately the preponderating influence of a sensuous and paganistic materialism precluded further understanding of the soul than a conceded abject and dependent portion of the human body. For this reason he represented its gross, corporeal operation merely as an empirical adjunct, and accepted this vitalizing essence, degraded of its spirituality, as a physical composition.

As hitherto stated, Galen admitted with Plato and Aristotle the triplicate faculty of the human soul, each of which was endowed with specific functions in propelling the sanitary operations of the body,[39] and upon the queried immortality of this principle refused to accept the Platonic ratiocination, and maintained an attitude of vacillating opinion.

Touching the efforts of the great medical scholar of Pergamus, to subordinate the movements of the soul to a subservient dependence on the human senses, it may be confidently asserted that the almost omnipotent authority of Galen, at a subsequent period conjoined with other causes arising from the Alexandrine

---

[37] Reynouard, Histoire de la Medécine, Tom. I., p. 329.

[38] Lessing, Geschichte der Medezin, Th. I., p. 102.

[39] Galeni, De Hippocratis et Platonis Placitiis, Lib. V., cc. 1, 2 and 3.

schools, largely promoted the transition to the Neoplatonic system, and opened an enlarging perspective to the application of remedies of assumed efficiency, whose entire system was an outgrowth of this medical psychology, and rested mainly upon the credulity of the sick.

In addition to pagan philosophy, Galen was well versed in the doctrines of Moses[40] and in the religion of Christ; but the partial obscurity of his superstitious deism induced him to sneer at their teachings and revile their neophytes.[41] So far as the historical value of this encyclopediacal writer is concerned, it may be confidently asserted that he has rendered as great service to this department of arts, as to the medical schools, especially when it is considered that he preserved the opinions of unnumbered writers on medicine from total loss, the treatises of whom have long since vanished before the progress of ages. Through this happy preservation, an excellent insight is given of the valiant struggles of the Dogmatists, Methodicals, and Empirics of the early centuries.

To what extent the treatises of Galen may be of practical service in modern times, they must be awarded the high commendation of securing subsequent medicinal art from total wreck during the turbulency of the Middle Ages, and as we shall hereafter observe, assisted at its revival into an embellished science through the mediæval Universities. From the time of Galen[42] to the close of the Sixteenth century,[43] the works of the Pergamic sage fully satisfied the demands of the practitioners of medicine, who depended on his surgical and anatomical writings, without questioning their authority. According to the concurrent attestation of writers of the Patristic

[40] Galeni, De Usu Pulsuum Corpor. Human., Lib. XI., cap. 3, queries whether Moses excelled Epicurus in the acuteness and utility of his reasoning.

[41] In the De Different. Pulsuum, Lib. III., cap. 3, Galen distinctly inculpates the followers of Moses and Christ as so rigidly sectarian as to be unworthy the name of physician and philosopher, and seizes another occasion to ridicule the slender intellect stock of these sects, Ib., Lib. II., cap. 4.

[42] Matter, École d'Alexandrie, Tom. II., p. 37.

[43] Friedlander, Geschichte der Heilkunde, p. 156.

era, he was an object of adoration almost divine[44]—a culture of worship barely shaken or modified down to the close of the Middle Ages,[45] through the introduction to Europe of Arabic medical science, which was based upon the Galenic system.

[44] Athenæus, Deipnosophi, Lib. I., cap. 2, asserts that the skill of Daphnus in medicine obtained the distinction of a "sacred art"—*ιερὸς τῆν τὲχνην*—which Galen equalled by the practice and the superiority of his treatises.

[45] Roskoff, Geschichte des Teufels, The. II., p. 100.

CHAPTER III.

The Alexandrine Schools, and How They Affected the Curative Art—Early Organized—Literary Aggregation of Alexandria—The Writings of Medical Sages Preserved in the Great Library—Collections for this Pursuit Made by the Ptolemies—Study of Natural History at Alexandria—Zoological Garden—Erudite Professor of Medical Science at Alexandria—Loss to this Art by the Conflagration of the Library there—Cleopatra's Skill in Medicine—Botanical Studies—Decline of the Alexandrine Schools, and Its Cause—Rival Sects of Christianity—Disastrous Effects Produced by These upon Medical Art.

WHATEVER may have been the immediate causes operating upon the successors of Alexander the Great, the institution of the several scholastic establishments in the Egyptian metropolis was an idea so unreservedly royal that it must ever receive in the interests of letters the most unstinted eulogy. It may have entered extensively into the governmental policy of the Ptolemies, to subjugate the people of Egypt by counter balancing the sacerdotal influences of Memphis, which as the phantom of an ancient power provoked unceasing inquietude to the Greek conquerors.

The population of Alexandria above all demanded special attention, in order to hold in proper subserviency the curiously amalgamated races, who either originally resident of the country as Egyptians naturally composed the larger element, corrupted by Hellenistic contact, but hopeful of withdrawing from foreign dominion, or other indigenous people still maintaining the characteristics of separate nationalities forced into companionship by the resistless power of a victorious army.[1] To these was joined a multitude of Jews whom Alexander or the Ptolemies introduced from Judea in pursuing a carefully defined plan of conquest. So numerous indeed was the Jewish populace in the time of Philo that he

[1] Matter, École d'Alexandrie, Tom. I., p. 71.

estimated them at the round figure of a million actually residing in the city of Alexandria.[2] In order to fuse the ideas, manners, usages and institutions of the principal nationalities thus forcibly united in the Egyptian metropolis, the Lagides sought to commingle the sciences and arts of the two nations, of whom the one gloried in inventing, and the other boasted in perfecting these inventions.

By the fusion thus provoked through the enlightened judgment of the Ptolemaic dynasty, Egypt preserved the illusions of their national religion, conjoined originally with a preponderating influence in the laws and usages, but liable to the seductive temptation of a brilliant and dominant race.[3] For this reason the first Ptolemies sanctioned the perpetuation of the sacerdotal colleges of Thebes, Memphis, and Hierophile, but as the sure fruition of an illuminated policy arose the Alexandrian Gymnasium.

Under all aspects the creation of the Museum by the successors of Alexander transcends all, in its important consequences upon art and science, including that of medicine, by the aggregation of vast numbers of works of priceless value; the writings of Egyptian sages, Jewish codes, the laws of Solon, the poesies of Homer and Orpheus, Platonic and Aristotelian treatises, and the careful preservation of the essays of Hippocrates, Galen, Oribasius,[4] etc. The origin of this library ascends to Ptolemy Soter, according to Irenæus,[5] and so largely were these collections made by Demetrius under the Lagides that they aggregated the enormous number of two hundred thousand manuscript volumes,[6] upon the accession of the librarian Zenodotus.[7]

---

[2] Aversus Flaccum, Lib. II., p. 523. At nearly the same epoch the Liberentinii Jews inhabited that portion of the trans-Tiberem in Rome, whose extensive area indicates great numbers. Ibid, De Virtitutibus, Lib. II., p. 568.

[3] Matter, op. cit., Tom. I., p. 74.

[4] Eunapius, Vitæ Sophistor., p. 498.

[5] Aversus Hæres., Lib. III., cap. 21, § 2.

[6] Josephus, Antiq., Lib. XII., cap. 1.

[7] Suidas, Lexicon, sub nom. Zenodotus.

Identified with and perhaps a portion of it,[8] was the Museum, unqualifiedly the most lasting in its influences on the development of science, and on the spirit of the period during this and succeeding ages. If the assertion of Philostratus[9] be accepted that this establishment was organized in the nature of a college or association of the learned, to which the erudite and illustrious men of the world were invited as resident members, it is evident the ancient Egytian sacerdoty must have contributed a certain element of hierarchial influences.[10]

Indeed this synod of the wise and scientific was presided over by a priest, which gave the organization a religious character.[11] To what extent this especial feature was uniform and so accepted by the denizens of the regal institutions, is confessedly obscure. But as Matter[12] justly concludes, in noting at the court of the Lagides a priesthood of three different religions which had in the time of Herodotus begun to assimilate, that at an early date the fusion of creeds and ceremonies, the astute policy of the new dynasty, was substantially proceeding,—an event which was repeated towards the decline of polytheism, and impressed the curative art with this irrational amalgamation for many centuries. On account of the valued privileges attached to membership in the Alexandrian schools, from a remote period this city became the object of general attraction to both scientific and art scholars.

Among these, the earliest to claim such royal franchises by prompt presence at the Egyptian capital were professors of medical science and mathematics—Herophilus, Eristatus,[13] and

---

[8] Athenæus, Deipnosophi, Lib. IV., cap. 83.

[9] "Est autem museum mensa Ægyptica, quae ex omni terrarum orbe honoratissimos viros convocat." Vitæ Sophistor., Lib. I., cap. 22, § 5. The paragraph cited, perhaps hyperbolical, indicates that in the time of Hadrian the Museum still maintained its ancient reputation. Apollonius of Tyana, the hero of Philostratus, occupied the seat of Helicon in the Museum. Vit. Ap., Lib. IV., c. 24, § 1.

[10] Strabo, Geograph., Lib. XVII., c. 1.

[11] Scholars maintained there at public expense. Philostratus, Vit. Sophist., Lib. I., c. 22, § 5.

[12] École d'Alexandrie, Tom. I., p. 97.

[13] Lessing, Geschichte der Medezin, Th. I., p. 53.

Euclid, the former of whom preluded most gloriously to the innovations in medicine.[14] In the collections of diversified manuscripts which added to the celebrity of Alexandria, eager zeal was displayed for faithful transcripts where the originals were not procurable. These transcribers, noted for calligraphic art, were maintained at public expense, and at a later date, under Domitian, called to Rome to exercise their perfunctionary duties for its libraries.[15]

Galen states,[16] that when the enthusiastic Ptolemies first sought to increase their aggregation of medical and other rare works, they were oftentimes imposed upon by worthless copies, but subsequently distinguished with the utmost care between valuable and useless transcripts. In many cases, of the books loaned accurate copies were made, and instead of returning the originals to their owners, these were retained, and the transcripts sent to the possessors. The original treatises were then deposited in the library with a memorandum, signifying an intention to have them critically examined by competent authorities. To such critics was entrusted the care of assorting all books not properly classified, and after being subjected to close inspection, they were suitably tabulated and permanently placed on the shelves of the library.[17]

Erudition has sought to maintain the hypothesis[18] that one of the earliest official acts of the successors of Alexander called into existence zoölogical gardens, where rare specimens of natural history were displayed for the advanced cultivation of the Alexandrine scholars,[19] and at the same time opened botanical parks to the eager research of medical professors and

---

[14] Matter, École d'Alexandrie, Tom. I., p. 127.

[15] Suetonius in Vita Domitiani, cap. 20.

[16] Comment. II., in Epidem. Hippocrat., Lib. III., p. 606 seq., Kühn.

[17] Galeni, De Dyspnœa, Lib. II., Ibid, Comment. II., in Epidem. Hippocrates, Lib. III., c. — p. 606.

[18] Schlosser, Univers. Histor. Uebersicht der Geschichte der Alten Welt., Th. II., p. 196 seqq.

[19] Athenæus, Deipnosophi, Lib. XIV., c. 77.

students. The Ptolemies, down to the very termination of their dominion over Egypt, appear to have encouraged the curative art, and for the purpose of restoring declining health, surrounded themselves with the most illustrious physicians of the age.[20] Under the son of Ptolemy II., who politely declined the offer of magnanimous Rome to aid him in the Seleucide conflict,[21] the explorations begun by his distinguished ancestor, to accumulate materials illustrating natural history, were vigorously maintained, and larger numbers of manuscripts added to the great library.[22]

The science of medicine of the period was fully represented at the Museum by distinguished professors, who according to Athenæus,[23] restored the knowledge of this art to the towns and islands of the Grecian Archipelago. Later events incident to the reign of Ptolemy VII., who revenged himself for the almost universal abhorrence of his infamy, made Alexandria nearly a desert,[24] assassinated the youth of the city assembled in the Gymnasium,[25] which caused the dispersion of many illustrious scholars from the metropolis, and among these the erudite scientists, disciples of Herophile;[26] but the scattered schools of the curative art, consequent on this tyrannical act, remained inferior to those of Alexandria.[27]

Towards the close of the second century before the Christian era, arose the embittered emulation between Pergamus and Alexandria, whose varied details were possessed of such fascinating interest to the people of antiquity. This literary war-

[20] Lessing, Geschichte der Medezin, Th. I., p. 52, and Matter, École d'Alexandrie, Tom. I., p. 160.

[21] Eutropius, Breviar. Histor. Rom., Lib. III., c. 1.

[22] Galeni Com. II., in Epid. Hippocrat., Lib. III., p. 606 seq.

[23] Deipnosophi, Lib. VI., c. 83.

[24] Justin, Lib. XXXVIII., c. 8.

[25] Valerius Maximus, Memorabil. Lib. IX., cap. 2, De Crudelitate Exter., § 5.

[26] Touching the dominant influences of Herophile over the medical schools of Pliny's time, vide Histor. Natur., Lib. XXIX., c. 5.

[27] Matter, École d'Alexandrie, Tom. I., p. 215.

fare gave rise to the invention of parchment, thus named on account of its manufacture at Pergamus in consequence of her rival Alexandria refusing to allow the export of papyrus or paper, upon which the scholastics of the oriental city wrote their literary themes.[28] The most serious result of this quarrel was the falsification of ancient writers, by the erudite of both cities. Through the salutary aid of an Indian prince, prisoner at the Ptolemaic court, familiar with the Greek tongue, an expedition was organized, which ended in the procuring of numerous spices from India.[29]

About the period of the absorption of the Egyptian kingdom into the expanding dominion of the Romans, the schools of Alexandria still continued to be the centre of medical studies; and notwithstanding the apparent dissidence between the demands of a strict science and public affairs, its professors exhibited, equally with their brother philosophers, a taste for diplomacy. Dioscorides[30] and Serapion, two physicians of Alexandria, were the envoys of the elder Ptolemy to Rome, and at a later date were bearers of dispatches from Cæsar to one of his officers in Egypt.

It is indeed noteworthy that such secular concerns received the attention of medical scholars at a time when the study of this science was pursued with ardor in the metropolis. Zophyrus, a wise and skilled professor, had there a school of medicine under his direct supervision, of which Apollonius of Cittium was so enthusiastic a pupil, that on returning to his adopted city he drew up a careful treatise on anatomy, and, as an indication of personal esteem for Ptolemy XI., dedicated the work to his royal patron.[31] In absence of historical proofs to the contrary, it may be assumed that the bitter and prolonged

---

[28] Ibid, Tom. I., p. 214.

[29] Strabo, Geograph., Lib. II., c. 3.

[30] Not the disciple of Apollonius of Tyana, of whom Philostratus describes the attempt to withdraw from the vengeful ferocity of Nero. He was also a physician, Vit. Apoll. Tyan., Lib. IV., c. 11, and Lib. V., c. 43.

[31] Matter, École d'Alexandrie, Tom. I., p. 28 .

struggles for supremacy between the Roman consuls, which by Cæsar's policy were transferred to Alexandria, necessarily retarded the progress of medical science in the scholastic institutions of the literary metropolis.

One of the severest, perhaps temporary hindrances to its uninterrupted development, was the direct catastrophe which it certainly sustained in the conflagration, by the forces of Cæsar, of the great library, among whose number, variously estimated,[32] aggregated in diverse sorts almost a million volumes, doubtless many valuable treatises on anatomy and medicine were included and totally lost.[33] Such portions at least as were preserved from entire destruction, consisted of collections made by Cleopatra in her palace, while it would seem that the books in general use by the scholars at the Museum were left untouched.[34] It is certain that some of the treatises orignally retained at the great library were extant in after ages, a convincing proof that this colossal institution was not totally burned.[35] Julius Cæsar evidently intended, when time and convenience should admit, to repair these disasters, touching which he maintains entire silence.[36]

When the young Egyptian queen united her fortunes with Marc Antony, and in the gracious confidence of a woman, stirred by the heroic valor of a conquering hero, surrounded him with the joyous charms of lavish expenditure and personal beauty, she displayed such passionate taste for fine arts and medical science,[37] that the new governor of Egypt, in deference to a zeal cultivated into elegant scholarship by a profound and practical knowledge of the languages of her kingdom, hastened to give to her the priceless collection of books,

[32] Aulius Gellius, Noctes Atticæ, Lib. V., c. 7.

[33] Ammianus Marcellinus, Gesta Roman. Histor., Lib. XXII., c. 16.

[34] Matter, op. cit., Tom. I., p. 243.

[35] Abulfagus, Histor. Moslem., p. 114.

[36] Cæsar, Bell. Civil., Lib. III., cap. 3.

[37] Galeni, Liber de Ornatu ad Achoras, Lib. I., cap. 7.

which the kings of Pergamus had previously bequeathed to the Roman Senate.[38]

The Roman emperors, upon the conquest of diversified nationalities, appear to have closely imitated Grecian scholastic institutions in such as were created by them at different points on the African coast, in which the Latin language was chiefly used, although it was the superb pride of the imperial dynasties to protect the scientific schools of Alexandria by public patronage and administrative encouragement.[39] Notwithstanding the concession by Nero that the Egyptian capital should have its own magistrates, natives of the country,[40] and the professed determination of Augustus to foster its institutions, who actually constructed an edifice whose appointments should attract the erudite scientist, the spirit of civil liberty had vanished, and with it ancient splendor, leaving the elements of gradual decay behind. Whatever may have been the character of Tiberius in the annals of the empire, Suetonius,[41] his biographer, unequivocally affirms his affection for Augustus, and a zealous admiration for the famed science of Alexandria—philology. He was moreover in close relations with the chief librarian of the literary capital, Cheremos, whom he summoned to Rome in order to superintend the education of young Nero.[42]

Claudius manifested the patronizing spirit of his predecessors by the construction of an entirely new Museum, the object of whose creation is abundantly set forth by the annalist of his reign. Each member of the Claudian establishment was required annually, at a fixed epoch, to read aloud before an audience, throughout their entire length, the twenty books of Etrurian history and the ten books of the history of Carthage,

---

[38] Plutarch, Vita Anton., cap 58.

[39] Matter, École d'Alexandrie, Tom I., p. 248.

[40] Tacitus, Historiar. Lib. I., c. 2.

[41] Vita Tiberii, cap. 70.

[42] Suidas, Lexicon, sub nom. Dionysius and Alexand. Ægе. His estimate of the brutal character of the royal pupil is delineated in this verbal sketch which he made of him: "Nero lutum sanguine maceratum," Ib.

which the Emperor had himself composed[43]—a species of public oratory current long before the age of Claudius, and formerly in vogue in ancient Rome.[44]

The object of this apparently bizarre function, seems to have been an attempt to establish a historical connection between the modern descendants of ancient Carthage and the origin of Roman laws and institutions, which should mould the minds of the Alexandrians into subjection on the basis of common ancestry.[45] During the emergencies of Vespasian in his conflict with Vitellius, his rival, the Emperor was so busily engaged in questioning the oracles of Egypt, and in aggregating sufficient funds for war, that the schools of Alexandria were not patronized by him. He was affable, but too eagerly occupied in coining money[46] to be affected by the sarcasms of the citizens, who at first believed him deeply pious on his consulting the temple of Serapis,[47] and afterwards found him using the sanctuaries for forging coin.

Indeed, so little attention was bestowed by Vespasian on scholars that he expelled the whole body from Rome excepting Musonius.[48] Domitian, who it is true exiled the philosophers during his sojourn in Egypt, appeared to be highly exalted over the religious affairs of its sacerdoty, instituted poetical and oratorical contests, with prizes for Greek and Latin prose,[49] and caused duplicates of the volumes then existing in the Egyptian metropolis to be made to replace those lost in the frightful conflagration at Rome.[50] The Alexandrine schools,

---

43 " Veteri Alexandriæ Museo alterum additum ex ipsius nomine; institutumque ut quotannis Τυρρηνιχῶν liber," etc. Suetonius, Vita Claudii, cap. 42.

44 Valerius Maximus, Memorabil, Lib. III., c. 7, § 16.

45 Horatii, Satira, Lib. III., v. 74.

46 Vespasian was a firm believer in magic art. Dio Cassius, Histor., Lib. LXXVI., cap. 8.

47 Suetonius, Vita Vespas., cap. 7.

48 Dio Cassius, op. cit., Lib. LXVI., cap. 13.

49 Sueton., Vita Domitiani, cap. 4. Xiphilin, Vita Domitiani, p. 254.

50 " Bibliothecas incendio absumtas impensissime reparare curasset, exemplaribus

whether of medicine, or arts and general philosophy, maintained, through the reigns of Nerva and Trajan, a fluctuating vitality, without, so far as historical records extend, imperial patronage, materially assisting to alter the vicissitudes which quickly prepared the way, towards the close of the ensuing century, for a rapid decline and total decay of usefulness. Polemon,[51] and other erudite professors in the literary and scientific contests at Alexandria under Hadrian,[52] were created Knights of the Roman Quirites.[53]

The immediate cause of the decline of these great schools of science, was the endowment at Rome of an Athenæum, and at Athens of a library.[54] The direct result of these foreign institutions was a tendency of the cultured scholars of Alexandria to congregate at the imperial metropolis, although royal favor still prevented the utter denuding of the scholastic organizations of Alexandria.

In their general situation the same categories of authors perpetually reappear: grammarians uniting the study of rhetoric with philology and criticism; historians also renowned as geographers; mathematicians professing the entire range of astronomy, mechanics, and arithmetic; and medical scientists, who joined to a knowledge of this art that of natural history and botany.[55] Naturally enough these varied schools of medicine, botany, and the philosophical studies in Alexandria, were on a much more enlarged dimension in members and numerical proportions, during the first two centuries, inasmuch as the amalgamation of foreign governments with the Roman Empire, necessitated that culture for which these scholastic insti-

undique petitis missis Alexandriam, qui describerent emendarentque." Sueton., op. cit., c. 20.

[51] Philostratus, Vitæ Sophist., Lib. II., c. 10, § 7.

[52] Touching his eloquence, envied by Gregory of Nazian, vide Suidas, Lexicon, sub n. Gregor. Naz.

[53] Jul. Capitol., Vita Marc. Antonini, cap. 4.

[54] The great culture of Athens at this period was recognized by Marcus Antoninus, Philostratus, Vit. Sophist., Lib. II., c. 10.

[55] Matter, École d'Alexandrie, Tom. I., p. 271.

tutions offered superior attractions, and which was demanded for political advancement.[56]

Learned professors proceeded directly to Egypt to acquire medical and other sciences, which they were to gloriously display in the Latin metropolis, particularly as at this epoch it was the custom, carefully followed, to struggle for celebrity in Alexandria, and if successful to proceed to Rome, where such distinction was readily conceded and largely compensated by wealthy citizens. Towards the termination of the reign of Hadrian a singular aggregation of philosophers had been formed in the literary metropolis of the world. In the first ages of our era, in exact proportion as the Christian doctrines advanced, the number of Cyrenecians, Epicurians, and frivolous Sophists, who usually assembled at the Museum, receded before Stoicians, Peripateticians, or Platonists, seeking in all earnestness teachings more sober and less trivial than those of ther predecessors.[57]

While Augustus withdrew his friend Arius, the Stoic, from the Museum, another of this sect was selected to fill the vacant membership: Theon, profoundly skilled in rhetoric and the science of physiology.[58] Sotion,[59] of Alexandria, master of Seneca, professed the principles of the Stoics in conjunction with those of Pythagoras. Peripatetic philosophy found its representatives in Boethius,[60] tutor of Strabo. In the person of Ammianus, whom Nero exiled from Alexandria to establish in

---

[56] The Latin idiom was peremptorily essential to office under the Roman government as early as the Republic. Valer. Maxim. Memorabil., Lib. II., cap. 2, No. 2. At a later date Claudius disfranchised a Grecian governor who was ignorant of the official language of the empire. Suetonius, Vita Claudii, cap. 16.

[57] Matter, École d'Alexandrie, Tom. I., p. 276.

[58] Eunapius, Vitæ Sophistor., sub. n. Ionicus, p. 499. The Theon referred to by Europius was of Gallic nativity, and thought worthy to rank with the skillful Oribasius.

[59] Eunapius, op. cit., Prefat. 2–5, p. 454, admits he had freely used the material collected by Sotion for his lives.

[60] On Boethius' Book of Anatomy, vide Galen, De Anatomicis Administrationibus, Lib. I., c. 2.

Athens, Peripatetism was united with the doctrines of Plato.[61] Plutarch, the disciple of Ammianus, may be taken as an illustrious example of the profoundly moral and religious tendencies of his preceptor and of the age.

During the uninterrupted continuance of these grave subjects of philosophic meditation, and while the zealous minds of their several professors were earnestly exercised over the possible solution of such sober problems, one of the most brilliant and mystic spirits of the time, Philo, surnamed the Jew, boldly unrolled before the erudite of Alexandria the Mosaic doctrines, slightly concealed beneath a gloss of Platonism, a method identical with that of Aristobulus,[62] who had hitherto disguised them under a Peripatetic exterior. In order that the city itself might become the chief center of a powerful movement in philosophy, and so disintegrate the older systems as to admit new ones, which should alter the prevailing tendencies of the human spirit, and open it to the acceptance and credulity of dogmas whose direct effect upon the teachers and disciples of the schools prepared the transition to Gnosticism, and inaugurated the calamitous decline of medical science, the presence and skill of a highly endowed dialectician were essential. Such personage was found in Enesedinus, who attacked the principles of Pyrrhonism, and directly leveled his argumentative doubts against the doctrines of the sensible elements and the medical studies resting upon these.[63]

This onslaught startled the whole school of Alexandria, and the more, indeed, since at this period a movement began to evince itself towards more exact sciences, such as reforming the calendar, or better knowledge of cosmography.[64] It is doubtless true that natural sciences, especially that of medicine and its associate branches, were no longer cultivated with that patient erudition of the time of Herophile and Erostatus,

---

[61] Philostratus, Vitæ Sophistor., Lib. II., c. 27, § 6.

[62] Bruckerii, Histor. Philosoph., Lib. II.; c. 2, § 33.

[63] Eusebius, Præparatio ad Evangel., Lib. XIV., cc. 7 and 18.

[64] Bailly, Histoire de l'Astronomie, Tom. I., pp. 170 and 76–122.

although the medical school of Alexandria yet maintained its ranking pre-eminence—so much so, indeed, that down to the time of the Christian Emperors, in the fourth century, it was sufficient for an adventuring physician at Rome to announce himself as an Alexandrian student, in order to acquire instant favor.[65] Soranus, as we have seen, a disciple of this school, upon an offer by the Archiatria, instantly abandoned his professorship in the Egyptian city to pursue the same duties elsewhere under Trajan and Hadrian.[66] Others, however, such as Heraclius, still taught this science there when Galen came to study anatomy and medicine in the illustrious city.[67] Upon the complete organization of the Athenian school instituted by Hadrian, the scholastic institutions of Alexandria ceased to be the center of Greek letters, that potent attraction which so strongly induced the Hellenistic youth to study abroad; and from this epoch the decadence of the Museum began to manifest itself.

Other puissant causes were operating to alter and modify the influence of these schools in the Egyptian city—causes which prepared obstacles to the advance of medical science, and laid the foundation for a retrocession of its economy throughout the entire Middle Ages. At this important crisis two new sects suddenly arose into recognized vigor in Alexandria, the one Gnostic and the other Christian, and made their appearance equipped with the glittering fascinations of a most singular novelty.

Notwithstanding Judaism had in a moderate form pioneered the way for the introduction of Christianity into Alexandria, the unceasing efforts and voluminous writings of Aristobulus and Philo,[68] directed to proselyting converts to their

---

65 "Pro omni tamen experimento sufficiat medico ad commendandam artis auctoritatem, si Alexandriæ se dixierit eruditum: et hæc quidum hoctenus." Ammianus Marcellinus, Lib. XXII., cap. 16. Same suggestion of Vopiscius, Vita Saturnini, cap. 1.

66 Suidas, Lexicon, sub nom. Soranus.

67 Galeni, Com. II., in Lib. De Natur. Humor., p. 22.

68 Bruckerii, Histor. Philosoph., Lib. II., cap. 2, § 33, and Matter, Histoire du Gnosticisme, Tom. I., p. 56 seqq.

new doctrines, adroitly hidden beneath Platonism, evidently quickened the sluggish indifference of its scholars, without obtaining numerous followers from the Museum. Philo's treatises, it seems, were consulted by Christian neophytes, in order to acquire free knowledge of paganism or polytheism, without being compelled to study the writings of heathen authors, where everything wounded their faith.[69] This use to which the written doctrines of Philo Judæus and Aristobulus were subjected, the latter of whom united the apostolic acts whose long usage, so closely assimilated throughout as to deceive converts, was suddenly transformed into catechetical form, and reappeared as expositor of the new faith in the hands of proselytes.[70] While these obtained a few notions of philosophy, of dialecticism, of polemics, and, as may be drawn from the controversy of Origen against Celsus,[71] of medicine, by which the doctrines of philosophers and paganistic theories might be combated, the ordinary evangelical minister sought to captivate the populace, and propounded a revelation, to those profoundly meditating, of an approaching social crisis.

The most celebrated of their scholastic institutes was directly in face of the Museum, and from its situation was accorded a superiority of science and dignity, and was known by the name of Didaskelon.[72] Originally used for tuition in the Christian faith, and presided over by either a Stoician or Platonist, it ultimately gloried in a more extended course of studies, which included history, philology, in a limited degree mythology, cosmography,[73] and, as it would seem, such knowledge of supernal interposition as aided in the cure of maladies, necessitated by the physicians still clinging to paganism, and in order that the neophytes might successfully vindicate the

[69] Matter, École d'Alexandrie, Tom. I., p. 287.

[70] Matter, École d'Alexandrie, Tom. I., p. 287.

[71] Origen, Contra Celsum, Lib. VIII., p. 416.

[72] Eusebius, Histor. Eccles., Lib. V., cap. 10. Nicephorus, Histor. Eccles., Lib. IV., c. 32, states that this institute had obtained a venerable repute for its scholastic excellence.

[73] Nicephorus, op. cit., Lib. IV., c. 32.

omnipotence of their Deity over Apollo or the divine Æsculapius, through whose intermediation oftentimes, anciently, the sick were supposed to be restored to health,[74]—by those divinities the wrath of whom caused sickness.[75]

While the Museum itself still pursued the entire range of literature and sciences, including that of medicine, the Didaskelon was essentially a religious institution for instruction in sacred things, and affected such acquaintanceship with science as was essential for proselyting purposes. The philosophical studies pursued there were the more dangerous to Polytheism on account of its eclecticism, and for a further reason that those who taught it had completely renounced the exclusive principles of paganism which they had abandoned. Clement, of Alexandria, educated in the very best schools of the Church in the second century, and abundantly nurtured in all the sacred and profane sciences of the Egyptian capital, openly proclaimed himself an eclectic.[76]

This system of selection for the moulding of the creed and ceremonials of the rising sect naturally enough recruited innumerable notions originally the undisputed patrimony of paganism, and adopted to great extent polytheistic doctrines themselves, especially such as related to the supernatural causation of maladies, but attributed them, as we shall presently discern, to a subordinate gradation of puissant demons that were subrogated to the offices of the paganistic divinities. At this epoch the Christians indeed formed a feeble minority, but the chiefs were little distanced by the learning of their antagonists. Of the leaders distinguished among the novel sect for learning should be expressly mentioned Origen, whose treatises aided in shaping their religious faith, and provoked the transition of heathen ideas touching the new rôle which medicine should

74 Effigy to Æsculapius typifying the descent of divinity into the human body to inquire of its ills. Callistratus, Descript. X., § 1.

75 "Morbos ad iram Deorum immortalium relatos esse." Cor. Celsus, De Medicina, Lib. I., p. 2.

76 Clemens Alexandr. Stromata, Lib. I.

assume for ages. At the early age of eighteen[77] he abandoned paganism, and allied himself with the school of Clement of Alexandria.

Polytheistic authority, and the menaces of the people,[78] compelled him to leave the city and retire into Arabia, where his great reputation for erudition had preceded him. Severe measures were useless to totally destroy this rising scholasticism of the Christians, especially as its learned professors resisted such efforts with physical suffering, and gladly taught the prescribed lessons of letters and sciences for a few coins daily, and gave instruction in matters of faith, contented to live unshod, fasting much on the grossest diet.[79] By the side of this Christian eclecticism, which the writings of Clement of Alexandria and Origen so clearly defined, another sect ascended into notice, offering superior attractions to the polytheists of the Museum, and excited at the instigation of the pontiffs the same rigorous treatment as leveled against the Christian school, and likewise opened itself to a bitter and uncompromising hatred of the sacred and profane authorities at Alexandria, as well as the philosophers, as may be gathered from the fragments of Origen's reply to the sharp and envenomed diatribes of Celsus.

This new rival, whose audacious asseverations elicited the bitterest denunciation of Tertullian,[80] was an amalgamation of elements purely Grecian and Christian, united with the theogony of Ancient Egypt and the strange cult of the Orient.[81] It seems to be established that these Gnostic schools, although of earlier origin, were first founded in Alexandria by Basilides during the reign of Marcus Aurelius,[82] and vitalized by Valentinus some years later, through the junction of the Ophites'

[77] Eusebius, Histor. Ecclesiastica, Lib. VI., cap. 3.

[78] Nicephorus, Histor. Ecclesias., Lib. IV., cc. 4 and 5.

[79] Eusebius, Histor. Ecclesias., Lib. VI., c. 3.

[80] Tertullianus, Adversus Gnosticos, cap. 1.

[81] Beausobre, Histoire du Manicheisme, Tom. II., p. 204; and Matter, Histoire du Gnosticisme, Tom. I., cap. 1., § 1.

[82] Vide Irenæus Adversus Hæresos, Lib. II., Præf. 1-2.

doctrines. These sects were quickly attacked by the polytheists, prior to assailing with violence the Didaskelon. At Alexandria they were confounded with the followers of Christ, and at Rome they passed for Jewish dogmatists. Celsus urged against the Christians so close an identity with the Basilidians as to be distinctly unrecognizable. The striking prominence of the Egyptian element among these sects may be inferred when it is stated that the sagacious Hadrian inculpated them with adoring Serapis. Before examining the evolutions arising from the Gnostic doctrines, so far as the same co-operated to modify the principles upon which the system of medical economy had been solidly based and provoked methods of cure of magical similitude, we shall doubtless observe from the declining efficiency of the Alexandrine schools, that the prostration of this science, begun by polytheistic proselytes to Christianity, was concluded with its triumph. Had it been possible, an obstacle to this frightful decay of the science of medicine might have emanated from the Museum of Alexandria, whose position was gradually becoming more and more embarassing.

Evidently, a total indifference to the existence of the rival sects, and uninterrupted continuance of profane studies by this scholastic institution, must necessarily weaken its influence and cause it to be abandoned by the reflecting spirits of the time. On the other hand, an attempt to dispute these new doctrines would cause it to advance upon strange territory, and to leave behind the study of letters and science, for an examination of moral teachings utterly subsersive of its organization and foreign to its creation. It is indeed true, that so far as the actual professorial functions of medical scientists were concerned, they, with the grammarians and mathematicians, pursued their ancient labors as though no changes had occurred in the Greek and Roman world,[83] while their colleagues of the Museum struggled, in this emergency, to oppose a new dogma to the Christian eclecticism of the one and the Gnostic syn-

[83] Matter, École d'Alexandrie, Tom. I., p. 294.

cretism of the other. Had the great school been able to maintain an uninterrupted existence, a salutary check would have delayed the entire downfall of medicine as a science; and instead of the curative art being abandoned to the doubtful remedies of supernatural elements as an integral portion of religious culture, or further degraded by impotent charlatans, the principles of the Galenic system must have survived.

Unfortunately, with the steady advance of sects inimical to polytheism, each day weakened this medical school, through the uncompromising hatred of proselytes to the paganistic system of therapeutics and its alleged causation of maladies, while other catastrophes prepared the way to its complete extinction. Marcus Antoninus undoubtedly possessed sincere affection for the culture of letters, and was animated by so unusual an interest in all matters pertaining to Greece that he caused himself to be made an initiate into the ancient mysteries while sojourning at Athens,[84] to whose schools he devoted his energies and imperial patronage almost exclusively. His biographer briefly states that he was clement to Alexandria in such affairs as brought him in contact with the citizens.[85] Commodus, the son of Aurelian, also visited Egypt, but his presence was sterile in benefactions to its schools.

The entire interest displayed by Septimus Severus in Alexandria seems to have manifested itself in collecting such documents and records as had escaped the Cæsarian conflagrations by storage in the sanctuaries of the city, and safely depositing them in the tomb of Alexander, which, with the Museum, was left untouched by the devouring flames.[86] Such action preserving the relics of remote antiquity ought naturally to have stirred a zealous interest in these venerable remnants of Egyptian archæology, but the profound insensibility of its scholars should be cited only for reprobation.

---

[84] O *αῦτοχράτωρ Μάρχος 'Αθήναςε ὑπὲρ μυστηριων εοτάλη*, Philostratus, Vitæ Sophistor., Lib. II., cap. 10, § 7.

[85] "Fuit Alexandriæ clementer cum iis agens." Julin. Capitol., Vita Antonini Philosoph., c. 26.

[86] Dio Cassius, Histor., Lib. LXXV., cap. 13.

Caracalla, affecting profound adoration for his hero, Alexander,[87] and professing credulity in an old tradition touching the complicity of Aristotle in the death of the Macedonian conqueror, in order to prosecute his nefarious schemes against the city and its scholars, ordered the deportation of all strangers from Alexandria, deprived it of all its privileges conceded by Hadrian, and suppressed the benefices to its erudite professors.[88] The books of the Peripateticians were burned, and all their immunities instantly revoked.[89] Heliogabalus neglected letters to devote himself to mysteries and magic, which, by the force of imperial example, received much inquisitive attention during his reign.[90]

The most lasting catastrophe to the scholastic institutions was provoked by the resistance of the city itself to Aurelian, who besieged that portion of it where his imperial rival had taken refuge, and where were located its professorial edifices. As a consequence of forcible conquest, Alexandria was subjected to pillage and incendiarism about the year 272.[91] Stripped of those elegant quarters, which so long had been the pride and resort of men of science and eminent scholars, its walls were overthrown[92] and its structures entirely destroyed.[93] For the future, the scholastic establishments of the great literary emporium were reópened in the suburbs and under the policy of Diocletian, who favored them as a potential adversary of the Christian schools, which he struggled to eradicate, the erudite professors of Alexandria again endeavored to combat the doctrines of their rivals.

---

87 Spartianus, Vita Caracallæ, cap. 2.

88 Ibid, cap. 6.

89 Ibid, cap. 6.

90 Dio Cassius, Histor., Lib. LXXIX., cap. 11. In these rites children were immolated in order to render the magic spell more effective: "Mactatis pueris adhibitis magicis artibus," ib.

91 Vopiscius, Vita Aureliani, cap. 32.

92 Ammianus Marcellinus, Histor., Lib. XXII., cap. 16.

93 Eusebius, Histor. Eccles., Lib. VII., cc. 18, 21.

The arena dividing the Museum and the Didaskelon had become the theatre daily of the great struggles between the defenders of polytheism and its enemies; and it is evident that this antagonism, which excited so lively an interest in polemical discussions, often ending in bloodshed, was not designed to foster that spirit of scientific investigation which emanates from quietude. Christian and Gnostic sects regularly established in Alexandria, with the avowed design of overthrowing polytheism to its very principles, were most perilous to the schools of letters and sciences in the city, and this menacing rivalry, so novel, modified almost radically their studies and literary tendencies

From the sphere within which they had hitherto confined their researches, with especial predilection for philosophical examinations which naturally included the science of medicine, they were now compelled to pass to the serious consideration, unwillingly, of moral and religious subjects. The direct consequence of this abnormal condition, so foreign to the splendid system established by the Lagides, revealed itself in the diminishing number of mathematicians, historians and medical professors, and attested the profound alteration in scholastic affairs, superinduced by the vicinity of their increasing rivals. For the future the entire body of Alexandrian scholars was suddenly transformed by imperious necessity into moral philosophers, now occupied with religious questions of the most serious importance, and brought to bear against their antagonists the most bitter opposition as the final refuge of declining paganism.[94]

With the rapid expansion of the Gnostic and Christian sects, the scientific propagation of medicine declined, and in its stead were substituted unnumbered practices foreign to the principles of reason, but eliminated, as the creeds themselves, from diversified and ancient forms of religious ceremonial and belief. By this method, the curative art receded as a science, in exact proportion as Christianity or Gnosticism progressed;

[94] Matter, École d'Alexandrie, Tom. I., p. 305.

and when the former triumphed, under the colossal support of secular power, with the new system of religion came remedial adaptations, absurd, irrational, and no longer dependent on the fragile imperfections of human reason, but elevated to celestial or divine manipulation. Touching medical studies still pursued in Alexandria toward the close of the third century, barely mention is made of an eminent scientist, subsequent to the epoch of Galen, Soranus, and Julian.

Although this culture was then object of attention in the Egyptian metropolis, its professors have left no trace in science behind them. Such branches of mental embellishment as mathematics, through the efforts of Claudius Ptolemus, Isidore,[95] and Diophantes, merit commendation, while the Grammarians appalled at the forbidding aspect of the new situation arising from the inroads of Christianity, quickly abandoned the city and sought preferment and larger compensation at Rome.[96] From the system or dogma pursued by Ammonius Saccus, which affected reflecting minds and aggregated great numbers of eminent reasoners of the age, such as Plotinus[97] and Origen, originated the elements which finally prostituted medicine to the level of charlatanism. Substantially an eclecticism, it was the design of Ammonius to closely unite polytheistic doctrine, including its cumbersome formulas, to the Christian creed, with its principal features. By this startling plan he formed a syncretism of the substantial portions of Grecian and Oriental faith,[98] to which Plotinus, as a profound thinker, exalted polytheist, and partisan of eastern creeds, and Origen, the eminent Christian philosopher and scrupulous athlete for

---

95 Voltaire, Essai sur les Moeurs et Usages, Tom. IV., p. 364; and Bossuet, Histoire des Mathematiques, Tom I., p. 147 seq.

96 Origen himself seems to have sought Rome on account of the superior opportunities for the display of his erudition, but subsequently returned to Alexandria. Nichephorus, Hist. Eccles., Lib. IV., c. 11.

97 Ammianus Marcellinus, Lib. XXII., c. 16.

98 Bruckerii, Histor. Philosophic, Lib. I., cap. 2, § 4.

the dogmas of Christ, each within the limits indicated, severally belonged.[99]

Amid such bitter polemical controversy, where each leader, stirred with exalted enthusiasm, sought to successfully vindicate the faith of his religious predilection—where each system of religion, whether old or new, was carefully scrutinized, and those elements most proper to captivate wavering minds selected with judicious eagerness, on the basis of a lofty eclecticism—it should excite little astonishment that the science of medicine fell before this whirlwind of impassioned discussion, and in its place gradually crept to vigorous existence those heterogenous principles of divinized remedies assiduously applied by ardent zealots, and astutely recommended by the sacerdotal authorities of the rising Church.

To resist this downfall of a progressive science, the Alexandrine polytheistic schools, borne along by the force of religious debates, were utterly impotent; and indeed it would appear that towards the conclusion of the third century the serious study of the curative art was in a measure abandoned by its professors, in order to confront increasing sectarians upon the identical plane of supernatural efficacy in the treatment of maladies.[100]

---

[99] Ibid, §§ 6 and 7, and Eunapius, Vitæ Sophistor., Præfat, and sub nom. Plotinus, p. 454 seq.

[100] Origen Contra Celsum, Lib. VIII., p. 416; and Bruckerii, Histor. Philosoph., Lib. II., cap. 7, § 9.

CHAPTER IV.

Belief in Direct Demoniacal Influences—Adopted by the Christian Church—Debasing Effect on Medicine—The Angelic Heirarchy and Its Special Attributes—Power Over Earth and Its Denizens—Satanic Potency and His Subordinates—Cause Sickness and Pain—Talmud and the Cabbala—Rabbinical Lore and its Effect on Medicine—Potential Forces of Words—Expel Disease—Development of Magic Cures—Incantations by Hebrew Letters.

IN the year 312, Constantine, surnamed the Great, by a decree issued from the city of Milan, declared the Christian religion to be the faith of the Empire. This edict, which gave immediate ascendency to Christianity, was the ruin of both the Museum and polytheism. One of the earliest transformations of belief consequent on the inroads of the new sect and its gradual advance to secular power, arose from the unalterable confidence in the potency of unseen spiritual forces, personified as good or evil. This system of extraordinary puissance was the amalgamation of several doctrines, doubtless perfected by the Christians and Gnostics of Alexandria and adopted substantially by the Fathers, and continued in active operation throughout the the Middle Ages.

The Jews from their Oriental captivity accredited the efficiency of demoniacal influences, and through the writings of Philo propagated the same to Christian converts; while the Gnostics, from their rigid syncretism,[1] quickly absorbed the notion of preternatural interposition through the agency of aeons or emanations.[2]

This dogma, accepted in all its potential ramifications by the new Church under the name of angelic beings, totally overthrew the science of medicine, and reduced its economy

[1] Beausobre, Histoire du Manicheisme, Tom. II., p. 204.

[2] Matter, Histoire du Gnosticisme, Tom. II., pp. 116–341.

to the most abject dependence on divine manifestations. Next to the widespread belief in the second coming of Christ,[3] whose followers marked their profession by the sharpest contrast with the pagans,[4] was the unqualified acceptance, from the first century, of a mighty spiritual world, whose unceasing operations upon the earth and its people stood forth as an article of Christian faith. This notion was common to both Christianity and Judaism, and at the same time Paganism rivalled these sectarians in its exaggeration of preternatural forces. The existence of spiritual beings—angelic hosts—was not only accepted with an unquestioning faith,[5] but constituted a most fascinating subject of controversy, unsettled by synodal decretals,[6] to the Patristic writers. In general arrangement, the Christian writers recognized among the angels a subordination as strict as existed with the sacerdoty.[7] Angelic nature was admitted to be of finer composition than humanity, on account of its element of immorality, an attribute of Deity, and consequently invisible.[8]

Their corporeal essence, modeled upon that of their divine Head, was a deft structure of light and fire of the most sublime splendor. Of unlimited freedom, they were munificent for good or evil.[9] That view of a spiritual being, which accorded to him divine power,[10] as contrasted with the theory of æons or emanations, ultimately gained the ascendency.[11] Touching the activity of these invisible entities, the Fathers were unanimous

---

[3] Tertullianus, Contra Marcianos, Lib. III., cap. 13.

[4] Tertullian, De Spectaculis, cap. 7; and Minutius Felix, c. 8.

[5] Origen, Contra Celsum, Lib. VIII., p. 401.

[6] Ibid, Principia, Prœm., § 10.

[7] Clemens Alexandr., Excerpta, cap. XI., §§ 8 and 9; and Ignatius, Ad Trallianos, c. 5.

[8] Fulg. Respuens, De Trinitate, cap. 8; and Justin Martyr, Dialog. cum Tryph. c. 57.

[9] Irenæus, Ad Haer., Lib. IV., c. 37, §§ 1 and 2. Origen, De Principia, Prœm. I., c. 8.

[10] Lactant., Instit., Lib. IV., c. 8.

[11] Justin Martyr, op. cit., c. 128.

that God himself exercises upon his creatures, through the mediation of angels, such intentions as pleased the divine will.

The earlier teachers of the Church maintained that to these was committed the supervision of all things appertaining to the earth and its inhabitants,[12] an opinion reiterated by subsequent dogmatists. Some of the Fathers designated the specific attributes and duties of angels. According to Origen, the splendid being Raphael had special care over the sick and infirm,[13] while Gabriel exercised superintendence over war, and Michael attended the devotional prayers of believers.

In the time of Hermes, an angel of penitents is mentioned, and as late as Tertullian,[14] and Origen,[15] the angel of prayer seems to have received a well defined outline as to duty and efficacy. Immovable and lifeless things of earth acknowledged the potential interposition of these mandatories of the divine Regent,[16] while the incarnate representative of Deity himself, from earliest infancy, was provided with a protecting spirit, whose dutiful care produced for Him beneficent pleasure, accorded answer to humble petitions, and created irresistible force against seductive temptations.[17]

In striking contrast to the beneficence of the guardian spirit, quickly followed the presence of a malevolent angel, whom Tertullian asserted to be in constant attendance upon each person.[18] Others maintained the doctrine, which gradually grew into an important element of mediæval faith, and aided in the servile subjection of medicine, that impure demons closely united themselves to man, and while using him as a habitation, made him believe they were good angels.[19] In their hidden

[12] Origen, Contra Celsum, Lib. VIII., p. 397 seqq.

[13] Ibid, De Principia, Lib. I., c. 8.

[14] Tertullianus, De Oratione, cap. 12.

[15] Origen, Contra Celsum, Lib. VIII. p. 400.

[16] Ibid., Lib. VIII., p. 398 seqq.

[17] Ibid., De Principia, Lib. III., c. 2.

[18] "Nam et suggissimus nullum pæne hominem carere dæmonio." Tertullianus. De Anima, Lib. I., c. 57.

[19] "Qui quoniam sunt spiritus tenues, et incomprehensibiles, insinuant se corporibus hominum." Lactantius, Institut. Divin., Lib. II., c. 15.

recesses of the human body they vitiated health and provoked disease.[20] Satan, himself, among the early Christian sects, excepting the Gnostics, was regarded as an angelic personage, whose freedom Deity had abused and thereby become evil.[21] The religious philosophy of Gnosticism seems to have rendered it essential to separate the sublimest idea of Divinity, in order to deduce the unfinished good of the Universe, from an imperfect being—the Demiurgos—opifex mundi, especially since the discussion in a polemical sense of evil was perpetually extant, as an integral portion of the system.[22] In its broadest acceptance, it may be stated that the Satanic notion, at this epoch, was certainly developed by such views as directly antagonized the creed of the dominant Church—the ponderous influences of its rival sect tended to modify these doctrines, and the impress they made was propagated uninterruptedly for centuries, and in their practical social application further burdened the curative art and rendered its scientific resurrection quite impossible. In the New Testament it is unequivocally stated that the death of Christ was a victory over the devil; but according to the Gnostic system, the Demiurgos, or Creator of the world, regarded His operations as a direct invasion of power,[23] and consequently, on the scheme of retaliation, the heretical divinity arrayed himself in mighty conflict against the Triune God, which resulted in the crucifixion of Jesus.[24]

To Irenæus may be attributed the subrogation of Satan to the personality of the Gnostic Demiurgos, and with it the translation of religious controversy upon a ground which rendered the argumentation of the Church so powerful, but intensified embittered differences, by which for many ensuing centuries nearly all manifestations arising from activity of natural

---

[20] "Valetudinem vitiant, morbos citant." Ib.

[21] Tertullianus, Adversus Marcion, Lib. II., cap. 10.

[22] Tertullianus, De Persecution. Haeres., cap. 7.

[23] Irenæus, Adversus Haeres., Lib. II., cap. 7.

[24] Roskoff, Geschichte des Teufels, Th. I., p. 225.

law, involving weakness of body or of mind, were directly referred to diabolical agencies.[25]

According to the enunciation of Irenæus, mankind, through trangression of divine command, fell absolutely from the time of Adam into the power of Satan.[26] Christ, in freeing man from this encumbrance of servitude, purchased this absolution with blood, but the Marcionites[27] and Gnostics urged that the Demiurgos, on account of his creating the human race, preserved the right of proprietorship, and consequently the Polemical Fathers admitted the lawful claim of the devil to man as a result of original sin.[28] That such right was of binding effect upon humanity, obtained ready credence from the Fathers during the early portion of the Middle Ages. Augustine acknowledged it as full and incontestible,[29] while Leo accorded it as a tyrannical and unjust claim.[30]

The representation of Satanic authority, personified as an independent ruler, with his avowed right, arrayed in opposition to Divine Will, had so far passed into the foreground that the conception of salvation was ultimately significant, in a dogmatic sense, as a means of emancipation from the power of the Devil. Eclesiastical writers of the first centuries generally admitted that all impure manifestations among the Pagans originated from illicit communication with subordinate angels of Satan, and from such admixture emanated pride, envy, and licentiousness.[31]

Since the good angels were declared to be corporeal, also

---

25 "Et occulte in visceribus operati, valetudinem vitiant, morbos citant, somniis animos terrent, mentes favoribus quatiunt." Lactantius, Divin. Instit., Lib. II., c. 15.

26 Adversus Haeres., Lib. V., c. 1.

27 Matter, Histoire du Gnosticisme, Tom. I., cap. 3.

28 "Ideo eum habuit in sua potestate." Irenæus, Advers. Haeres., Lib. V., c. 21, § 3.

29 "Quibus universus autem mundus subjectus est." August., Lib. Arbitr., Lib. III., c. 32.

30 Sermo XXII., c. 3.

31 Lactantius, Divin. Institut., Lib. II., c. 15.

the evil ones were assumed to be of a grosser nature, because Satan himself was endowed, from his fall, with a physical body,[32] but these angelic forms of Deity were of a far finer essence than that of man.[33] Origen, in his celebrated treatise and polemical discussion with Celsus, asserted the prescience of demoniacal personages, as infinitely superior to human intelligence, and that such knowledge was obtained by a correct interpretation of the stars.[34] But the most significant attribute conceded to these demoniacal beings was their recognized ability, in common with Satan, to engender sin and largely propagate among humanity the unconditional stipulations of misery and vice, which prerogative incorporated the principle by which the systematic use of medicaments and cures of maladies, during the Middle Ages, were universally administered.[35] Early Christian writers boldly asserted that all the disorders of the world originated with the Devil and his sinister companions,[36] because these were stirred with an unholy desire to obtain associates in their miseries.[37]

Demoniacal æons or emanations, portraying this diabolical principle of evil, were acknowledged to be the primitive source from which arose the multifarious elements of sorrow and pain, including earthly sufferings, pestilence among men, sickness, and other bodily afflictions,[38] but inflicted with consent of Divinity, whose messengers they were. The Fathers of the early Church were fully persuaded that these beings took possession of the organism of the human body, and ridiculed

---

[32] Origen, Com. in John, Lib. XX., cap. 22.

[33] Origen, Contra Celsum, Lib. VII., p. 334.

[34] Ibid., Lib. IV., p. 167.

[35] Irenæus, Adversus Haeresos, Lib. V., c. 24, §§ 2 and 3.

[36] Athenagoras, Legat. pro Christ., Lib. II., c. 27, avows the supreme control of these beings of the earth's inhabitants: "Vicesque et ordinem omnium—elementa, cœlos, mundum—moderarent."

[37] Cyprian, De Vanitat. Idol., Lib. III., § 8.

[38] Origen, Contra Celsum, Lib. VIII., p. 416, and Lib. V., p. 132. "Itaque corporibus quidem et valetudines infligunt et aliquos casus acerbos." Tertullian, Apologetic., cap. 22.

the solemn asseverations of surgeons that many of these alleged demoniacal infirmities were attributed to material agencies;[39] and Cyprian charged that demons caused luxations and fractures of the limbs, undermined the health, and harassed with diseases.[40] In the practice of magical art, evil spirits often, it was claimed, provided cures for sickness.[41]

To these most positive and unequivocal utterances of the Fathers, that infirmities assigned by pagan physicians to scientific causes were, on the contrary, produced by malevolent angels, was added the allegation that the devilish hosts were inventors of astrology, necromancy and magic.[42]

The most fleeting examination of the writers of the period before us attests the high importance of this doctrine touching the supernatural gifts accorded Satanic beings, which had so profoundly permeated the ecclesiastical fabric that a scientific explanation of natural events was absolutely impossible; and so far as the direct association of this teaching with the cause of physcal ills extended, it will readily permit the conclusion that the unquestioned triumph of the Church, whose adherents marked the appearance of corporeal afflictions as produced by demoniacal influences[43] arrayed in combat with the forces of Deity, must of necessity banish medicine, except so far as it abandoned its scientific attitude and assumed the form of administering medications upon a sacerdotal system.

New converts to Christianity were seriously informed that contact with a pagan exposed them to the most favorable on-

[39] Origen, Com. in Matthew xvii. 5, and Ibid., De Principia, Lib. II., c. 2, and Lib. III., c. 2.

[40] "Membra distorquent, valetudinem frangunt, morbos lacessunt." Cyprian, De Vanit. Idolat., Lib. III., § 8.

[41] "Venefici plane et circa curas valetudinem." Tertul., Apologet., c. 22. Tertullian, with characteristic boldness, does not hesitate to say: "Æsculapius medicinorum demonstrator"—Æsculapius, with demon aid, etc., Ibid., cap. 23.

[42] Tertullianus, Apologetic, cc. 21 and 23. "Eorum inventa sunt astrologia, et aruspicina, et necromantia, et ars magica," Lactantius, De Divin. Institut., Lib. II., cap. 17.

[43] Tertullian, ut sup., cap. 22.

slaught of unseen demons, alone subjugated by the name of Jesus,[44] and that in their daily intercourse with the outside, the heathen world, each paganistic touch was virulent with diabolism, and must entail damnation! How narrowed in morals and dwarfed in mental conception the Christian populace finally became, may be gathered from the indignant assertion of Tertullian,[45] that whoever, in the pursuance of his usual handicraft, worked for the construction and embellishment of heathen idols, by this act retrograded to paganism, and stood as a despised and proselyted image-worshiper; but what frightful debasement of human reason is attested by his fervid proclamation, that the offices of Ludi Magistris and Professores Literarum were incompatible with and repugnant to Christianity, for the reason that these functionaries under the empire required a description of pagan deities, an explanation of their mythology![46]

Development, or even preservation, of medical science was therefore impossible, when it is considered that such system required the exercise of dispassionate ratiocination, whose operations necessarily must trace bodily infirmities to natural causes; but ecclesiastical authority had declared these to be diabolical, against which it was futile to struggle: contact with science, as with the pagan, involved possible damnation; to believe otherwise was heresy, and the person thus believing was liable to exorcism.

To this colossal development of an unshaken faith in the existence of unseen potent spirits, presented as the punitive messengers of Deity,[47] operating upon humanity through

---

[44] Origen, Contra Celsum, Lib. III., p. 133.

[45] "Nulla ars, nulla professio, nulla negotio, quæquid aut instruendo aut informandis idolis administrat carere potuit titulo idololatriæ." Tertul., De Idololatria, cap. 11.

[46] "Primum quibus necesse est Deos Nationum prædicare nomina, genealogia, fabulas, ornamenta, honorifica quaeque eorum enuntiare tum solemnia festaque eorundem observare." Tertullian, De Idololatria, cap. 10. Converts forbidden to carry gems with idolatrous images on them. Clemens. Alexandr. Pædagog., Lib. II., c. 12.

[47] Ibid, Recogniti., Lib. IV.

grievous maladies and physical infirmities, the Talmud and Cabbala severally added powerful influence in extending this doctrine to infinity, and largely aided in selecting remedies so eagerly sought during the Middle Ages. In the more remote times, a well-grounded fear prevented the Jews from making written explanatory comments upon the revered text of the Old Testament, because, as alleged, these would degrade the Sacred Scriptures from their exalted rank. Increasing, in some cases contradictory interpretations, induced the Rabbi Jehuda, a native of Tiberias, in the third century, to undertake the task of codifying these Hebraic scholia. This collection of what was previously the oral transmission of interpreted law received the name of Mishna or Second Law.[48] From this epoch the Mishna was the central point around which all rabbinical studies concentrated, designated Gemara, inasmuch as these claimed to contain the genuine essence of Mosaic teachings.

Towards the close of the fourth century an unknown scholiast collected the exegetical elucidations, explanations and interpretations produced by the Gemara, and united them to the Mishna, as a commentary out of which arose the Talmud.[49] The word Cabbala, whose original signification was used in the sense of "reception," or transmission, obtained at a later period the meaning of secret lore, because the metaphysical and theosophic idealities which had been developed in the Rabbinical schools, were communicated only to a few, and consequently remained the undisputed property of a limited and close organization.[50]

Venerable elements of ancient religions emanating from Egypt, Zoroasterian teachings imparted from Babylonish captivity, Greek thought, especially in high repute through the weighty influence of the Alexandrine schools, each in order

---

[48] Pfeiffer, Critica Sacra, p. 388; and Buddeus, Introd. ad Philos. Ebraeor., p. 91 seq.

[49] Pfeiffer, op. cit., cap. 15, De Talmuda, p. 386.

[50] Bruckerii, Histor. Philosoph., Lib. II., cap. 3, § 2.

deliberately appropriated by adroit Rabbins, ultimately exercised powerful control over both the material itself as well as the method of instruction, imparted by teachers only to their most skilled and able disciples.[51] From the system of religious culture originated a theosophic scheme, the operation of which was perpetuated for centuries. The plan of these mystical interpretations, oftentimes in direct antagonism to the letter of the record, and finally transferred to the Talmud, was used by Philo himself with eminent power, to whom indeed the Cabbalists attribute the chief features of their curious doctrines.[52] As an influential precursor of these mystical devotees, Philo doubtless may be regarded as a scholastic deeply learned in Platonic-Pythagorean puissance of numbers and their symbolical forces, which he was accustomed to regard as a moralistic prototype; but when observed according to form and gradation these letters, to uninitiates as lifeless, contained the secret essence of vitality and were emblems of supreme truth.[53]

Philo's enunciation of a hidden and concealed Divinity, as contrasted with a tangible, revealed Deity, whose vital spirit suffused the universe and linked back humanity, through this revelation, from the dark, invisible and primal base of existence, closely resembles the Sephiroth of the Cabbalists, with its omniponent head and succeeding gradation of divine forces.[54] According to these idealists, the Deity created all things by the effective operation of the Word, whose subdivisions the *Logii*, are vitalized acts of God, designated as his angels, repose in their atmospheric abodes beneath the world or in heaven, as servants and executive instruments of the Superior Divinity or mediators and impassible judges of men.

The Cabbalists assert their system is an exact analogy of this

---

51 Vide Bruckerii, op. and loc. cit., p. 408.

52 Buddeus, Introduct. ad Histor. Philos. Ebraeor., p. 59. Sometimes interpreted to signify: Secretum Legis, Ibid., p. 152.

53 Buddeus, op. cit., § 18.

54 Bruckerii, Histor. Philosoph., Lib. II., cap. 2, § 9.

scheme. Many devotees of this lore pretend to trace the origin of their mysteries back to the time of Adam; but the frequent association with the people and customs of Egypt, the land of mysticism and contemplative life, where many Israelites had been forcibly conveyed after the conquest of Palestine, furnishes a more satisfactory derivation of the system.[55] Uninterrupted intercourse between the Egyptian and Palestine Jews, propagated to the latter such secret learning possessed by the former, which ultimately grew into a regular cult of erudite and mysterious teachings.[56] It was boldly asserted that the mere expression of the words of Holy Scripture was verbal only, and that beneath these reposed a genuine signification, which was forever concealed from the profane and divulged to initiates alone. This asseveration was insisted upon as a uniform, unequivocal principle of the system.[57]

The Cabbala was potent to explain each secret meaning with which Deity had endowed the letters and points of the Sinaitic code. This mystic deciphering was performed by means of Gematria, which consisted of letters, lines, figures and numbers, etc.,[58] the latter of which, in the Cabbala, were particularly powerful; or by means of Notarikon, which was a system of important words composed of initial and terminal letters.

Themorah taught the suitable collocation of an indefinite alphabetical arrangement.[59] These letters, punctuations, and other visible signs, which collectively made up the Holy Writings, stood in closest correlation with the divine and celestial emanations of Deity himself, whose operations they with absolute certainty elucidated; and by the mere utterance

[55] Bruckerii, op. cit., § 4.

[56] Buddeus, Introduct. ad Philos. Ebraeor., § 11, p. 28 seq.

[57] Ibid, p. 59.

[58] Bruckerii, op. cit., Lib. II., cap. 3, p. 411. "Gematria est arithmetica explicatio vocis e numeris, quos juxta valorem literarum suarum Arithmeticum continet." Pfeiffer, Critica Sacra, p. 209.

[59] Ibid. p. 213.

of a visible sign within which was a concealed force, the spirit beings, over whom the uttered symbol had especial power, were at once started into activity—a movement largely intensified, if the Cabbalist were able to fix the mystic type upon his mind.[60] In these arts remedies were found to be of sovereign puissance to expel diseases.[61] As a direct result of such potential influence on spiritual hosts, each wish of the human heart could be satisfied. These pious practices, exercised in strict accord with the Sacred Scriptures themselves, affected not merely the material world, but in their mighty and searching manifestations influenced the higher gradation of invisible spirits, and were thus endowed with the property of harmonizing the heterogenous things of earth upon a system which involved the propagation of the Universe. Man himself as the exact prototype of the world in minature, with his corporeal and spiritual endowments in the lower sphere, stands in a fixed and determined relationship to the upper sphere, even to the Divine Head, to whom all things are subjected.[62]

In close union with Sephiroth, which consisted of ten subtle forces, were brought the properties of Divinity, ten omnipotent names, ten orders of angels, three heavens with seven planets, and ten principal members of the human body.[63] This system, adapted to use during mediæval times on an enlarged scale for the treatment of diseases and bodily ailments, combined with the equally superstitious practices fostered by ecclesiastical authority for the cure of maladies, aided in debasing medicine from its scientific dignity, and reducing it to the level of a magic art.[64]

One of the most serious results of the extending application

---

[60] Roskoff, Geschichte des Teufels, Th. I., p. 248.

[61] "Censent enim Judæi, per artes Kabbalisticas e Scriptura petendas averti mala, pelli morbas," etc. Pfeiffer, op. cit., p. 209.

[62] Buddeus, Introduct. ad Histor. Philosoph. Ebraeor., p. 345.

[63] Ibid., p. 277.

[64] "Duplicam esse, continentem nomina Angelorum ac Spiritum variorum, ac docentem quomodo morbi curandi," etc. Buddeus, op. cit., p. 352.

of the Cabbala, and which coöperated with the saintly idolatry of the Church and demoniacal influences to banish medical science, was the logical transformation to which the Cabbala itself was subjected. Instead of maintaining the exercise of sound reason in the development of their doctrines, the Cabbalists gradually receded from the philosophical character of their investigations, and personified the whole of Nature, the causes of physical phenomena, the psychic manifestations; and identical with the demonology of the Romish Church, introduced an unlimited number of good and evil demons, whom they conceived as permeating the most remote regions of earth, heaven or man, and believed themselves necessitated to the exactest surveillance of action in order to attract the favorable interference of the good and avoid the malevolence of bad spirits. By what methods these results were accomplished, the Cabbalistic theurgist instructed his disciples.

The conjuration of these rival beings was performed by the vocalizing of certain verses or single words taken from the mystic Script which expressed the diversified names of Deity and his angelic hosts,[65] or were composed of different collocations of the Hebraistic alphabet, and by means of amulets on which rhymes, certain phrases or words arranged upon the canonitical scheme of divine or angelic nomenclature, and illustrated with various figures. To these names the Cabbalists attributed irresistible potency to provoke disease of any character, and to cure maladies the most dangerous and mortal.[66]

More recent devotees to the Cabbala fully recognized the resistless force of these incantations for the cure of diseases,

---

[65] "Qui spiritus corporeos esse, rebusque corporeis delectari credunt, quive litterarum characteribus occultam quandam reconditam vim." Buddeus, Introduct. ad Histor. Philosoph. Ebraeor., p. 352.

[66] "Nomina Angelorum ac Spiritum variorum, ac docentem quomodo morbi procreandi iidem iterum curandi, civitates evertandae, terræ motos excitandi." Buddeus, op. cit., p. 352. According to Maimonides, More Nevochim, Pars. I., caps 61, p. 108, there were forty names used for such purposes: "Amuleta sive chartas experimentales conscribentibus."

provoking ills, etc., and warned against their use; others, equally persuaded of their efficacy for good or evil, absolutely interdicted them, particularly as the most trivial error in arrangement, form or utterance, would not only cause the most frightful convulsion in the upper regions where these invisible beings reside, but render the enchanter himself liable to grievous injury, of which the Talmud furnishes notable examples.[67] The immensity of space, similar to Gnosticism and Christianity, was peopled by the Cabbala with beneficent or malicious angels, graded in rigid subordination to leaders on whom specific duties devolved, such, for instance, as collecting the prayers of men and weaving them into a crown for Omnipotence.[68]

Of the number of malevolent spirits, constantly provoking diseases and infirmities upon man, it was impossible to fix a limit; they were alleged to surround mankind so densely that each person had a thousand to his right and ten thousand to the left of him. Endowed with the subtlest activity, they were able to reach the remotest points of earth in the twinkling of an eye, and by their great prescience, were eagerly sought after on account of their cognizance of future events.[69] As a potential means of preservation and duration through the Middle Ages, the secrecy of instruction imparted to initiates was of especial importance, and resembled the methods adopted by the Gnostics.[70]

Although the origin of cabbalistic lore lies concealed in the darkness of distant ages, its effective existence was recognized by the sacred and profane society of the first centuries, and doubtless such recognition developed from the writings of Philo and the mysticism of the Essenes.[71] A thirst for secret sciences was a mighty propelling force towards cabbalistic sources, whose fascinating forms were greatly embellished and

---

[67] Buddeus, Introduct. ad Histor. Philosoph. Ebraeor., p. 275.

[68] Ibid, p. 347.

[69] Delrio, Disquisition. Magicar, Lib. I., cap. 4, Quest. 4, p. 28 seq.

[70] Matter, Histoire du Gnosticisme, Tom. II., p. 491 seq.

[71] Bruckerii, Histor. Philosoph., Lib. II., cap. 3, § 4.

enlarged, when the more ancient Aristotelian philosophy had survived its usefulness, and the Alexandrine schools were waging bitter warfare against multiplying sects and the Christian Church, particularly since the elements of the Cabbala closely assimilated to the amalgamation of Oriental doctrines with the Platonic-Pythagoreanism.[72] The mania for mystic erudition which swept so strongly through the Roman Empire in the early ages of the Christian Church, aided in degrading the science of medicine in the second century, to such extent that its most eminent professor complained of this debasement arising from enthusiasm for these rites and ceremonies.

The embittered denunciations of the Fathers against the use of magic attested the fervid zeal manifested by the leading minds of the period to become initiated into the mysterious secrets claimed to be imparted within closed sanctuaries.[73] During the time of Hadrian and the Antoninii, a public proffer was made by the Jews and Pagans at Rome of initiation into these occult sciences, formerly the exclusive property of the Egyptian priesthood, whose possession it was asserted gave an undisputed control over the world of demons and by the potential efficacy of amulets, talismans, and uttered spells, procured for the possessor a mastery over nature.

From the opening of the Christian era, adoration was unqualifiedly given to magical forces whose assumed potency was hidden from vulgar inquiry by the restrictive power of obligations and impressive rites.[74] Under the charm of serious investigation, and influenced by religious principle, this science was yet admired by many philosophers. Cabbalistic mysteries at Alexandria[75] doubtless in their most comprehensive significance aided in moulding the thoughts of inquiring scholars

---

[72] Bruckerii, Histor. Philosoph., Lib. II., cap. 3, § 4.

[73] Clemens. Alexandr. Cohortatio ad Gentes, cc. 1 and 2; and Tertullianus, Apologetic. Adversus Gentes, cap. 23.

[74] Salverte. Sciences Occultes, p. 87.

[75] Beausobre, Histoire du Manicheisme, Tom. II., p. 203.

and religious enthusiasts, to an examination of the power of rites whose knowledge was only to be obtained under the attractive form of secrecy. The distinguished Judaico-Platonic writer of the second century, in according his unstinted admiration of this singular art, boldly announced it to be a science which discloses the veiled forces of nature, and leads to a direct contemplation of celestial power.[76] Although in his day the notion of magus seems to have received currency to express the highest form of reliance upon Divinity, properly approached by certain secret methods, a century and a half later the biographer of Apollonius of Tyana hastens to disclose that his hero was not a magician, and in disclaiming such nomenclature for his hero, compares him to Plato, who likewise was instructed in Egyptian arcana without incurring this reproachful epithet.[77]

---

[76] Philo Judæus, De Specib. Legibus.

[77] Philostratus, Vita Apollonii Tyan., Lib. I., c. 1, §§ 1 and 2.

CHAPTER V.

Christian Philosophers Influenced by the Cabbala—The Chaldaic System and Magic Art Avowed by the Fathers—Treatise on Magic by Noah's Son—Used to Avert Pestilence—Schools for Such Instruction in Alexandria—The Curative Power of Apollonius the Magician—Spirits Invoked by Occult Rites—Cure Bodily Ills—Care Prescribed in these Operations—Theurgic Arts—Chaldaic Soothsayers Accorded Profound Insight into Metals, Plants, etc.—Resemble Mediæval Alchemists—Egyptian Incantations of Special Force Against Sickness—High Charges of these Practitioners—Such Curatives the Basis of Subsequent Saintly Remedies—Power of Names—Of Angels—Translated Chaldaic Names Lose their Force—Jao or Jehovah—Pagans Use it to Cure.

IT is little surprising that the most profound and erudite philosophers of the early ages of Christianity sought the pretended disclosures which were professedly in the custody of the ancient mysteries, as a possible solution of the grave and serious matters which so deeply exercised their minds. These secret associations, especially the Bacchic, Egyptian and Grecian mysteries, originally of close identity if not absolute unity,[1] maintained a fluctuating existence down to the time of their utter extinction by imperial Christianity,[2] and to some extent may have aided in moulding the monastic organizations of a subequent period—traces of which influence it is claimed are discernible.[3]

According to Ammianus Marcellinus, Zoroaster, the great conservator of magic through his devotees, only added large portions of this occult art to the Chaldaic system.[4] One of the early Fathers of the Church, in admitting as did all thoughtful

[1] Gail, sur le Culte de Bacchus, p. 82 seq.

[2] XVI. Codex Theodos., Tit. X., Lex 14.

[3] Fosbroke, British Monachism, p. 35.

[4] Rerum Gesta, Lib. XXVI., c. 6.

scholars of that period the undisputed existence of magic and its malevolent or beneficial influences,[5] asserted that in the more remote combats which Zoroaster, King of the Bactrians, sustained against Ninus, each of the mortal contestants used the secrets of this science with the same utility as their weapons of war.[6] The holy and sainted Epiphany narrates that Nimrod, in establishing the foundations of his realm, introduced the magic arts of which the invention was afterwards attributed to Zoroaster.[7]

In the fifth century it was publicly announced that a treatise of this science, written by Chem, the son of Noah, was in current use,[8] and composed by such illustrious authority, obtained no doubt the honors of obedient admiration, as well as abject imitation. When it is considered that Arnobius himself, in faithfully delineating the peculiar belief of his age, maintained that the enchantments and potential efficacy of this art ascended to the time of Seth, a son of Adam, it may be regarded as a logical conclusion that the possibilities of magic were well understood and agreed to with unquestioning faith.

Justin admits that the Israelitish youth, Joseph, carried as a slave into Egypt, obtained there so profound a knowledge of magical arts as to satisfactorily explain the prodigies presaging famine and pestilence to the people, who, without his succor thus procured, must have perished.[9] Disbelieving pagans or skeptical Jews, in acknowledging the puissance of Christ by which he manifested his divine mission, deliberately charged that in transcending the miracles performed by native magicians, He had perfected himself in clandestine arts stolen by him from the sanctuaries of Egypt,[10] and used illicitly the names and

[5] Salverte, Sciences Occultes, p. 89.

[6] Arnobius, Adversus Gentes, Lib. I., cap. 5.

[7] Adversus Haeres., Lib. I., cap. 1.

[8] Salverte, Sciences Occultes, p. 88.

[9] Lib. XXXVI., cap. 2.

[10] "Magus fuit, clandestinüs artibus omnia illa perfecit; Ægyptiorum ex aditis angelorum potentium nomina, et remotas furatus est disciplinas." Arnobius, op. cit., Lib. I., cap. 43.

secret rites of potential angels.[11] Apollonius, in defending himself from the appellation of enchanter, denounced the practitioners of these occult arts and sciences as *artisans* of miracles, who, upon failing to produce the result or cure of maladies which they had confidently predicted, loudly insisted upon the accidental omission of certain substances.[12]

In the Egyptian metropolis it was no unusual event, subsequent to the proclamation of Christianity as the religion of the Roman Empire, to find venerable sacerdotal institutions completely transformed into a school for the instruction of magic,[13] which was the object of eager research. Such practices were by no means restricted in their extension to those professing an admiration for declining polytheism, or devoting themselves as enthusiastic Israelites to the culture of the Cabbala and Talmud—for independent of the practical admission of the use of an elevated magic by the Christian Fathers, nearly all the philosophical schools of the epoch were addicted to magical arts.[14]

The bitter incrimination of Apollonius against the blundering enchanters of his day was graciously less severe when he announced himself as professor of a science which Divinity had bestowed upon him as a recompense for austere virtues; and further, to perform successively these miraculous cures where the ignorant charlatan exposed his mechanical appliances and failed, he required no elaborate preparations or sacrifices, but with sublime confidence in his temperance and piety, such startling manifestations of superior power were of easy procuration.[15] Cheremon, thoroughly persuaded of the practibility, taught the art of invoking divinities, and even in defiance to their resistance compelling them to operate the prodigy demanded.

---

[11] Arnobius, Adversus Gentes, Lib. I., cap. 43.

[12] Philostratus, Vita Apollon. Tyan., Lib. I., c. 2.

[13] Matter, École d'Alexandrie, Tom. I., p. 319.

[14] Matter, Histoire du Gnosticisme, Tom. II., p. 170.

[15] Philostratus, op. cit., Lib. I., c. 2.

In undertaking to dispute the assumed logical position of this great Egyptian sage, Porphyry affirmed that the gods themselves had established such formulas and methods of invocation, by which their omnipotent interposition might be secured.[16] Touching the essence of this controversy, doubtless the distinction is merely designed to signify that an altercation is here revealed between the scholiasts of rival systems of occult arts.[17] Expressing the means by which man has the empire over these spiritual beings whose unlimited resources were invoked in the cure of bodily ailments, Iamblichus distinguishes them into two classes, one of which is the Divine type, from whom nothing can be obtained except by the humility of prayer and the practice of ennobling virtues.

The other class of invisible emanations, corresponding to the obedient remedial deities of Cheremon, were defined by the Theurgist as spirits entirely divested of reason, discernment and intelligence, and endowed with a puissance of action transcending that possessed by man, each gifted with a virtue or force destined to accomplish resistlessly its certain and specific object, forced to exercise this especial function when commanded by man, inasmuch as reasoning and discernment elevate him above these invisible entities, and render them subject to his superior power, the result of higher intellectuality.[18] Much of this presumed exercise of extraordinary puissance may have originated in the chemical knowledge of these skilled magicians or Thaumaturgists.[19] The divinized beings thus described possessed a unique property which they exercised without consciousness or comprehension. Acting unintelligibly, they readily became the blind instruments for the production of miraculous events and cures in the hands of

---

[16] Eusebius, Præparatio ad Evangel., Lib. V., cc. 8 and 11.

[17] Salverte, Sciences Occultes, p. 106.

[18] The operation to secure this subjection proceeded through the gradation of spirits: "Semper enim in sacrarum operationum ordine per superiora numina inferiora vocantur." Iamblich., De Myster. Ægypt., p. 170.

[19] Salverte, op. cit., p. 107.

men whose intelligence and science acquired the methods of mastering them, and of judiciously applying their energies.

Iamblichius also clearly states that any one experimenting to obtain control of these puissant beings, if ignorant of the process necessary to be followed, must infallibly terminate his labors in useless efforts if he should fail to employ a single substance in conformity to the prescription of sacred rites.[20] Of these divinities, thus subordinated to magical power, some must be invoked in the Egyptian language, and others in the Persian tongue,[21] but such names lose their efficacy if changed to another dialect.[22]

If the miracles, especially the astounding cures of maladies, alleged to have been performed by Apollonius of Tyana, are admitted unreservedly by a Christian Father as genuine,[23] it may be accepted as correct the inculpation of Celsus that the Presbyters in the new Church used magic books containing the names of powerful demons for purposes of incantation.[24] According to Maimonides, the magical knowledge of Chaldaic soothsayers included a thorough insight into the secret properties of metals, plants, and animals, in this essential point resembling the mediæval alchemist, which was subordinated to the manifestation of skill touching the science of the seasons, atmosphere, and temperature.[25] The age which received unquestioned the possibilities of resurrecting the dead by evoking their spirits,[26] or admitted, as Lactantius, that there were enchanters ever ready to confound the incredulous by the subtile exhibition of such supernatural powers,[27] was, it may be concluded, fully prepared to witness the complete prostration

[20] Iamblich., De Myster. Ægypt., Dist. II., p. 10.

[21] Origen, Contra Celsum, Lib. I., p. 30. Iamblich., op. cit., p. 97 seq.

[22] Origen, op. cit., Lib. V., p. 261.

[23] Justin Martyr, Questiones, Qu. XXIV.

[24] Origen, op. cit., Lib. VI., p. 302.

[25] More Nevochim, Lib. III., c. 37.

[26] Justin, Apologia, Lib. II.

[27] Divin. Institut., Lib. VII., cap. 13.

of medical science, and to devote inquisitive enthusiasm to the potential efficacy of magic, disdaining the contact of reason in deducing the cause of diseases from the operation of natural laws.[28]

Profoundly impressed with a belief which was of universal extension, that human sickness originated through the direct influence of evil demons, as hitherto explained, theurgic art, in the time of Origen, divided the body into thirty-six diverse parts, the care of each being placed under the supervision of a like number of divinized beings of immortal types and resistless force; over whom the sacerdoty exercised domination, and through invocations in proper form procured effectual remedy for the diseased member from its particular *Gnome* or Divinity.[29]

Galen bitterly complained that notwithstanding the admitted fact of the derivation of prescription formularies in his day from Egyptian sources, these characters, which taught the usage of simple medicaments in infirmities, were regarded as containing within themselves the property of magical cures, and that these medical enchanters, in collecting their herbal medicines, murmured upon them Egyptian incantations to render them more potent,[30] and whether successful in their treatment or otherwise, these practitioners charged enormous prices, which Clement, of Alexandria, severely denounced.[31]

In its earliest phases the contest between the fervent sectarian disputants, either in Alexandria or other great cities of

---

[28] Philostorgius, Histor. Ecclesiast., Lib. VIII., c. 10.

[29] "Ex Ægyptiis, dicentibus humanum corpus in trigenta sex partes distributum, et suam cujusque potestatem habere, sive dæmonem, sive deum quendam aethereum. Quidam autem plures dicunt, eosque dæmones propria lingua nominant, etc., et invocati sanant morbos quisque suarum partium." Origenes, Contra Celsum, Lib. VIII., p. 146.

[30] "Præstigas quasdam deliras Ægypticas, junctis nonnullis incantationibus, quas quum herbas colligant admurmurant. Pleraque vera ista herbarum nomina aut Ægyptica aut Babylonia, quaeque nonnulli aut privatim, aut notæ gratia illis imposuerunt." De Simplicium Medicam. Temperament, Lib. VI., Prœm., p. 792 seq.

[31] Clemens Alexandrin., Cohortat. ad Gentes, cap. 1 and 2.

the Roman Empire, and prior to the substitution of Christianity in the place of Polytheism, seems to have largely reposed upon the asserted superior omnipotence of either the Pagan gods or the Divine Heads of the Christian religion, and particularly the power of each to cure disease. Out of this evidently developed the alteration of both social and religious fabrics of the times, which accorded the most unlimited potency to antagonizing Divinities, but mutually relegated these forces for provoking bodily ills to the inspiration of impure spirits, whose influences might be conjured by magical rites. In the second century, the emperor Hadrian attributed his cures of aqueous congestion, which for a prolonged period had affected him, to the succor of enchantment.[32]

If, therefore, such remedies were accepted as practical by so enlightened a ruler as Hadrian, it serves as a valuable example from which to conclude their universality among the people in Rome. One of the defenders of Christianity, towards this epoch, questioned not the genuineness of miraculous cures performed by paganistic hierarchy or polytheistic divinities. He explained them upon the general charge of invocation of malevolent demons, so often resorted to by the mutual adherents of rival sects.

The interpretation given these wonderful restorations to robust health, by the author[33] alluded to, substantially establishes the entire system on which the Romish church throughout the Middle Ages founded the practical introduction of the use of saintly remedies for aggravated infirmities. Tatian in commenting on these astounding cures, urged that the divinities, veritable demons, first carried the disorder into the body of a healthy man, and, having notified the suffering person that they would cure him provided he implored their aid, obtained

[32] "Interim Adrianus aquam intercutam curavit magicis artibus." Xiphilin., Vita Hadriani, p. 295. A peacock's tongue was regarded by Heliogabalus as a remedy against epilepsy: "Lingua pavonum—ab epilepsia tutus diceretur." Lamprid., Vita Heliogabali, cap. 19.

[33] Tatian. Assyr., Oratio ad Gentes, p. 157.

the glory of working a miracle by causing an infirmity to cease which they themselves had provoked. A few months previous to his death, Hadrian, then ill of the serious malady which finally terminated a most valuable existence, was confronted with a medical enchantress, who professed undoubted ability to effectually cure his disease. In urging the purity of her divine mission she alleged that a dream warned her of the suffering Emperor, and directed her to assure him of a speedy convalescence, but resisting the solemn mandate, she was afflicted with loss of sight. Upon being again ordered by the celestial vision to appear in the imperial presence with the soothing tidings of future health to the illustrious sufferer, she came to fulfill the mission, and it was claimed, received an instant restoration of unimpaired vision;[34] but the prodigous remedy prophesied failed, and the august patient died soon after the charlatan's visit, exclaiming: "Many physicians destroyed the king!"[35] The imperial city seems to have quickly become the centre of operations of practitioners of supernatural cures, and indeed was a favorite resort for Chaldaic soothsayers,[36] who combined the prophetic voice with the practical pecuniary benefits of medicine; and Sully himself did not hesitate to consult such magicians touching the significance of certain physlcal malformations, which appeared on the surface of his body.[37]

Diocletian, in the year 296, when the Egyptians were organizing their discontented factions for a revolt against the imperial authority at Alexandria, not only caused a frightful slaughter of many eminent scholars and illustrious men of the city, but ordered by mandate such books collected and burned as treated on the artificial composition of gold,[38] a secret still

[34] Spartian, Vita Hadriani, cap. 23.

[35] "Multi medici Regem sustulerunt." Xiphilin., Vita Hadriani, p. 296.

[36] Chaldaic haruspices and medical charlatans infested the Roman metropolis in the time of Cato: "Haruspicem Chaldæum ne quem consuluisse velit." De Re Rustica, cap. 5.

[37] Vellius Paterculus, Histor. Rom., Lib. II., cap. 24.

[38] Suidas, Lexicon, sub v. X ημια.

remaining in custody of the Egyptian sanctuaries. This order was promulgated for the purpose of depriving the Egyptians of a means of procuring money with which in future to wage war against the Romans.[39]

In addition to Chaldaic magicians professing the accomplishment of wonders and miraculous cures at Rome, as late as the time of Alaric, king of the victorious Huns, when the armies of this nation menaced the metropolis with a siege, Etruscan enchanters offered to repulse them by directing against that army and its chief a thunderbolt; and as a sufficient attestation of their prowess publicly vaunted the performance of this prodigy at the city of Norma when similarly besieged, which ended in the enemy's discomfiture.[40]

The Episcopal authorities of Rome were disposed to essay the possibilities of executing the promises of the Etruscans, but, according to Zozimus, the populace of the city displayed such repugnance against the proposed miracle that they were politely dismissed, and the metropolis capitulated.[41] From the preceding statements it will perhaps clearly appear that throughout the diversified gradations of social and religious life during the early ages of the Christian Church a belief in the existence of unseen, invisible beings, endowed with attributes of power for the causation or cure of maladies, was so firmly interwoven with the faith of sectarians, whose converts were proselytes from the Jews or Polytheism, as to render the administration of medicine upon a basis of science quite impossible.

The progress of this debasement of the curative art from the time of Galen was rapid and uninterrupted. Methods of curing disease by the practiced survey of scientific inquiry, quickly passed from the domain of an exact science, where events were explained within a logical circle, and entered upon the sombre pathway of direct demoniacal production, whose remedial

---

[39] Delrio, Magicar. Disquisit., Tom. I., p. 30.

[40] Sozomen, Hist. Eccles., Lib. IX., cap. 6.

[41] Hist. Rom., Lib. V., cap. 42.

pathology, it was unanimously agreed, transcended the skill of the physicians, and consequently became the undisputed prerogative of divine or magical interference. As urged, the Cabbalists maintained that through the collocation of certain letters in multiplied figures the invincible power over angelic hosts was assured.

In theurgic operations, names having some fancied association with the unseen forces constituted a most important element. Thus, for instance, in Lucan's day Grecian or Roman magicians threatened these invisible demons with the invocation of some redoubtable name, in order to quicken their lagging movements.[42] In the celebrated treatise of Origen, embodying his curious controversy with the Epicurean,[43] Celsus, enemy of the Christian faith, the polemical writer frankly admitted there were names naturally endowed with great and vital virtues, such as the Egyptian sages and more enlightened Persian Magi used.[44] While Origen accorded the existence of magic as not entirely chimerical or impotent, and as a system regulated by strict rules and known to few, he boldly declared the names of Sabaoth and Adonai, when arranged in suitable form, to be irresistible.[45]

One asseveration of this writer is of high importance in its immediate relationship to these causes, so actively at work at this epoch to mould into shape elements which constituted for centuries the exclusive system by which bodily diseases were treated through the assumed efficiency of the sainted emissaries of Deity. He states that persons sufficiently skilled in these matters would find other mysteries in the names of such pure angels as Michael, Gabriel, Raphael, etc., and that to this philosophy of nomenclature is to be referred the name of Jesus,[46]

---

[42] Lucan, Pharsalia, Lib. VI., v. 748.

[43] "Celsus Epicurius," Origen Contra Celsum, Lib. II., p. 97.

[44] "Nominum efficacium quorum aliquot utuntur Ægyptiorum sapientes, aut Persarum magi doctores." Origen, op. cit., Lib. I., p. 19.

[45] Voltaire, Essai sur les Moeurs et Usages, Tom. I., p. 17.

[46] Origen, Contra Celsum, Lib. I., p. 18 seq.

which so often had manifested its divine puissance in expelling demons.[47]

Chaldaic names when translated lost totally their magic force.[48] From whatever source these names were derived, there seems to have been a unanimity touching their unlimited subtle and remedial powers. Names of Cabbalistic deities, to a great degree drawn from the older Persian system, were endowed with extraordinary potency.[49] To Jah was attributed wisdom; to Jehovah, prudence; and to Adonai, unbounded empire.[50] Their possession does not appear to have been restricted to particular sects of the early Church; but was eagerly sought after by all, and when found to exhibit a magic or curative force through material representatives, these divinities were used by sectarians indifferently. Of the names anciently admitted to be charged with divine power, that of the Jewish God, Jehovah, was the most adjured, both by the Cabbalists and other religious bodies, whose systems assimilated with the Hebrew faith. Consequently, in the doctrines of the Cabbala, this name representing the Divine Essence was of exalted type, and figured as a means of obtaining a fulfillment of human wishes, as well as a powerful auxiliary in curing maladies. Other religions, for example Polytheism, recognized the inherent merits of correctly pronouncing the word Jehovah. In the Valentinian system, one of the revolted elements, Sophia, or wisdom, as a deified emanation, was forced to recede into her proper limitations, by virtue of the mysterious name Joa.[51]

To what extent the adoration of the mystical Hebraistic Divinity's name was carried on account of its presupposed puis-

[47] "Qui autem potuerit de nominium secreta ratione philosophari, multa facile inveniet et de appellationibus Angelorum Dei quorum alius Michael, alius Gabriel alius Raphael." Origen, op. cit., Lib. I. p. 20.

[48] Ibid.

[49] Beausobre, Hist. du Manicheisme, Tom. II., p. 800 seq.

[50] Matter, Histor. du Gnosticisme, Tom. I., p. 100.

[51] Matter, op. cit., Tom. I., p. 101; and Tom. II., p. 198 seq.

sance to vanquish disease, may be inferred from the following curious facts: Theosebius, a Pagan philosopher, espoused a woman who appeared ultimately to be possessed of a demoniacal spirit—a species of nervous disorder, universally admitted to be the production of an evil being. In order to obtain this demon's departure from its feminine habitation, he employed, to begin with, the most pious adjurations and gentlest exhortations; but the obstinate and malevolent angel gibed and scoffed at him. At length, with exhausted patience, Theosebius conjured him in the name of the Hebrew god—Jao, under the attested invocation of the rays of the sun. The demon thereupon instantly departed, protesting that although he revered all the gods, he was especially reverential towards that one whom the Israelites adored.[52]

This word, when properly arranged, was irresistible in its operations, and had at its command the powers of earth and heaven;[53] when, however, its exact pronunciation[54] and collocation had perished, the enthusiasm to recover the same was increased in proportion to the marvellous properties attributed to its material form.[55] In the second century, the Synhedrin directed a repronunciation of this word, as a necessary innovation, in order to counteract the expanding deification of Jesus among Israelitish converts to Christianity, and to have a distinctive sign by which the Jewish nation might be disintegrated from the Christianized Hebrews.[56]

The Christians having adopted the Adonaite substitute for Christ, the Synhedrin enacted that the quadrilateral name should be again uttered as in more ancient times, and that

---

[52] Beausobre, Histoire du Manicheisme, Tom. II., p. 67. The original authority may be found in Photius Cod., 242, col. 1037, sub nom. Damascus.

[53] Voltaire, Essai sur les Moeurs et Usages, Tom. I., p. 157.

[54] Ibid., Tom. I., p. 107.

[55] Buddeus, Introduct. ad Histor. Philosoph. Ebraeor., p. 43 seq.

[56] Graetz, Hist. of the Jews, p. 114.

each should salute the other by it.[57] As a talisman of medicinal property, it was carried about the person in tubes, or more generally on parchment.[58]

---

[57] Ibid., p. 115.

[58] "Amuleta sive chartas experimentales conscribentibus." Maimonides, More Nevochim, Pars. I., c. 61, p. 108. Maimonides asserts that evil and designing men sought to collocate the letters of the word for sinister purposes. Ductor Dubitant, Lib. I., cap. 60, folio 24.

CHAPTER VI.

Apollonius Claimed as Inventor of Magic Cures—His Marvellous Success—Amulets Introduced as Preventatives Against Disease—Engraven with Figures as Remedies—Gnosticism Developed this System—The Abraxas Gems—Potency Increased by Ephesian Letters—Raphael as an Angel of Cure—Medical Property of Abracadabra—Metrical Treatise on its Puissance—Remedial Power of Certain Minerals—How Used and When Worn as Charms—Decline of Classical Letters Provoked a Deterioration of Arts and Sciences.

APOLLONIUS of Tyana was claimed as the inventor of these powerful adjuncts of the curative art, and practised his system of medicine upon the theory that no cures could be made successful without a patholgy for the soul.[1] From the empirical sagacity of paganistic docrines touching talismanic remedies, to the incorporation of an identical faith into Christian theology, the advance was rapid and the transition unimpeded. Apollonius, the polytheistic philosopher and medicist, had professed unexampled cures by the agencies of talismanic influence;[2] and a Christian Father readily followed the route thus opened, to like vindication of the puissance of his Deity.

Synesius, one of the most erudite philosophers among the early Christians, was persuaded that the art of making amulets and talismans, the invocation of spirits and the use of their prowess, was neither vain nor criminal. On the contrary, he never suspected other than the most natural event in these operations, a belief shared uniformly by the most enlightened followers of Christ in that distant age. He says that as there is a certain sympathy and affinity between bruised and afflicted

[1] Philostratus, Vita Apollon. Tyan., Lib. III., cap. 44, § 1, claims for his hero, in this system, a species of divination: "Ejus donum esse medicam."

[2] Philostratus, op. cit., Lib. III., cap. 45.

parts of the animal frame, although not contiguous, which in the most remote distances one member feels the pangs of pain when its fellow member is suffering, likewise an identical affinity exists between parts of our terrestrial world and unseen beings of exalted excellence for good or evil, who reside within the unbounded limits of the celestial and sublunary sphere. By the selection of suitable plants, metals or minerals, to which specific figures and words are to be added, these superior beings are quickly influenced by that sympathy which they have for such material types.[3]

He also avows that the celestial creatures dwelling above the terrestrial world, having an incorporeal nature and exempt from affections, are beyond the reach of enchantments or talismanic influences, and cannot be evoked by any means; but the spirits resident in the atmospheric regions, created from corporeal substances, possess sympathetic senses, through which they are moved by human infirmities and affinities.[4] The Basilideans and other sects developed from the Gnostic systems accorded the mightiest power to stone talismans[5] prepared for initiates into these mysterious sanctuaries as a ready means of recognition.[6] These gems, endowed with omnipotent curative and talismanic power, quickly acquired a celebrity undiminished for ages, and whose possible interpretation even yet attracts erudite attention, and were generally known under the denomination of Abraxas.

Basilides, the founder of the sect from which these emanated, so far as scholastic research can establish his identity, lived under Trajan and his immediate successor, from about the middle of the first to the beginning of the second century. He was of Syrian[7] nationality, and taught in the literary metropolis of the world,[8] where, as a neophyte in the Christian

[3] Beausobre, Histoire du Manicheisme, Tom. II., p. 49.

[4] Ibid.

[5] King, Gnostics and their Remains, p. 93.

[6] Bellermann, Drei Programmen ueber die Abraxas Gemmen, Th. III., p. 12.

[7] Matter, Histoire du Gnosticisme, Tom. II., p. 57 seq.

[8] King, The Gnostics and their Remains, p. 78.

religion, he declared himself to be a disciple of Matthew, and gloried in having for his preceptor a scholar of the apostle Peter.[9] As the propagator of the system of Simon the magician, whose thaumaturgic skill was widely known in the days of the first evangelists, he seems to have been attracted by the oriental doctrines of the Gnostics, and struggled to combine pure Christianity with the cosmologic and aeon theories of Gnosticism.

In order to render his teachings of readier comprehension to converts, he selected tangible representatives and images from numerous systems in Alexandria, where it is probable that he finished a remarkable career in peaceful quietude.[10] In the annunciation of his mystic principles touching Divinity and divine properties, works and creations, their influence on spirits and worlds, the demiurgos or opifex mundi, and the manifold forces of nature, he appears to have followed the scheme of the Syrian Saturninus, a contemporary. The construction of this dogma was an amalgamation of Christian, Judaistic, and Polytheistic religions, and especially of oriental Gnosticism. Influenced largely by the theurgic practices of his predecessor, Simon the magician, he boldly taught the irresitible puissance inherent in the Abraxas images when properly understood. Such knowledge was communicated to converts similar to Gnostic mysticism, under the solemnity of secret instruction.

Whether these gems were originally designed as a means of recognition for the Basilidean catechumens, or, from the first, used as a remedy already possessed of resistless force to cure maladies, or prevent ills of diversified types,[11] is not clear perhaps for each. Irenæus charged upon the Basilideans the use of images, invocation of deities, and incantations, as an important feature of their religious creed,[12] and that the forces of a

---

9 Matter, op. cit., Tom. I., p. 186.

10 Matter, op. cit., Tom. II., p. 58, No. 3

11 Bellermann, Drei Programmen ueber die Abraxas Gemmen, Th. I., p. 29.

12 " Exorcismis et incantationibus utuntur." Adversus Haeresos, Lib. I., cap. 23, § 4.

plurality of worlds were appropriately named under the denomination of angels. The gems or stones used by these religious enthusiasts, were composed of various materials—glass, paste, and other minerals, and sometimes of metal.[13] Through the irresistible might of Abrax, their supreme divinity, the Basilideans were protected amid persecutions, and evaded the searching inquiry of imperial investigations.[14]

On account of the potential and resistless power of this word, it was compared to the magical and curative puissance of Ephesian letters and formulas, largely applied in the early ages of Christianity for such purposes.[15] As talismans and amulets for the cure of diseases, these stones were of extensive use. For the purpose of giving these additional energy, short twigs and pellets were thrown upon a designated place, and, according to the form assumed in their fall, a sage or augur interpreted the significance, and engraved upon the Abraxas stone as of especial potency.[16]

Thus prepared, these curious gems were admitted to possess an efficacy for hygienic practices, and extensively used by the Gnostics, and perhaps other sects. The illustrious Alexandrine scholar, Clement, stricly interdicted the use of gems for personal ornamentation, with evident allusion to the Abraxas stones.[17] The oft-recurring figure of a serpent on these talismans was specially designed to be used among the faithful as a curative of or preventative against diseases,[18] and in this essential point exactly harmonized with the Divine principle underlying the serpent system of Æsculapius, by which sick-

---

[13] Bellermann, op. cit., Th. I., p. 29.

[14] Irenæus, op. cit., Lib. I., cap. 24, § 7.

[15] Suidas, Lexicon, sub v. Ephes. Grammat.

[16] Bellermann, op. cit., Th. I., p. 39.

[17] Pædagog., Lib. II., cap. 12. He also makes the sweeping inculpation that much evil had invaded the world through woman's greed of pearls: "Maximi autem precii margarita mundum muliebrem per summam lasciviam mirandum modum invasit." Ibid.

[18] Bellermann, Drei Programmen ueber die Abraxas Gemmen, Th. I., p. 60.

ness was anciently cured—a method of extensive adaptation.[19] In its alternative significance the serpent effigy accords with the Egyptian notion of an all-pervading spirit, thus faithfully reproducing the Abrax, and oftentimes engraven together. Some of them were worn as a safeguard against both vice promotive of bodily infirmities, and error productive of spiritual disorders. The figure 5 cut with greater or less skill on the surface of the amulets appears to have especially related to the forces of the unseen and natural worlds.

On the principle admitted by modern scientists, that the botanical system is a development of this number, it may be assumed to represent a higher appreciation by this sect of that science which is closely conjoined with the curative art. The name of Raphael, the beloved patron angel of early Christians for the cure of disease, was appropriated by the Gnostics with all his fancied energies. This word, lettered in the Hellenistic dialect, among other names of well-known or unusual angelic beings, is frequently met on the Abraxas gems, and in this form was anciently used as a medicinal remedy and preventative of physical suffering.[20] One of these is engraven with Armenian letters, and contains a standing invocation for fruitful delivery, and in its medicinal property was evidently a cure for sterility.[21] Under what specific circumstances these amulets were obtained by the filiates into these closely-organized religious bodies, it is perhaps impossible to state.

It would appear, however, to be a logical deduction to assume that they were quickly passed to neophytes, impressively charged to avoid the slightest indiscretion which would attract the profane authorities and aid them in discovering the locali-

[19] Plinii, Histor. Natur., Lib. XXIX., cap. 24, § 8. Arnobius, Adversus Gentes, Lib. VI., cap. 25, says of him: "Æsculapius cum baculi," or serpent-twined staff. Æsculapius is declared to have obtained his knowledge of medicaments through dreams sent him in Apollo's Temple. Philostratus, Vita Apollon., Lib. III., cap. 44.

[20] Bellermann, op. cit., Th. II., p. 30.

[21] Bellermann, Die Drei Programmen ueber die Abraxas Gemmen, Th. II., p. 37 seq.

ties where the Gnostics met in secret conclave. Oftentimes these amulets were evidently conferred upon younger members, by the more aged Basilideans, an action doubtless sanctioned by the governing hierarchy. This formal transmission was usually accompanied by a holy invocation to the substitute name, to be particularly gracious to the adolescent devotee.[22]

The Abracadabra, derived from abrax, when repeated several times and written in pyramidal shape on parchment, as early as the Third Century was solemnly recommended by a pagan versifier as a sovereign remedy in cases of intermittent fevers.[23] This sagacious writer was Quintus Serenus Samonicus, who appears to have attained high rank and illustration, but favoring the unsuccessful partisans of Caracalla's brother, was with others assassinated while enjoying the hilarity of a Roman banquet.[24] He composed a metrical treatise on the salubrious precepts of medicine, and thus chants the magical and health-giving properties of Abracadabra:

> "Inscribas chartae quod dicitur abracadabra
> Saepius et subter repetis, sed detrahe summam, etc.
> Et magis atque magis desint elementa figuris," etc.[25]

He also asserted that sleep might be superinduced in the most desperate cases of insomnia by the incineration of lettered parchment and, mixed with tepid water, drank as a potion.[26] The science of Galen was not independent of urging the use of amulets as medicinal cures, and advised a trial of them for headache[27] and inebriety,[28] and pronounced them sovereign against fevers.[29]

---

[22] Ibid., Th. III., p. 12.

[23] Beausobre, Histoire du Manicheisme, Tom. II., p. 55 seq.

[24] Capitolinus, Vita Caracall., cap. 4.

[25] De Medicinæ Præcepta, entitled Hemitritæo Depellando, p. 96 seq.

[26] "Charta igitur variis quam pinxit littera verbis, Uritur inde calido potatur in amni." Seren. Samon., De Medecinæ Præcepta, p. 98.

[27] Galen, De Compos. Medecam., Lib. II., c. 2.

[28] Ibid., De Remed. Parabil., Lib. I., cap. 1.

[29] De Morborum Causis, Lib. I., c. 2.

Jasper, hematite and hieratite stones were strongly recommended for unusual sanitative virtues,[30] but the sapphire excelled as a remedy for scorpion bites.[31] These incautious counsels were rigidly adhered to and enlarged upon throughont the Middle Ages. Notwithstanding the efforts of the leaders of the Christian Church during the first three centuries to subject their followers to a discipline which should promptly distinguish them from the Judaizing-Oriental sects surrounding them, as well as from other polytheistic adversaries, it is evident that absolute prevention of the use of these curious talismanic figures by the Christians was quite impossible.

From the statement by enlightened scholars of the Church that there was an efficacy in certain literal collocations whose proper adjustment was able to set in motion one or more of the invisible demoniacal forces, it may be readily concluded that actual efforts of believers to control these beings were early essayed. Towards the close of the second century Clement Alexandrinus, in his treatise on matters of immediate interest to converts, directed that the faithful should avoid carrying stones on which idolatrous figures were engraved.[32] It was also forbidden the neophyte to gaze on such effigies.[33] Other sects more or less closely identified with the Basilideans, or perhaps further removed from the unadulterated doctrines of Christ, adopted images to represent their religious system, and to which excessive potency was ascribed. The Carpocratians[34] and Ophites used such figures, including a rampant serpent, as an emblem of their secret faith.[35]

It is beyond dispute, as may be judged from the serious caution and censures of Clement of Alexandria, that the

---

30 Ibid., De Composit. Medic., Lib. IX., cap 2, § 19.

31 Ibid., § 29.

32 Pædagogi, Lib. II., cap. 12; and Lib. III., c. 11.

33 Bellermann, Drei Programmen ueber die Abraxas Gemmen, Th. II., p. 17.

34 Irenæus, Adversus Haeresos, Lib. I., cap. 24.

35 Origen, Contra Celsum, Lib. IV., p. 202.

Christians themselves were largely addicted to these superstitious usages in the cure of diseases, or for potential protection against the machinations of demons by whom the believer was compactly surrounded, according to the admission of the Fathers. Inasmuch as the earlier converts and their successors accepted the new faith with all its diverging oddities, and professed an unqualified credulity touching the doctrine of the emanation of physical infirmities from demoniacal sources, sanctioned by the ecclesiastical guides, oftentimes direful necessity compelled the faithful to resort to tangible remedies for grave maladies, where frequent invocations were ineffectual.

The Clementine diatribe attests unequivocally a numerous portion of the followers of Christ in hot pursuit after Gnostic talismans and amulet cures. Doubtless the faith of Galen in such methods may have rallied large numbers of both Christians and Polytheists to their adaptation; but the extinction of medicine as a system regulated in harmony with an exact science, and its degradation to the administration of simple medicaments[36] directed by talismans, endowed with a divinized efficiency, impelled sectarians to remedies which the hierarchy was powerless to prevent—remedies which were the material types of that subtle force, whose evolution rendered celestial or demoniacal beings docile to the will of the conjurator. From the Milanese edict, in the year 312, Christianity obtained not merely the recognition of legal sanction to an uninterrupted existence, but an illustrious victory over Polytheism, by being subrogated in the venerable place of its embittered rival.

Notwithstanding the signal triumph of the new faith, the downfall of paganism was yet retarded, and its principles unextinguished. It is indeed true the first Christian emperor, influenced by the alteration of public affairs, solemnly proclaimed the death penalty against all persons proffering sacrifices to heathen gods,[37] which shortly before had received the

[36] Lessing, Geschichte der Medezin, Th. I., p. 118.

[37] Codex Theodosianus, XVI., Tit. X., Lex. 2, an. 341.

divided honors of an Empire on the one hand quivering with anxious solicitude for their material representatives, while on the other compliance with hated laws against proselytes yielded most unwilling obedience.

This rescript forced the summary conclusion of heathen rites and ceremonies in the temples of the Empire. Although thus highly favored by imperial legislation, and protected in the undisturbed celebration of their faith, the professors of Christianity were at first unable to vanquish the numerous adherents of polytheism. Many of these indeed preserved their paganistic worship of images in secret, while the heathen proselyte recruited into the ranks of the church militant in numerous instances, through a necessary policy of the pontifical authorities, brought with him fragmentary forms and ceremonies which in their ancient application added to the pompous service of Jupiter Maximus or Venus Dea, were now suffered to vindicate the majesty of the religion of Christ, and increased the splendor of its expanding ritual.[38] To this invariable tendency of Christianity prior[39] and subsequent to its imperial establishment, may be fairly attributed the perpetuation of numerous mystical properties claimed for heathen deities, and sanctioned under the adjustment of new names or altered relations.

Other serious and important circumstances contributed to the lasting debasement of medicine as an exact science, following the era of Constantine the Great. When it is considered that the fundamental principles upon which rested the fabric of medicinal art for many ages, involved the highest credulity of the human mind, and a species of mythological gradation of puissance hitherto sanctioned by the Fathers, and now admitted under the garb of saintly worship or a practical adoption of the demoniacal doctrine as a conceded antagonism to the rapidly increasing idolatry of martyrs and blessed rel-

[38] Beausobre, Histoire du Manicheisme, Tom. II., p. 41; and Origen, Contra Celsum, Lib., I., p. 32; and Lib. VI., p. 301.

[39] Origen, Contra Celsum, Lib. VI.

ics, it will excite little surprise that the Manicheian theories of the fourth and fifth centuries powerfully assisted in maintaining more enlightened minds among the Christian sacerdoty to so firm and unshaken a belief in the dualistic teaching of Manes, typical of eternal rivalry between supremest divinity and the no less potential Satan, with its unremitting warfare and angelic powers against the diabolical retainers of the arch enemy. Amidst these restless circumstances the Teutonic invasion provoked an inextricable confusion in social and ecclesiastical affairs.

The most deplorable result of these frightful disorders, which swept through the fairest portions of the Roman Empire like a relentless storm of death and desolation, was the utter prostration[40] of scientific culture, driven with fanatical contempt from the Church.[41] The sudden withdrawal from profane and sacred society of those influences which strengthen the reason and fortify it against the encroachments of superstitious exaltation during the fifth century, quickly attested the debasement into which the Christian leaders had descended.

For example, Saint Basil, under the stinging reproach of a conscience hastened into ripe luxuriance through the somnolent mortification of dreary solitude, feelingly lamented the days of his youth—not as may be supposed from recollections of frailties incident to adolescence, but for the reason that while young the Christian hero had nourished his mind with an abundance of classical literature now the object of profound contempt.[42] The placid life of monasticism, with its complete ignorance of all things not contained within the mythical Septuagint, lives of the Martyrs, or homilies of holy predecessors, was the subject of Basil's most exalted commendation.[43]

---

[40] Cassiodorus should be gratefully distinguished from the degradation of his age under examination, as one urging the importance of physical tests in medicinal treatment, Edicta Reg. Ostrogoth., No. XIX.

[41] Roskoff, Geschichte des Teufels, Th. I., p. 259.

[42] Basil, Epistolæ, Ep. 223.

[43] Ibid.

Even the illustrious Jerome had so far become inoculated with the poisonous miasma, slowly perverting pontiffs and priesthood, that he openly proclaimed an unfading belief in a dream which solemnly warned him against the terrible crime of perusing the writings of antiquity, and threatened him with a punishment reserved for unbelievers. This awful alternative the saint evaded by promising never to read pagan books again.[44] Even Gregory the Great, to whose vigilant efforts the Anglo-Saxon dynasties of England owed their conversion to the doctrines of Christ a century later, boldly announced a stultified pride in his ignorance, and declared a knowledge of grammar even for a layman to be indelicate, while for a bishop such familiarity was disgusting.[45] For several centuries succeeding the triumph of Christianity, so long as the Pontiffs and Episcopacy glorified in their ignorance as stated, the vulgar mind divested of solid ratiocination, accepted tradition as an authority equivalent to the Scriptures, which rapidly advanced the clearly defined antagonism of Good and Evil, arrayed in unceasing struggle between unlimited, invisible hosts, and finally developed the systematic origin of diseases by demoniac production, and their cure by angelic or saintly remedies.

The doctrines of Manes, strenuously contested with polemical zeal in the fifth century by Augustin, materially added to the propulsion towards peopling earth, air and heaven with invisible spirits, engaged in a struggle for the humble and superb, the affluent and indigent Christian. Gnostic and Basilidean teachings united with the Cabbala, had so far influenced popular belief prior to the full development of Maneсheism, as to accept without hesitation the possibility of physical ills and infirmities originating, under divine permission, from demon causes.

To these, doctrines universally accredited by ecclesiastical teachers, and servilely submitted to by the less enlightened flock, the more accurately defined dogma of Manes touching

[44] Hieronymus, Epistolæ, Ep. 31, ad Eustach.

[45] Gregor. Maxim., Epistol., Lib. IX., Ep. 48.

Persian dualism, should be added as finally establishing the mediæval faith in the fluctuating success or discomfiture of the benevolent or malevolent principle, distinctly embodied as angel, saint or demon, which relegated the practice of medicine to the sanctuaries as an article of creed, or abandoned it to the charlatan and empiric, whose principal skill consisted in magic or cabbalistic conjurations. Manes, in harmony with the dualism of ancient Persia, constructed his religious system on the theory of an eternal antagonism between the powers of light and darkness.[46] From these sharply contrasted elements developed an elaborate faith which assigned to Omnipotent Deity attributes of beneficence, brilliancy and happiness, while, per contra, to his rival was conceded almost equal puissance, with the sombre features of gloom and misery.[47] To the prince of despair was given humanized form, with the factors of increase.[48]

Manicheism, from the first regarded as the arch enemy of Christianity, immediately, subsequent to its triumph over polytheism, was subjected to a most sanguinary persecution by the more successful rival. Laxity of discipline and morals among the followers of the ecstatic Manes may have contributed to this crushing animadversion. Nothwithstanding the general acceptance of the dogma of good and evil as irreconcilable antagonists enunciated by Lactantius[49] and the Christian Fathers, with its curious ramifications of spiritualized emanations and unlimited power to provoke and cure diseases, the initial point was the great arena of controversy against the Manicheans.

In their ultimate effect upon medical culture, these ecclesiastical polemics, in solidifying the doctrine of maladies and other

---

[46] Augustin.,Contra Faustum, Lib. XI., c. 1. On the Fetichism of Manes vide Beausobre, Histoire du Manicheisme, Tom. II., p. 369; and at so late a date as the ninth century, Voltaire, Essai sur les Moeurs et Usages, Tom. I. p. 502 seq.

[47] Augustin, Contra Faustum, Lib. XXI., cap. 1.

[48] Ibid., Lib. XX., c. 14.

[49] Instit. Divin., Lib. II., c. 12.

physical disorders, evils in the world, as a direct penalty, or as invaluable aids, to saintly advancement, cannot be overestimated.[50] Gregory Nazien himself chants the pains of body as provoked by demons,[51] and intimates the uselessness of medicaments to cure such diseases.[52] He asserts the frequent cure of sickness thus created, by an imposition of hands.[53]

---

[50] Gregor. Nazien. Oratio, Lib. XIV., c. 31.

[51] Ibid., Carmina, LXXXIII:

> " Et multos morbis ac dæmonum vinculis
> Laboravit."—V. 27.

[52] Ibid., " Morbus compressus medicamentis non opportunis." V. 17.

[53] Ibid., L.:

> " Capitibus earum, qui mihi sese inclinant,
> Et morborum suorum me curatorem vocant."—V. 104.

CHAPTER VII.

Antagonism of Angels of Light and of Darkness—All Diseases Spring from the Evil Principle—Magic Avowed as a Science by the Church—Potency to Cure of Cross Sign—Metrical Panegyric of this Curative—Early Use of Reliques for Remedies Against Maladies—Puissance of a Wax Pellet—Amulets Written on Parchment by Saints—Formula of Exorcising the Principle of Disease—Amulets Against Bodily Infirmities Transplanted from Paganism—Good and Evil as Attributes of Angels Applied to in the Sortes or Hazards—Rescripts Forbid Chaldaic Art, etc., in the Cure of Maladies—Imperial Ordinance Affords Security to Practitioners of Magic Medicine—Laws of the Wisigoths Recognize the Force of Magic to Cause Disease.

OUT of these enthusiastic utterances grew the grave theory that as all disorders and aggravated maladies were sent upon the body or mind by the hosts of darkness, under Divine sanction, they should be accepted as a means of final salvation, as inducing patience in terrible suffering. In the opinion of theologians, sickness was preferable to insolent pride,[1] and leprosy was asserted to be a sacred disease.[2]

During the controversial conflict between the church and Manicheism, a belief in the corporeal substance of demons gradually assumed a tangible shape, and when these were designated as invisible it was alleged to be on account of their possessing a finer body than mankind,[3] and that prior to the fall they were clothed with a bodily texture of more delicate composition.[4] Before an imperial rescript had established the Christian church, sacrificial offerings to idolatrous images were

[1] Gregor. Nazien., Epistolæ, Ep. XXVI.; Augustin., Civitat. Dei, Lib. I., cc. 8–10; and De Morib. Eccles., cc. 8, 11, substantially agrees with this view of the origin and spiritual effect of human suffering.

[2] Gregor. Nazien., Oratio, Lib. XIV., cap. 6.

[3] Cyril Hieros. Catac., XVI., c. 251.

[4] Augustin., De Genes., ad Lib. III., c. 10.

merely denominated heathenish, but subsequently were apostrophised as demoniacal offerings. Consequently, by legitimate progression, impure spirits came to be regarded as the founders of Paganistic culture, aptly compared to a worship of the devil, who had instituted false oracles and deceptive miracles.[5]

Magic, frankly avowed as a possible science, was the especial property of demoniac spirits, and showed the fate of polytheism as a manifestation of diabolical puissance. Successive synods of the church, one in Spain, prior to the edict of Milan. as early as the year 305, and another held in Laodicea, A. D. 343, enacted that the exercise of magical arts should be evidence of intercourse with demons.[6] At the same time, the use of magic was interdicted as a cure for diseases,[7] and especially declared to be a lure of the devil.[8] A decretal of the fourth century, issued by pontifical authorithy, commanded the bishops to labor with assiduous zeal to exterminate utterly from their Dioceses damnable magic and soothsaying usages invented by Satan; and wherever a man or woman should be found exercising these dangerous gifts, to promptly expel them from episcopal territory.[9]

To the undisputed swiftness of demons to traverse remotest distances,[10] was conjoined omnipotent power, an opinion sanctioned by no less a personage than the Pontiff Gregory Maximus himself.[11] Arnobius unequivocally asserts that the most irregular passions of the human heart are caused by dia-

---

[5] Eusebius, Præparat. ad Evangel., Lib. III., c. 16; and August., De Civit. Dei, Lib. II., c. 24.

[6] Burchard, Decreta, Lib. VI., c. 26.

[7] "Incantationibus quibus libet infirmitatibus hominum nihil posse remedii confere," etc. Ibid., Lib. X., c. 40.

[8] "Insidias antiqui hostis." Burchard, Decret., Lib. X., c. 40.

[9] "Episcopi, ut perniciosam a diabolo inventam sortilegam et magicam artem ex parochiis suis penitus eradicent." Gratian, Decret., Pars. II.; Causa XXVI.; Ques. V., c. 12.

[10] Hilar. Pict., Tract. in Psalm 67.

[11] Gregor., Max. Moral., Lib. XXIV., cc. 19, 20; and Lib. XXXII., cc. 12, 15.

bolical powers.[12] Thus arrayed against the mighty army of the Satanic realm, the Christian, when beset by bodily or spiritual disorders, without question accepted as the creations of impure angels, possessed a remedy of Cabbalistic similitude, but of infinite curative force. The sign of the cross and invocation of the name of Christ,[13] relentlessly and with magic power caused the demoniacal hosts to recede.[14] In a Latin poem of the fifth century the puissant forces of this symbol are fully set forth in tolerable metre, describing a colloquy in which a certain Tityrus is asked to divulge the cause that exempts his herds from those virulent disorders to which neighboring animals are subject:

> Dic age Tityre,
> Quis te subripuit cladibus his Deus?
> Ut pestis pecudum, quae populata sit
> Vecinos, tibi nulla sit.[15]

To this inquiry the following answer is made, which sets forth the marvelous properties of the cruciform sign:

> "Signum quod perhibent esse crucis Dei,
> Magnus qui colitur solus in urbibus
> Christus, perpetui gloria numinis
> Cujus filius unicus.
> Hoc signum mediis frontibus additum
> Cunctorum pecudum certa salus fuit.
> Sic vero Deus hoc nomini præpotens
> Salvator vocitatus est.
> Fugit continus saeva lues gregis,
> Morbis nil liciut. Si tamen hunc Deum
> Exorare velis, credere sufficit:
> Votum sola fides juvat.
> Signum prosit idem perpete saeculo,
> Quo vis morbida vincitur?"[16]

---

[12] Advers. Gent., Lib. IV., c. 7.

[13] Orig., Contra Celsum, Lib. III., p. 133.

[14] Athanas., Contra Gentes, cap. 1; and De Incarn. Verbi, cap. 47.

[15] Severus Sanctus, Carmen De Mortibus Boum, v. 104. Diseases cured by the sound of Christ's voice. Arnobius, op. cit., Lib. I., cap. 48.

[16] Severinus Sanctus, Carmen. De Mortibus Boum, p. 27 seq.

In addition to this potential remedy, maladies of the body or of mind thus provoked through Satanic agencies, baptismal water, the Holy Ghost, extreme vigilance, were soberly recommended as of an infallible efficacy when all others failed.[17] At this epoch curative methods were introduced, which affected uninterruptedly medical economy, with occasional variation, to the close of the Middle Ages.

As early indeed as the time of Gregory of Tours, bishop and historian of the Frankish kings in the sixth century, application was made of sainted reliquaries as a remedy against the devil, his demons and their recognised force. The Turonese pontiff narrates the miraculous efficiency of a small pellet of wax, taken from the tomb of Saint Martin, in extinguishing an incendiary fire, started by his Satanic majesty, instigated by malicious envy, that this omniptotent talisman was in the custody of an ecclesiastic![18]

In the sixth century the usual method of exorcising the king of darkness was performed by a written formula. Whenever a person appeared to be stricken with a grievous malady which failed to yield under ordinary invocation and true magic of the Church, accompanied perhaps with simple medicaments, the sacerdotal authorities instantly proclaimed the sufferer possessed of the Devil. As in the case previously cited of Theobasius' wife, whose infirmity obstinately refused to recognize the conjuring power of paganistic deities, the resistless exorcism of Holy Eugendus was oftentimes resorted to, when lesser saints were confessedly impotent, and invariably ejected the Arch Fiend from the Christian believer.

Such amulets were frequently written on parchment or

---

[17] Gregor. Nazien., Oratio. XI., cap. 3. "Desperatis omnibus remediis." Ibid., op. cit., Lib. XXIV., cap. 10.

[18] Gregor. Turones., Miraculæ Martini, Lib. II., cap. 26. Holy dust was at this period used in quenching flames. Beda, Historia Ecclesiastica, Lib. III., c. 10. Meinwerck, in the eleventh century, forbid the foolish practice of throwing the corporale Dominicum into fire in order to stay their progress: "Ad extinguendum incendium temeraria præsumptione in ignem projiciant." Vita Meinwercki, cap. 76, § 5.

other substances, and hung about the neck. The formula of Saint Eugendus may be taken as a prototype of those in general use at this or earlier periods of the Church, and reads as follows: "Eugendus servus Christi, in nomine Dei nostri Jesu Christi patris et Spiritus Sanctus, præcipio per scripturam istam spiritus gulæ et iræ et fornicationis et amoris et Lunatice et Dianitice et meridane et diurne, et nocturne et omnis spiritus immunde, exi ab homine, qui istam scripturam secum habet. Per ipsum te adjuro verum filium Dei vivi, exi velociter, et cave ne amplius intrœas eam. Amen. Alleluia."[19] The existence in this conjuration of Dianitice and Lunatice, evidently warrants the conclusion that this formula followed those of a more ancient period. Notwithstanding the pleasing theory adopted by the earlier Christian writers, that the powers of darkness were unable to harm the faithful without permission of divinity,[20] to whom demoniacal spirits were ultimately subject,[21] unlimited puissance was conceded to those beings who existed under divine sanction, and according to the celestial scheme by which virtue should behold its highest reward as a contrast to the debasement of vice,[22]—consequently satanic omnipotence was permitted to exist as a standing menace against the commission of overt sin.[23]

The use of amulets for the cure of disease, or talismans to preserve the wearer from bodily ills, was taken directly from paganism, and adopted by the new converts after their profession of Christianity. Other equally superstitious usages current among polytheists survived to the new Church. Among these was a custom of opening the Bible, and, according to the first lines seen, chanted or spoken on entering a chapel, the issue of any future enterprise was oracularly prophesied.

---

19 Acta Sanctorum, Tom. I., Jan. I., p. 52; Vita Eugendi, cap. 7.

20 Clemens. Alexandr. Stromata, Lib. VI., c. 3; Origen, De Principiis, Lib. III., c. 27.

21 Chrysosth., Epistolæ, II., ad Timoth., cap. III., Homil. 8.

22 Lactantius, Instit. Divin., Lib. II., cap. 9; Lib. V., c. 7.

23 Cyril, Hierosal. Catech., VIII.

When Chlodwig the Wisigothic ruler had determined on waging war against the Gauls, in order to forecast the result of the martial campaign, he petitioned Deity to make manifest a sign by which the happy conclusion of the conflict should be known, on entering the edifice dedicated to Saint Martin, the tutelary and patron of the converted Franks. Passing into the sanctuary, certain words of a psalm being sung were interpreted to be the prophetic signal of his subsequent victory.[24] Numerous edicts of synods and ecclesiastical councils endeavored to crush out by the terrors of sacerdotal and secular punishment these and unnumbered practices which had become engrafted into the social fabric of converted pagans, rigidly retained and openly avowed. The graves of the saints or martyred dead, from a date so early as the epoch before us, were favorite places for the exhibition of rites similar to that of the Gothic king. Here indeed the sacred Scriptures were opened, and, amid pious prayers and fastings, the credulous neophyte sought out the letter or word of particular relevancy to his actual wants of body or future condition, through which material type the saint invoked designated an answer of a cure or promise of prolonged life to the humble petition of the devotee.

As sortes sanctorum, this species of sortilege took a lasting hold upon the minds of proselytes, to such extent that repeated enactments of synods and councils were powerless to extirpate it.[25] Touching this survival of paganistic customs to Christian converts these statements are of importance, but so far as their influence extended to introduce the system of invoking dead saints to whose relics magical or divine power was attributed, such facts constitute valuable attestation to determine the possible era when the irreconcilable conflict between the great antagonists of good and evil, approached the usage of that idolatrous adoration which maintained its existence

---

[24] Gregor. Turon., Histor. Francor. Regum, Lib. II., c. 37.

[25] Capitulare Tertium, Anno 789, Can. IV., apud Baluz., Cartular. Carlovingiani, Tom. I., col. 243.

throughout the middle ages, and provided the most salutary elements of curing the sick and infirm, by debasing medical science and elevating the resistless potency of relics!

Other circumstances of especial weight confirmed the vulgar mind in an unshaken faith that these invisible forces, in mortal opposition to the hosts of Satan and his agencies, were vastly superior to medical or surgical skill in the treatment of human disorders. Ecclesiastical decretals and secular rescripts provoked popular credulity, and unequivocally vindicated the faith in the appliance of supernatural arts, although directed against them as magical and paganistic. By order of Constantine the Great, in the year 319, the earliest legislative interdict, apparently under the pressure of the Christian hierarchy, such practices were totally forbidden.[26] Violation of this statute was threatened with severest punishment.[27]

The only exception from the sweeping penalties of the decree, permitted the use of magic to prevent destruction by tempestuous hail storms, denuding rains, and in its relation to medical economy of greater significance, to cure diseases.[28] Supernatural or occult sciences for the purposes indicated, were doubtless tolerated as a just system of remedies gradually unfolded from assenting doctrines of the Christian Fathers, and from the rapid increase of idolatrous reverence by the people, of saintly relics,[29] or may have been suffered to exist as an indulgence which canon and secular law were alike powerless to repress.

In the year 357, the highest penalty of imperial legislation was invoked to prevent the usage of Chaldaic or magic art, auguries, soothsayings and astrology, to determine future

---

[26] IX. Codex Theodosian., XVI., Lex. 3.

[27] "Concremando illo Haruspice." Ibid., Lex 1.

[28] "Nullis criminationibus implicanda sunt Remedia humanis quæsita corporis." Ibid., Lex. 3. Remedies by incantation, Alex., Trallian, Lib. XII.; and Ammian. Marcellinus, Rer. Rom., Lib. XVI., cap. —; and Lib. XXIX., cc. 1 and 2. Vide Origen, Contra Celsum, Lib. VI., p. 301; and Lib. VIII., p. 417.

[29] Beausobre, Hist. du Manicheisme, Tom. II., p. 658 seq.

eventualities.[30] Thirty-five years later Theodosius was obliged to enlarge the scope of the preceding laws, so as to more closely determine the extent to which magic art should be deemed malevolent, especially since in the year 389 Valentinian and Orcadius had interdicted the freedom of soothsaying. The Emperor decreed that any person endeavoring to elevate himself above the laws of Nature, inquiring into forbidden things, seeking to explain the occult or hidden, searching for the illicit, evoking damage upon another, should be apprehended and treated as the most ordinary criminal[31]—thus leaving the original law of medicinal or curative enchantment untouched.

From the preceding summary of the Theodosian rescripts, it is palpable that the practice of the rites indicated, when essayed upon matters forbidden by the policy of ecclesiastical government, was assumed to be a direct recognition and invocation of demoniacal spirits, and consequently so far polytheistic as to necessitate the repressive force of secular authority. The demand for this edict accurately reproduces the widespread influence of such usages, and the extension of them among the people of the empire. Of far greater value, however, in its connection with those causes precipitating the downfall of the curative science, is the admitted distinction between diverse practices of magic, carefully set forth by the rescript of Constantine in the year 327.

It is there distinctly affirmed the person accused of enchantment shall be tried according to the intention with which he exercised this art; and in case of benevolent design, there was no infraction of law, but where a contrary purpose was established, the accused should be punished.[32] Therefore, the practice of magic under legal sanction, within certain prescriptions, was a lawful avocation, especially when applied to the

---

[30] Codex Theodos., cit., Lex. 4. Touching the Chaldean soothsayers, vide Claudiani, De IV. Cons., Honor., v. 147; and Montalembert, Les Moines d'Occident, Tom. II., p. 170.

[31] XVI. Codex Theodosianus, Tit. X., De Paganiis Sacrific., Lex. 12.

[32] IX. Codex Theodosian., Tit. XVI., Lex 3.

8

cure of bodily suffering; but when incantation was used for the determination of those secrets regarded as the exclusive province of Divinity, it was deemed unlawful and punished as a crime. In the beginning of the fifth century all magicians of the empire classified as mathematici[33] were interdicted the pursuit of their craft by Honorius, who ordered them expelled from all cities, and their manuscript books committed to fire.[34] In the same age treasure hunting, with sacrificial accompaniments and magic practices, was forbidden, under severe penalties. Ecclesiastical policy, after the Christianization of Teutonic Pagans, was naturally directed to assimilating the doctrines of the church with the customs of their new converts. In dealing with the universal belief in the efficacy of incantations and sortilege among the Germans, the sacerdoty proscribed the use of criminal spells, which emanated from Satan, and were heathenish, and consequently laid under synodal ban, but encouraged the sort of magic or adjuration of saintly relics, which idolatry was sanctioned by Divinity.

A law of the Spanish Wisigoths threatened the malefici, or operators of evil arts against any one, or his cattle, vintage, or other personal possessions, whether performed by ligation or script, with unstinted cudgelling, shaving of the hair, and disgraceful perambulatory exposure; and like penalty was inflicted upon those who by blood tests provoked destructive hail storms, or by the invocation of base demons blinded the senses of men, and made nocturnal sacrifices to these spirits, or conjured them by magic.[35] At the same epoch the legislative authority of this nation was compelled to enact a decree against rifling sepulchres of their skeleton contents, which were to be used as remedies against diseases.[36]

---

[33] Ibid., Lex. 8. Touching their presence in Rome, vide Montalembert, Les Moines d'Occident, Tom. II., p. 170.

[34] IX. Codex Theodos., Tit. XVI., Lex 12.

[35] Lex. Wisigoth., Lib. V., Tit. II., Lex 4.

[36] "Si quis mortui sarcofagum abstulerit, dum sibi vult habere remedium." Ibid., Lib. XI., cap. 2; apud Canciani., Leg. Barbar., Tom. IV., p. 181. Heinecceius, Elem. Juris. German., Lib. II., art. 341; where the reason of this rifling of tombs for curative remedies is sketched out with his usual learning.

Theodorick the Gothic king published an edict which adjudged the death penalty against such as operated in black arts, interpreted signs, or prophesied by shadows.[37] A notable exception to the universal belief of these times touching the omnipotence of demoniacal powers may be found among the Langobardic laws, which expressly deny the possibility of the human body being destroyed by gradual decay or wasting diseases superinduced through magical means, and peremptorily interdicts the death of young women charged with the serious crime of witchcraft.[38]

---

[37] Edicta Theodorici, cap. 108; ap. Pertzii, Monu. Germ., Tom. V., p. 164.

[38] Leges Langobard, Lib. I., Tit. 2, Lex 9.

CHAPTER VIII.

Schools of Medicine in Alexandria After Galen—Professors of this Art Engage in Imperial Politics—Are Befriended by the Emperors of Rome —Altered Condition of Alexandrine Art and Scientific Institutions— Medical Culture Pursued there to the Mohammedan Conquest—This Art Maintained to a High Degree—Scientists in the IVth Century Vivisect Criminals—Treatises of Professors in Constantine's Time—Pharmaceutical Knowledge of the Illustrious Ionicus—His Surgery—The Eclecticism of the Great Oribasius—Poisons—Strange Malady or Mania Described by Oribasius—Opium Used as a Narcotic by Polytheistic Physicians—Cabbalistic Conjurations Favored by Professors of Medicine—Formal Division of Magic into Medical or Curative Branches —Curative Properties of Gems, etc.

THE edict of Milan, by which Christianity obtained imperial recognition, was nowhere throughout the extensive domains of the colossal empire more keenly realized than in the city of Alexandria, the chief seat of literature and science,[1] inasmuch as the controversy between the old and new religions was here most bitterly agitated and maintained with great erudition.[2] Increasing scholastic institutions of enlarging importance elsewhere, particularly those of Constantinople and Athens, objects of royal favor, gradually undermined the litetary celebrity of the Egyptian metropolis. Scientific culture necessarily declined in the leading polytheistic capital, where the adherents of paganism were compelled to apply their erudite energies to the defence of venerable mythology.

One of the first imperial acts of Julian upon acceding to the government was an endeavor to resuscitate ancient institutions in Alexandria. The attempt was apparently successful, and the mission entrusted to the careful judgment of a physician

[1] Lactant., De Mort. Persec., c. 48; and Eusebius, Histor. Eccles., Lib. IV., c. 5.

[2] Matter, École d'Alexandrie, Tom. I., p. 314.

of Cyprus, named Zeno,[3] who arrived on the territory already prepared to accept imperial overtures in consequence of a revolt against the Christian pontiffs, and at a time when Polytheism had been revived amid the splendid pomp of its ancient ceremonies. Zeno, having been deprived of his puissant patron, was sufficiently fortunate to obtain an oblivious inattention in this city, where a majority of its inhabitants, in defiance of imperative decrees, had declared themselves Christians, and as an illustrious professor of medical science was enabled to surround himself with numerous disciples, among whom may be distinctively mentioned Jonicus, Magnus, and Oribasius.[4]

The Serapeum, one of the leading schools of Alexandria, preserved a fluctuating vitality down to the time of Theodosius in the ensuing century, on account of a superstitious reverence which repressed the violent exhibitions of religious hatred among Christian proselytes.[5] In order to enforce the enactment of the Emperor, directing polytheistic temples to be closed,[6] it became essential for the Alexandrine Christians to make especial demand upon the zeal of the illustrious Theodosius, who granted the Episcopal authorities of the city some of these scholastic edifices, which were remodeled into churches.[7] The Serapeum was demolished by direction of Theophile in the year 391, when the Nilometre, which anciently was kept there, became the ornament of a Christian church.[8]

A limited number of paganistic schools were permitted by ecclesiastical policy to maintain in Alexandria a devitalized existence, such for example as offered no absolute antagonism with the dominant faith, and appear to have maintained so great sagacity and prudence in their demeanor that the decree

---

[3] Eunapii, Vitæ Sophistor., s. nom. Zeno.

[4] Eunapius, Vitæ Sophistor., p. 497 seqq.

[5] Zozimus, Hist. Rom., Lib. III., c. 11.

[6] XVI. Codex Theodos., Titul. X., De Pagan. Sacrif., Lex 4.

[7] Sozomen, Hist. Eccles., Lib. VII., c. 15.

[8] Rufinus, Lib. XII., c. 22.

of the year 529, closing the Athenian establishments, excepted those of the Egyptian capital from its operation.[9] Down to the incendiary fires of Moslem fanaticism in the seventh century, the appearance of scientific culture in mathematics and medicine was still pursued, so far as the altered state of religious and secular changes permitted. It should be added in justice to the declining studies of these sciences, that nowhere were they more seriously investigated under the light of Hippocrates and Galen, or the writings of these sages commented with greater zeal, down to the destruction of the city by the Arabs.[10]

Galen's influence, entirely confined to polytheistic elements, with varying efficiency continued to excite an interest in the study and practice of medicine among the disciples of this art, and claimed such attention for many centuries. As the metropolis of literary and scientific excellence and original seat of anatomy, Alexandria, where Galen warmly urged the science to be studied,[11] necessarily possessed irresistible attractions for those desiring instruction in curative and surgical art down to the expiration of its cultured usefulness in the year 643. Whether the inculpation of Tertullian be correct, or regarded as the accusation of an enraged zealot, that medical scientists of his day resorted to vivisection in the interest of anatomy, and so charges Herophilus,[12] it is evident that so long as the practice of the science by such as maintained a devotion to polytheism, was not placed under the prohibition of canonical interdict, this branch of medicine was certainly pursued for ages subsequent to the time of the Pergamic sage. Eastern Jews of this age appear to have given some attention to acquiring such knowledge of comparative anatomy as to

---

[9] Matter, École d'Alexandrie, Tom. I., p. 331.

[10] Ammianus, Marcellinus, Rer. Rom., Lib. XXII., c. 16.

[11] Galen, De Anatomicis Administrationibus, Lib. I., c. 2.

[12] "Herophilus ille medicus aut lanius, qui sexcentas exsecint ut naturam scrutaretur, qui hominem odit ut nosset," etc. Tertullian, Liber de Anima, c. 10.

aid in the cure of diseases of animals,[13] a system, however, of ancient application.[14]

Among the medical practitioners and professors at Alexandria subsequent to Galen, about the middle of the fourth century, deserving of distinctive illustration, Zenon, as the emissary of the Emperor Julian, is the most eminent.[15] Of the treatises of this scholastic, whose principal labors were circumscribed by the reign of Constantine the Great, nothing has survived to modern times. His biographer describes him lauded as the most famous teacher and practitioner of the curative art in his day,[16] although he frankly avows that the principal cause of the perpetuation of Zenon's celebrity arose from the eminence of his disciples,[17] of whom mention has been made. Of these Ionicus of Sardianus, according to the unstinted eulogy of Eunapius, who asserts that he died just before his panegyric was completed, was descended from a parent himself an illustrious physician, and that the son was equally skilled in the science and practice. Through personal experiments he acquired remarkable distinction for anatomical knowledge.

So great was the profundity of Ionicus in pharmacy, it was asserted, that this valuable art had no secrets to withhold from him. He appears to have signalized his dexterity in surgery by inventing ligatures and appliances valuable to this portion of medicine.[18] Magnus, of Antioch, iatrosophista, or teacher of healing art, renowned for the singular accuracy of his medicinal qualifications, and as famous for a contentious spirit, which provoked a doubt in his mind whether physicians were of undisputed service in curing maladies, was possessed of the Aristotelian attributes to so great extent that in argumentation

---

[13] Grætz, History of the Jews, p. 231.

[14] Galen, op. cit., Lib. I., c. 1.

[15] Eunapius, Vitæ Sophistor., sub nom. Zenon.

[16] Eunapius, op. cit., sub nom. Zenon.

[17] Ibid.

[18] Ibid., sub nom. Ionicus, p. 499.

he sealed the lips of other medical professors with unbroken silence.[19]

The pungent satires of Magnus captivated the admiration of his disciples, but appear to have been equally distasteful to professional rivals. At this epoch, Theon,[20] who appears to have sojourned for a prolonged period in Alexandria and acquired a reputation for laborious study and industrious examination into the principles of this science, abandoned the city and returned to Gaul. A portion of his medical treatises are said to have been extant as late as the ninth century, but the authority for this declares their loss of slight importance.[21]

Of the polytheist philosophers whose research was mainly directed to medicine in the Alexandrine schools toward the end of the fourth century, none obtained the exalted distinction of Oribasius of Pergamos.[22] This scientist, who performed a part so important in the history of neoplatonism and polytheism during the apostasy of Julian, although a disciple of Zenon and personal surgeon of the Emperor, who discovered the future sage in his adolescent prominence,[23] was a close imitator of Galen.[24] So great indeed was his fame, that divine honors were actually paid him by foreign princes whose lives he had saved by medicinal skill at the very entrance to the tomb.[25] At the instigation of the Emperor, Oribasius prepared an abridgment (now lost) of the writings of Galen, in four books, for practical use by perplexed practitioners, and wrote a treatise of seventy-two parts, dedicated to his royal friend.[26] Among other compendious volumes by this cele-

---

19 "Doctores cogebat medicos tenere silentium." Ibid., sub nom. Magnus.

20 "Theon non admodus ingeniosus fuit nec acutus, sed studiosus ac laboriosus, si quis alius. Callebat ideo poetas et oratores." Photius, Bibliotheca, p. 368.

21 Photius, Bibliotheca, p. 368 seq.

22 Eunapius, Vitæ Sophistor., sub nom. Oribasius, p. 498.

23 "Quum vero illustris ejus esset ab adolescentia fama," etc. Ibid.

24 Oribasius, Libr. ad Euporist., p. 284.

25 "Barbaris ut numen quoddam eum colentibus," etc. Ibid., p. 499. This seems like fulsome adulation, but the biographer wrote it in Oribasius' lifetime.

26 Suidas, Lexicon, sub n. Oribas.

brated professor, he addressed a medical work of nine books to his son, Eustathius, and was the author of an essay entitled "De Regno et Affectibus."[27] Having completed the treatise to Julian, on the principles of medical science, which was purely a compilation, and realizing it to be too comprehensive for useful purposes, he drew up what unqualifiedly must have been a valuable addition to historical knowledge of the science, and doubtless equalled the history of Soranus on the same subject.[28] In his pathological system, music or incantation and rhetorical declamation were seriously accredited, and as rigidly enforced.[29]

Among other excellent services rendered to contemporary physicians was an elaborate compilation of prescriptions or receipts for the practical compounding of unguents, etc., which he had gleaned from venerable sources and found by experiment be of value.[30] As an eclectic in its most enlightened and logical signification, Oribasius selected with judicious care, the remedies of Erasistratus, Galen,[31] Dioskorides, etc., his predecessors, and arranged them in alphabetical order to make the same a practical cyclopædia of medicaments. In the exercise of professional judgment, this author in describing poisons proceeded with the utmost caution, so that criminal information might not be gathered from his compilations and used for illicit purposes characterizing the last days of declining Rome; but in the treatment of these by counter-toxicants or antidotes, Oribasius entered into the most minute details, with great skill and erudition.

Specific directions are given in the diversified works of the Pergamic scholar for the sanitative use of sand, oil, and sea-

---

[27] Ibid.

[28] Fabric., Biblioth. Græc., Tom. XI., p, 714.

[29] The practical use of music or incantation for cures is attested by the law of Constantine, IX. Cod. Theodos., XVI., Lex 3. Modulation of the Voice as Sanitative. Oribas., Tres. Lib., ad Euporist., p. 285.

[30] Oribas., In Tres Libr., ad Euporist., p. 243.

[31] Ibid., p. 284.

water baths,[32] and careful suggestions touching unguents composed of chalk and arsenic, largely applied as a hair restorative. A curious frenzy appears to have attracted considerable attention in his day, which preserved an existence until towards the conclusion of the middle ages. This grievous malady usually appeared in midwinter, when it assumed the most aggravated form and swelled to the proportions of an epidemic. Laboring under the agony of a nervous exasperation, those afflicted with this awful disease persuaded themselves that they were transformed into dogs or wolves.[33] Abandoning their habitations, an unaccountable mania precipitated them into the most secluded solitudes, and for this reason tombs of the dead were most persistently sought, and from these sepulchral domiciles the suffering invalids struggled to express their anguish by the sounds of those animals into which they seemed to be metamorphosed.

Under the treatment of polytheistic science, opium seems to have been used to alleviate, as a usual remedy,[34] but when the progress of that abnormal exaltation, consequent upon the religious fervor which crept through the empire during the three first centuries, had abandoned the deduction of natural ratiocination as an unsafe guide, such maladies were expressly denominated as diabolical visitations, to cure which by sagely compounded medicaments was regarded as profanity, and an invasion of the sacred prerogatives of Deity. While the efforts of the compiler, in his close servility to Galen, may merit the commendation of the historian as illustrating the condition of medicine at that period, impartial justice demands the severe condemnation of Oribasius for

---

[32] Ibid., p. 246.

[33] "Qui morbo lupino sive canino appelato corripiuntur in febrioris mense noctu exeunt, per omnia imitantes lupos aut canos." Aetius, Tetrabili, Lib. II., Serm. 2, cap. 11. Vide Petronius, Satyricon, c. 62.

[34] Evident use of narcotics in the empire, as Valentine drank absinthe after his bath. Epist. Vind. ad Valent., ap. Fabric. Biblioth. Græc., Tom. XIII., p. 448; and Philostratus, Vita Apollon., Lib. II., cap. 36, claimed for his hero the skilled preparation of sleep-producing medicaments—evidently opium.

accelerating the decay of the science and debasing it to the place of impotent magic and cabbalistic conjurations. This renowned professor, as narrated, was distinguished for his Neoplatonic and mystical philosophy. Having followed with fidelity the fortunes of his imperial friend Julian to the year 363, he was made the object of persecution under Valens and Valentinan, after the apostate's death. His intrigues under Jovian caused him to be exiled to a foreign country, where he signalized his expatriation by a display of heroic virtues which acquired him the unstinted admiration of the people.[35] Subsequently restored to the favor of Valentinian, he received honorable distinction. According to Eunapius, he was fond of that display and splendor which the possession of vast affluence only provides. It appears that Oribasius, in the pursuit of such social embellishments, hesitated not to increase his wealth by marriage with a lady noted for her birth and immense riches.[36]

It is unknown whether he was privileged to pursue the unimpeded practice of his profession among polytheists, which is indeed probable, inasmuch as he was possessed of that enthusiastic activity of zealots, who with unequalled devotion to a declining cause shook the sanctuaries and stirred the empire;[37] doubtless the concluding eulogy of his biographer would warrant such inference.[38] By the side of the practical polytheistic scientists, a class of paganistic mystics such as Plotinus, the commentator of Plato, sought to vindicate the claim of sacerdotal transmission of the curative art, which it was alleged was alone procurable through the solemn preparation of initiatory rites.[39]

The founder of the Manichean system of religion, similar to

---

[35] Eunapius, Vita Sophistor., sub n. Oribasius, p. 498.

[36] "Uxorem duxit divitiis et genere claram." Eunapius, Vita Sophistor., sub. n. Oribasius.

[37] Matter, École d'Alexandrie, Tom. II., p. 38.

[38] Eunapius, op. cit., s. n. Oribasius, p. 499.

[39] Matter, op. cit., Tom. I., p. 352.

the erudite of his day, exhibited an extended acquaintanceship with medicine; and from the attestation of credible writers the practice of this art at that epoch was so highly esteemed as to warrant the conclusion of a close union between medicine and religious faith, down indeed to the fifth century.[40] Plotinus endeavored to check the rapid spread of Christianity through the disciplinary school of high antiquity, and in this attempt assumed it possible to resuscitate the sanctuaries, with their authority over oracles, ancient mysteries, and the art of cures.[41] It was claimed that miraculous restoration to health had been performed from the days of Apollonius of Tyana down to the time of more recent philosophers in the fourth century.[42]

This art was especially rich in its diversified branches, and was at the period under examination divided into Theocracy, Goetic, Magic, Pharmacy, Theurgy and Theosophy. Several sects in Alexandria, more particularly the Neoplatonists, Gnostics and Manicheans,[43] were in consequence largely given to this system of magical cures, and sought to derive their art from the ancient Therapeutæ of Egypt and Orpheus respectively.[44] The excessive use of occult science by the followers of Manes opened the sect to the sweeping inculpation of magicians, and full of mysteries and devoted to those arts forbidden by the civil law. This accusation[45] subjected them to the animadversion of an imperial edict, repeated in the Theodosian code.[46]

From this singular amalgamation, not wholly confined to the polytheistic or Gnostic sects, arose a most perplexing task

[40] Beausobre, Histoire du Manicheisme, Tom. I., pp. 81 and 159; and Tom. II., p. 804.

[41] Matter, op. cit., Tom. II., p. 39.

[42] Philostratus, Vita Apollonii, Lib. IV., cap. 45. Cattarhal diseases in Apollonius' day, and temples sought for cure. Ib., cap. 44.

[43] Beausobre, Histoire du Manicheisme, Tom. II., p. 799 seq.

[44] Matter, École d'Alexandrie, Tom. I., p. 353.

[45] Beausobre, op. cit., Tom. II., p. 799.

[46] IX. Cod. Theodos., De Malificiis, Tit. XVI., Lex 3.

for the scholars of the rising Church. As a necessary consequence of the elevation of Christianity to the pedestal forcibly vacated by the ancient faith, an effort was made in some degree to clothe science and art in a Christianized garb.

On this principle certain treatises elucidating medicine, conformable to the precepts of the new religion, with such paganistic mythology as shocked proselyte sensibilities eliminated, were drawn up and obtained limited circulation. Increasing idolatry of martyred dead and saintly relics, in conjunction with the expanding belief in the potency of angelic hosts and demoniacal forces, provided abundant substitutes for the vanishing splendors of Polytheism. Obliged thus to adapt the declining principles of several sciences to new teachings, the same influences forced an outward conformity with the accepted ideas of cosmography and geography, but divested of the most insignificant vestiture of paganism.[47] In the prosecution of such indispensable modification, Christian efforts yielded homage to pagan science, and oftentimes invoked the venerable authority of writers of the most remote epochs.

The period of the rule of the Lagides dynasty was universally accepted as the most elegant, and therefore, possessing superior attractions to the transforming proselyte, was freely used for the selection of authoritative names with which to fortify effeminate compositions. The domain of medicine was not exempt from this species of literary falsification. A medical professor converted to Cristianity digested a volume from the aphorisms of Hippocrates, which he boldly announced had been drawn up under Ptolemy Evergetes and by his order.[48]

This compilation has been attributed to Oribasius. Among other authors whose writings were used for curative purposes, the poems of Homer appear to have obtained great celebrity.[49]

---

[47] Matter, École d'Alexandrie, Tom. II., p. 39; and Bossuet, Histoire des Mathematiques, Tom. I., p. 160.

[48] Matter, op. cit., p. 40.

[49] Hirschel, Geschichte der Medezin, p. 95.

Oribasius himself was far more deeply skilled in theurgic cures than the practical details of medicinal remedies.[50] This tendency to the use of thaumaturgic art for the cure of maladies developed rapidly among the professors of medicine in Alexandria subsequent to the time of Galen, and was a natural outgrowth of the strange controversies engaging the undivided attention of renowned savans and scientists in the Egyptian city. As late as the middle of the sixth century Aetius compiled a compendium of medical practice, in the form of selections from his predecessors, enriched indeed with personal observations and fragments of a treatise by Demosthenes of Marseilles on ophthalmic diseases, but displaying blind credulity in the puissant force of charms, amulets and talismans,[51] to cure grievous maladies when applied in accordance with the strict regulations of magical instruction identical with Goetic and Theurgic arts.[52]

This author attributed great obstetrical properties to the lapis ætites, and gagates stone.[53] The sapphire when taken as a potion pulverized in milk, cured internal ulcers and checked excessive perspiration.[54] The smargdine was recommended for strabismus, and spider webs, when prepared in a certain method, were declared a panacea for external ulcers.[55] Of the successors to Galen in popular estimation at the Roman capital, Alexander of Tralles may be designated as the most celebrated. In his earlier years this medical scholist enriched a highly-cultivated intellect with the elegance of extensive travel through Europe, the Spanish provinces, Northern Africa and Italy.

His renown as an expert surgeon caused him to become permanently domiciled at Rome, where he lived to an advanced

---

[50] Matter, op. cit., Tom. II., p. 40.

[51] Ætii Tetrabili, I., Sermo. 2, cap. 35.

[52] Matter, École d'Alexandrie, Tom. II., p. 40.

[53] Ætii, op. cit., cap. 24.

[54] Ibid., cap. 38.

[55] Ibid., cc. 39 and 165.

age, towards the termination of the sixth century.[56] Among the remedies urgently advised by the Hellenistic professor as a curative for diversified fevers, was an amulet prepared from an oil-tree leaf with this lettered incription, Καποια, the magical potency of which was asserted to be irresistible.[57] John of Alexandria, Paul of Ægina, and Palladius, the final representatives of that medical school which had hitherto illustrated the city of Egypt, were perhaps less superstitious, but almost entirely denuded of inventive power. Of these the first published,[58] was a careful commentary on the Hippocratian epidemics of which, however the original is no longer extant, while the translation survives in the Saracen language,[59] of which a Latin version was preserved and used during the Middle Ages.[60] Paul of Ægina wrote a practical abridgment of medicine in all its departments, including surgery, in whose preparation the treatises of his predecessors were liberally used.[61]

The third of the Alexandrian professors alluded to, was apparently contemporaneous with Alexander of Tralles, and attempted in a work on the phenomena of fevers to assimilate his theories of these infirmities to that of Galen, but is principally famous for the preservation of his oral discourses on certain portions of the writings of Hippocrates, evidently written out after their public delivery.[62] It admits of little doubt that the practical discipline so essential to the preservation and progress of medicine as a scientific cure of diseases, during several centuries preceding the destruction of the city of Alexandria by the Arabs, maintained an enfeebled vitality

---

56 Tirabaschi, Storia della Litteratura, Tom. III., p. 63.

57 Lessing, Geschichte der Medezin, Th. I., p. 164.

58 Matter, op. cit., Tom. II., p. 41.

59 Joannicii Arabis Artiscella, Venet. ed 1483, fol. apud Matter, École d'Alexandrie, Tom. II., p. 41.

60 Lessing, Geschichte der Medezin, Th. I., p. 169.

61 Matter, op. cit., Tom. II., p. 41.

62 Ibid., and Lessing, op. cit., Th. I., p. 169.

among both polytheists and Christians, but accompanied by the system of amulets and remedial gems. So far, however, as an exact physiological or anatomical knowledge extended, it necessarily diminished in proportion to the advancement and solidification of Christianity, whose dogmas especially eschewed the dissection of the human body.

The most serious catastrophe to medicine, exclusive of the tendencies of the age to accept disease as provoked by demons, certainly originated with the limited number who, while affirming an enervated faith in its scientific character, conjoined with the practice the least spirit of inquiry. The division of the empire was more favorable to the Greeks for the culture of medicine, and aided in preserving for many centuries the outlines of a science in the practical application to cures.

Even with the Hellenistic professors, converts to the Christian religion, anatomy and physiology, which it had been the pride and glory of the Egyptian metropolis to create,[63] in the seventh century passed from the domain of scientific system, to be examined almost entirely as objects of pious admiration touching the wonderful mechanical structure of the human body; and thus abandoned to holy curiosity, it was impossible to arrest the downfall which the progression of Christian faith accelerated—an inquisitiveness indeed only resulting in an impassioned declamation of the motives inducing the Divine Mind to construct this organism on its existing plan, and why the limbs, vision, etc., were organized and adapted to such diverse parts. Theophilus, a medical officer of the Byzantine Court under Heraclius, seriously elucidated the system of anatomy from a Christian standpoint, in his enthusiastic zeal for the handiwork of its Divine Author.[64]

---

[63] Matter, École d'Alexandrie, Tom. II., p. 22.

[64] Lessing, Geschichte der Medezin, Th. I., p. 170.

CHAPTER IX.

Edicts Touching the Practice of Medicine in Rome—Laws of Valentinus of the Fourth Century—Their Influence in the Western Empire—Impotent to Revive the Science—Treatise of a Gallic Professor—Avows Preternatural Cures—Other Gallic Medicists—Belief in Potency of Words—Disciples of the Æsculapian Art—Prostration of Medical Science at this Epoch—Curious Attestation of this Downfall—Charlatans Obtain Royal Favor—All Maladies Traced to Supernatural Sources—Babylonian Characters of Great Force—Era of Theodoric the Gothic Ruler—Paucity of Famous Professors at this Time—Gothic Disposition to Favor Medical Organization—Schedule of Charges Allowed—Penalty of Death for Stupid Surgery—Ecclesiastical Medicists—Organization of Hospitals.

NOTWITHSTANDING the frequent legislation by Christian Emperors in the interest of medical professors and their science, of which, like their polytheistic predecessors on the throne, they were deeply solicitous, the curative art almost ceased its legitimate functions before sacerdotal indifference, and was as a rational system apparently extinguished in the Western Empire by the destructive and subversive Gothic invasions. Although the transfer of the empirical metropolis to Byzantium was a severe blow to Rome,[1] which subsequently only survived as a pontifical municipality, associated with Constantinople by a slender thread of obedience,[2] the regulations established by authoritative edicts of paganistic rulers prior to the time of Theodosius, teaching the practice of medicine in this venerable city, were designed to inspire admiration of the enlightened policy which promulgated them.

The laws of Valentinus in the year 368, regulating the selection of a public surgeon salaried for gratuitous attendance on the poor,[3] and in case of his death prescribing the duties of

[1] Eutropius, Brev. Rom. Hist., Lib. X., c. 4.

[2] Montalembert, Les Moines d'Occident, Tom. II., p. 115.

[3] XIII. Codex Theodosianus, De Medic. et Profes., Tit. III., Lex 8.

summoning collegiate members in electing a successor,[4] were subsequently rëenacted and ratified under Theodosius and Justinian, who incorporated them in the codification of the civil rescripts. To this edict of the fourth century, Symmachus, Theodosian proconsul in the Italian provinces, alludes in a letter to his imperial patron, which narrates the circumstances under which a convocation of the college of surgeons in the municipal districts was agitated by the election of a public physician, and in adjusting the controversy the scholastic perfunctionary directed them to remember that the annual stipend conceded them by a generous government for medicinal services among the impoverished sick and infirm, should spur them to more faithful attendance upon the suffering poor, rather than assist the affluent through shameless greed. Finally, that they were only at liberty under legal sanction to accept from the diseased what these, when in good health, might offer, and not what was proffered amid the aggravated danger of their maladies.[5]

Favoring legal enactments,[6] confirming ancient and valuable privileges and immunities, were unable to infuse into the body of medical science, decaying under the pressure of increasing fanaticism, sufficient vitality to produce a person eminent by his services in the practice of this art. Rescripts were impotent to revive the essential principles of a science entombed beneath the ponderous weight of ignorant zeal which condemned its operations as an intrusion of the sacred mysteries of divinity.

To this envenomed antagonism must be added the unhappy condition of the Occidental Empire, especially repugnant to the necessary quietude of scientific investigation. Among the Romans of this age no names appear which justly rise to the dignity of professors of medical science;[7] and of Latin writers

[4] X. Codex Justinianus, Tit. LII., Leg. 9 and 10.

[5] Q. Aurelius Symmachus, Epistolarum, Lib. X., Ep. 40. The concluding part of this cautionary missive is a direct reproduction of civil law.

[6] Codex Theodos., cit., Lex 3; and Cod. Justin., cit., Leg. 6 and 9.

[7] Tiraboschi, Storia della Litteratura, Tom. II., p. 455.

on such subjects none remained as permanent residents in the ancient capital.

Before the close of the fourth century, Vindicianus obtained some distinction as the personal physician to Valentinus I.; but, although a native of Africa, he seems to have passed the whole of his professional existence at Rome, according to the laudatory narrative of Saint Augustin touching the excellence of this practitioner.[8] Of like nationality was another surgeon of high distinction, whose medicinal treatises are claimed to be of slight scientific value, and exclusively tend to the boldest empiricism, exhibiting a constant effort at the introduction of simple medicaments in place of a system of medicine. Equally subjugated by the magical and demoniacal tendencies of the epoch, his remedies partake largely of the credulity which followed quickly in the footsteps of an extinct science, and among these he solemnly attests the sovereign potency of the loadstone for a cure of headache.[9]

Toward the opening of the fifth century, Marcellus of Bordeaux, surnamed the Empiric, surgeon to the Emperor Theodosius the Great,[10] and magister officinum, in writing upon medicine, evinced the most abject superstition.[11] In a work entitled De Medicamentiis Physiciis, Empiriciis ac Rationalibus, this empirical physician was so completely under the baleful influences of his age, that he boldly avowed the remedial properties of preternatural or magic formulas. His compendium of curatives was largely drawn from the simple prescriptions of rude and illiterate peasants—agrestes et plebeii.[12]

---

[8] Augustini, Confession., Lib. IV., cap. 3; and Lib. VII., c. 6.

[9] Lessing, Geschichte der Medezin, Th. I., p. 120.

[10] Tiraboschi, op. cit., Tom. II., p. 455.

[11] Lessing, op. cit., Th. I., p. 120.

[12] In this he seems to have had the example of Oribasius before him, who unequivocally asserts that the most potent medicaments have thus been secured: "Virtutes medicamentum quae facile invenientur in ægris per varia loca, ubi docti minime inveniuntur medicii, qui curam impendere possint." Oribas., In Libros ad Euporist, etc., p. 243.

Frequent application is recommended of Oriental theorems for exorcising diabolical principles of maladies, and especially the use of redoubtable Christian formulas—a systematic adaptation of remedies which attests most unequivocally the profound degradation to which, under the dominant faith, medical science had descended. Few names of practitioners of this art arose above the social inundation of the fifth and sixth centuries[13], sufficiently distinctive to merit illustration; beneath the frightful wreck of art provoked by the destructive impulse of Teutonic invasions, medicine as a rational system, throughout the west of Europe, was submerged, and only revived under the scrutinizing curiosity of monastic inquirers after the lapse of ages. Saint Jerome mentions a physician of his day, by the name of Flavius, who had written voluminous medical books in Latin metre, but gives no clew to his nativity or permanent domicil.[14]

Occasional notices appear in the writings of proconsul Symmachus, of Roman practitioners, and of these he accords the most unstinted panegyric to Disarius, asserting that with impartial justice this professor, among all physicians in his day, was awarded the highest place.[15] Born in Aquitania according to his own statement, Disarius, after having attained to great eminence by following the avocation of medicine in the Latin metropolis, decided to return to his native province, much to the regret and lamentation of his proconsular friend and numerous patrons.[16] Saintly aid appears to have entered extensively into the practice of Disarius, who, before applying curatives to suffering patients, demanded celestial assistance.[17]

---

[13] Fabricius, Bibliotheca Latinit., Lib. IV., c. 12.

[14] In this connection he adds on the portentous force of words: "Quæ hæc portenta verborum, etc., Hippocratis vinculis allegandum," Hieronym., Contra Jovian., Lib. I., cap. 2.

[15] Q. Aur. Symmachus, Epistolar., Lib. III., Ep. 39.

[16] "Disarius medicinæ professor patrem tuum spe commodi uberioris in Galliam secutus fuit." Symmachus, Epistolar., Lib. IX., Ep. 44.

[17] "Et ante medicus manus opem sanctos coeli clementioris expectat." Ibid., Lib. III., c. 39.

Additional and trustworthy attestation touching the repute in which this Gallic professor was held by Roman citizens, is vouchsafed in the flattering eulogy of Macrobius, who introduces him among the interlocutors of his dialogues. Immoderately praised, in harmony with the epoch, almost to adulation, Disarius is proclaimed to possess all the secrets of creative nature possible for human intellect to comprehend.[18] Eusebius, a physician of this age, is rescued by Symmachus from oblivion, perhaps a just reward for medical mediocrity, although the scholastic panegyrist declares him equal to the most dexterous of his confréres.[19] To another, named Dionysius, a resident of Rome, the imperial representative urgently recommends a certain youth whom he qualifies as a future disciple of the Æsculapian art.[20]

In the letter addressed by Symmachus to his friend Theodosius, the names of John and Epectitus are especially mentioned, without such information as would lead to the presumption of their having written treatises on medicine meriting commendation. At this period Italy and its great metropolis failed to produce a professor of this science, leaving behind him a monument worthy of honor by posterity.[21]

A retrospective survey of the curative art from the era of Galen to the downfall of the Western Empire, and its complete prostration before the resistless forces of the Gothic armies, will vindicate the allegation of the terrible debasement of a science essentially progressive, and which under the enlightened investigation of the Pergamic scholar had advanced to great excellence. Since the third century, from the operation of causes hitherto specifically detailed, theurgic arts were dominant in all departments of this science; and by a curious

---

[18] Macrobius, Saturnalia, Lib. VII., c. 4.

[19] "Certe Eusebius medicorum peritissimus." Symmachus, op. cit., Lib. II., Ep. 18.

[20] Ibid., Lib. IX., Ep. 4.

[21] Tiraboschi, Storia della Litteratura, Tom. II., p. 456.

misfortune these occult forces were stoutly maintained to be a branch of learning, and as such, obtained the patronage of both polytheistic and Christian emperors.

Frequent and unquestioned facts attested the baneful inquiries of the Roman rulers into these mystical sciences, and by their illustrious example, powerfully aided in undermining the solid structures of scientific systems, which finally receded almost unrivalled into the custody of charlatans and vendors of magical formulas, whose puissant mandates vanquished the principles through which the causes of maladies were previously traced. We have stated the universal acknowledgment of extraordinary power claimed by Apollonius of Tyana.

A statue of this magical medicist and philosopher studded the walls of the Larario of the Emperor Alexander Severus, who rendered homage in like manner to Abraham, Christ, and Orpheus.[22] By the amalgamated influences of the Alexandrine sophists and the Neoplatonist schools of Ammonius Saccas, magical medication absorbed the more ancient philosophy, and confounded this with Oriental and Christian dogmas. All the operations of nature, especially its visible manifestations under the form of sickness and disease, were attributed to supernatural or demoniac sources,[23] which existed in the closest sympathetic relationship to each other, over which the truly wise, through a preparation by ascetic meditation, was able to render himself undisputed master. For this reason the Pythagoreans were confessedly so dexterous as to banish or eject spirits.[24] Basilideans, as skilled thaumaturgists, united their mystical rites with Christianity, and claimed to exercise the most unlimited power over unseen forces.[25] To Plotinus, the companionship of an invisible demon or diabolical spirit was accredited, through whose mediation he was not only able to use the prophetic vision,

---

22 Ælius Lamprid., Vita Alex. Severi, cap. 28.

23 Porphyr., De Abstinentia ab Esu, Lib. II., p. 210.

24 Lucian, Satyra, 347.

25 Salverte, Sciences Occultes, p. 513.

but readily cured the most distressing maladies,[26] which preternatural puissance was obtained through unimpeded absorption of his soul into the contemplation of Deity; by which means absolute dominion was procured over the world of unseen beings.[27]

By this unnatural potency he resurrected a cadaver, and conferred with him privately touching celestial matters.[28] Magic itself was divided into specific branches, to each of which individual properties were attributed; the ordinary, or Goëtic, controlled the operations of evil demons, consequently under the expanding system of ecclesiastical preventative and cure of bodily ills, was eagerly sought; Pharmacy, which through properly prepared medicaments subjected these demoniacal causes exciting sickness, while the secret or Mystic magic possessed irresistible rule over the most elevated spiritual hosts.[29]

Others separated this system, by which miraculous cures were wrought, into Theosophism, or the magic to which Divinity himself had accorded omnipotence; Theurgy, by which angels were manipulated; and Goëtism, which commanded the malevolent action of impure spirits.[30] It was of the use of Babylonish and Egyptian names for this purpose that Galen complained, and charged such practice to the medical theurgists of his day.[31]

Symbolic effigies, when combined with certain words properly collocated, exercised the greatest power on demoniacal diseases, and when written in the Chaldaic or Hebrew lan-

[26] Porphyr., Vita Plotini, cap. 10. His Egyptian birth, Eunapius, Vitæ Sophistor., p. 456.

[27] Porphyr., op. cit., cap. 23.

[28] Eunapius, op. cit., sub nom. Porphyr., p. 456.

[29] Matter, Histoire du Gnosticisme, Tom. I., pp. 186 and 214; and Matter, École d'Alexandrie, Tom. I., p. 353.

[30] Porphyr., De Abstinentia ab Esu, Lib. II., p. 210; and Eusebius, Præparat. ad Evangel., Lib. IV., c. 10.

[31] *Ονόματα ταῦτα Αἰγυπτιαχὰ Χαὶ Βαβυλώνια.* Galen, De Simplic. Medicamentor, Temper. ac Facultat., Lib. VI., Prœmium, Tom. XI., p. 793.

guage, this puissance was intensified,[32]—a system of typical images, as we shall hereafter discover of extensive application for cures among the early Teutonic converts. With such precursors it will be readily understood how, conjoined with the deplorable effect of Germanic invasions upon art and science, the belief in supernatural wonders quickly increased, and medical culture passed from the hands of the skilled and erudite into the reliquaries of martyrs and the sainted dead. Incredulity exhibited touching the alleged curative properties of these sacred remains, was equivalent to obnoxious heresy, under the ban of both canonical and civil law.

Thus, for example, Gregory of Tours avows being afflicted with severe pains in the head, and sought relief for his suffering by means of blood-letting or cupping. Fearing, however, that the malady might be too promptly cured by this remedy, he touched the disordered spot with the sombre pall of Saint Martin's sepulchre, and petitioned forgiveness of the holy martyr for applying profane medication.[33] The same writer states that an archdeacon, Leonastes, through the efficacy of fasting and prayers at the tomb of the Turonese saint, succeeded in restoring light to his blinded eyes; but having submitted himself to the surgical treatment of an Israelitish physician, who applied herbs and medicaments to the injured organs, the infirmity returned, which caused him to seek the skill of ambulatory physicians.[34] From the preceding fact the Pontiff of Tours deduced the following conclusion: that he who rendered himself worthy of celestial medicine needed nothing of earthly physicians.[35] From the sixth century the exercise of medical art was almost exclusively appropriated by cloisters and monasteries, whose occupants boldly vended the miraculous remedial

[32] Iamblichus, De Myst. Ægypt, p. 97 seq.; Ib., p. 170, on invocation of suitable demon, and superiority of diabolical rank to that of man. Ib., Dist. II., p. 10.

[33] Gregor. Turones., Miracula S. Martini, Lib. II., cap. 60. This pall cured obstinate pustular diseases. Ib., Lib. I., cap. 3.

[34] "Qui ambulans per multos medicos." Ib., Histor. Francor., Lib. V., cap. 6.

[35] Gregor. Turonesis, Miracula S. Martini, Lib. II., cap. 32.

properties of relics, chrism, baptismal fluids, holy oil,[36] rosy crosses, etc., as of unquestioned virtue.

At this era, in the civilized portions of Western Europe, and especially in Italy, the deplorable degradation of social life permitted slight hopes of an early resuscitation of medical science. That faint vestiges of an organized system of the practitioners of this art still maintained a feeble existence during the fifth and sixth centuries in the Italian metropolis, admits of historical proof; but the statutory regulation of the Gothic rulers, to which we shall presently return, must vindicate the inculpation of frightful debasement of lay medicists, and the near absorption of the science into the complete control of charlatans and monkish physicians.

Theodoric, king of the Ostrogoths, by his earlier residence at the court of Theodosius, had acquired a taste for liberal arts, which, when the changed circumstances elevated him to the perfunctionary duties of monarch of Italy, manifested itself in preserving the remains of fallen Rome. One of the first official acts of this ruler was the creation of a magistrate especially empowered to safeguard such relics of classical antiquity as had escaped the Teutonic destroyers, designated centurio nitentium rerum.[37] Other laws preserving public and private property,[38] were re-enacted by the Gothic ruler. Through the increasing activity of Cassiodorus, secretary to Theodoric, these efforts were largely rewarded in preserving from total destruction the relics of a glorious past. This scholastic, with the style of exuberant rhetoric inaugurated by Bœthius and himself, exhibited an ardent zeal for the preservation of medicine in an imperial order, where he indulges his fondness for hyperbole, and urges that the skilled Archiater should be able to judge the sufferings of nature by the throbbing pulse and urinary scrutiny.[39]

---

[36] Ammian. Marcellinus, Gesta, Lib. XVI., cap. 6.

[37] Ibid., Lib. XXII., cap. 4.

[38] XVI. Codex Theodos., De Pagan. Sacrific. et Templis, Tit. X., Lex. 15.

[39] "Offerentur occulis urinæ, ut facilius sit vocem clamantis non advertere,

So far as the substantial evidence of Theodoric's desire is concerned, to place the practitioners of this art resident within the city of Rome, and in other municipalities, through the solicitation of his confidential adviser, this was abundantly attested. The Gothic monarch re-established the dignity of Comes Archiater, or president-general of the surgical guilds; inasmuch as this distinctive title is mentioned by the monkish patron of polite letters among other formal investitures.[40] In alluding to the immunities of this ancient office and its franchises, he affirms a prerogative of official primacy among physicians of rank, the undisputed right of deciding litigated questions arising within their unions, and the uninterrupted access to the royal court.[41]

No names, however, of medical professors of high illustration, are referred to in the eulogistic allusions of Cassiodorus. Petrus was personal surgeon, or Archiater, to the Gothic monarch,[42] although another, and perhaps more justly celebrated physician of this king, was Elpidius, styled Rusticus, who does not appear to have surrendered himself up entirely to medicine, but wrote a dogmatic poem.[43]. It appears that Theodoric, himself, manifested a praiseworthy interest in medical matters, and enjoined their study.[44] In the year 554, after his campaign against the Franks, the emperor Justinian issued a rescript, by which the state of Italy, as established under the Gothic king, should be preserved, especially such laws as were enacted to continue perquisites and compensation of professors of medicine, in order, as the statute concludes, that students might have maintained for them suitable methods of instruction.[45]

---

quam hujusmodi minime signa sentire." Formulæ etc. Edicta Regum Ostrogothor., No. XIX., ap. Canciani, Tom. I., p. 31.

[40] Cassiodor., Formulæ, etc., No. XIX.

[41] Cassiodor., op. cit., No. XIX.

[42] Du Cang. Glossar., sub v. Archiater; and Baronius, Annales, sub an. 444.

[43] "Elpidius, Medicus Theodorici Regis," etc., Labigne, Bibl. Max. Patr., Tom. V., p. 462.

[44] Baronius, op. cit., sub an. 441, § 47.

[45] "Ut annona minstretur medicis et diversis. Annonam etiam quam et Theo-

In the first decade of the sixth century, the decrees of the Wisigoths indicate a disposition to favor an organization as yet propagating an uninterrupted existence in the provinces subjugated by them, although the singularity of these ordinances betrays the lamented decay of professional dignity among the devotees of the curative art. These regulations of the year 504 substantially survived to the eleventh century, as legislative guides in establishing the practice of medicine in the kingdom of Jerusalem, so valiantly won by the Crusaders. It was ordered that no physician should presume to cup or bleed any nobly-born woman without the presence of her father, mother, brother, etc., and in their absence, the attendance of a relative or neighbor of similar standing was peremptory, unless the emergency demanded instant attention, when the menials must attend.[46] The cause alleged for this stringent law,[47] is a positive attestation of the debased condition of the medical men of the period, who apparently preferred to wander from the footsteps of Hippocrates and Galen.

It may be questioned with candor whether this edict was originally designed for the professors or practitioners legislated for by Theodoric and Justinian, or for the Teutonic ambulatory medicastres, who indeed aspired no higher than charlatans; but a clause of this ordinance most unequivocally contemplates a high grade of surgical skill, transcending the dexterity of the peripatetic herbal venders.

For removing an ypocismata (a cataract?) from the eye, and restoring sight, the surgeon by law was allowed a large payment.[48] It was further decreed that any medical professor

---

doricus dare solitus est, et nos sicut etiam Romanis indulgissimus," etc., "quatenus juvenes liberalibus studiis eruditi per nostram rempublicam floreant." Pragmatica Sanctio, Lib. I., cap. 22, ap. Pertizii, V. 174.

[46] "Nullus medicus sine præsentia patris, matris, fratris, filii, aut avunculi, vel cujuscunque propinque, mulierem ingenuam flebotomare præsumat." Lex Wisigothorum, Lib. XI., Tit. I., Lex 1.

[47] "Quia difficilimum non est, ut sub tali occasione ludibrium interdum adhaerescat." Ibid.

[48] "Si quis ypocisma de occulis abstulerit, et ad pristinam sanitatem perduxerit

called in to cure a malady should first furnish satisfactory guarantee for the undertaking, and agree by contract upon the price for which restoration to health was to be compensated, and in case the disease terminated fatally, the agreement was vacated.[49] If the physician blundered in blood-letting or phlebotomy, where the patient was of noble birth, by cupping so freely as to debilitate him, he should pay a fine of heavy damages; but when a mortal ending followed the operation, the surgeon was to be immediately delivered over to the nearest relatives of deceased, who, according to the usual provisions of Germanic law, were thereafter the absolute custodians of his life or death.[50]

When the blundering or impotent medicist killed a serf, he was merely compelled to make restitution in kind[51]—a regulation enforced by the ordinances drawn up and published by the Crusaders at Jerusalem in the year 1090.[52] The humility with which this class of personages was invested may be inferred from the fact that they often assumed monkish vestments, as the appropriate raiment of the profession, as early as the epoch before us, and in this garb had unimpeded access to the presence of royalty.[53] The statutes of the Wisigoths accorded inviolability to physicians so far as arrest was involved, excepting in case of the homicide noted; in matters of debt,

---

infirmum v. solidos pro suo beneficio consequatur." Lex Wisig., Lib. XI., Tit. I., Lex 5.

[49] Ibid., Leg. 4 and 7.

[50] "Si per flebotomum ingenuus vel servus mortem incurrat, si quis medicus dum flebotomum exercet, ingenuum debilitaverit, c. solidos coactus exsolvet, si vero mortuus fuerit, continuo propinquis tradendus est, ut quod de eo, facere voluerint, habeant potestatem." Ibid., Lex 6.

[51] "Si vero servum debilitaverit aut occiderit, hujusmodi servum restituerat." Ibid., Lex 6. No physician was permitted to enter a prison without official accompaniment, in order that a prisoner should have no opportunity through fear of his crime—"per metum culpæ suæ"—to seek death at the hands of complaisant or corruptible practitioners. Ibid., Lex 2.

[52] Assisse et Bone Usanze del Reame de Hyerusalem, cap. 218.

[53] "Habitum monachi suscipiens * * * et se medicum fingeris." Rog. de Wend., Flor. Historiar., an. 497, Tom. I., p. 51.

when by the Roman code the debtor was liable to be held on a civil process, the follower of this avocation obtained his freedom upon furnishing security.[54]

Following the example of the civil law, these rescripts made abundant provision for gratuitous medical service among such as were in custody.[55] After the withdrawal of Cassiodorus from secular affairs in the year 528, consequent on his profession of monastic life,[56] his attention was directed without variance to such studies as comported with clerical vows. In the close vicinity of the Ravenna Archate, he constructed a monastery at private expense, where as a hermit he domiciled himself for the reception of anchorites.[57]

Cassiodorus was unquestionably the earliest Christian monk who realized the necessity of preserving the writings of profane authors, and in order to render such desire of practical utility, vigilant research was instituted in diverse localities for manuscripts, which were faithfully transcribed into numerous exemplars.[58] To exhortation this erudite cenobite added the force of personal example in such labors, by diligently comparing and collating several manuscripts of the Scriptures, to obtain a perfect copy.[59] With rare judgment for the period, Cassiodorus urged familiarity with polytheistic works in order the more exactly to comprehend the significance of prophetic and evangelical utterances.[60] From his devotion to conventual seclusion he manifested an ardent desire that the clerical brethren should acquire a skillful knowledge of medicine, so that efficient services might be given their infirm and disabled confréres. In this connection the celebrated scholastic speci-

[54] "Nullus medicus nauditum, excepto homicidii causa, in custodiam retrudat. Pro debito tamen sub fidejussore debit consistere." Lex Wisigothor., Lib. XI., Tit. I., Lex 8.

[55] Ibid., Lex 2.

[56] Muratori, Annali d'Italia, Tom. V., p. 492.

[57] Montalembert, Les Moines d'Occident, Tom. II., p. 77.

[58] Cassiodorus, De Institut. Divin. Litter., cc. 8, 30.

[59] Ibid., Præfat. ad Institut. Divin. Litter.

[60] Cassiodorus, De Institut. Divin. Litter., cap. 28.

fically designated various medical treatises which he had judiciously aggregated for the abbey library.

He fondly refers to the Herbarium of Dioskorides, "who had with the most scrupulous exactness described and portrayed the diversified qualities of rural herbs." In addition to this, he recommends as integral elements of medicinal instruction and discipline, that the recluses of his hermitage should vigilantly and studiously peruse the works of Hippocrates and Galen, of ready access, on account of Latin versions.[61] The therapeutics of the Pergamic scientist were especially commended to the notice of the monks, which contained the suitable details of the curative art proper to be known to monasteries. Another but unknown compendist was also honorably distinguished as having digested numerous treatises into a compact form.

Added to these he alludes to the works of Cornelius Celsus[62] and a Hippocratian treatise on herbal curatives, together with other medical books, collected for the monastic library, through divine assistance.[63] It may be inferred from the urgent commendation of the writings of earlier professors of this art, that down to the middle of the sixth century, there still existed a feeble recognition of a possible system adapted to the cure of maladies, so far, perhaps, as the practice was restricted to municipalities. Rapid advancement of saintly remedies, as previously used with their assemblage of baptismal waters, consecrated oils and other puissant articles of ecclesiastical appliance, enabled numerous deacons of the Church to exercise the Æsculapian art. An early priestly physician has survived to fame, by the name of Elpideus, oftentimes confused with Elpidius Rusticus,[64] previously alluded to. He was both a deacon of the Church and skilled surgeon, as may be gathered

[61] "Legete Hippocratem, atque Galenum, Latine lingua conversos," 560†8, Muratori, Scriptor. Rer. Ital., Tom. III., p. 930.

[62] Cassiodorus, op. cit., cap. 31.

[63] Ibid.

[64] Labigne, Bibl. Maxim. Patr., Tom. V., 9, p. 462 seq.

from an epistolary correspondence principally written by St. Ennodius, who expressly mentioned him as a personage of fine culture, in that erudition embellishing the mind.[65]

Touching his medical skill, it would seem he was sufficiently dexterous to heal the Gothic ruler, Theodoric, of a grievous illness.[66] He seems to have been upon such intimate terms with the king as to receive his confidence touching the causes inducing him to execute Symmachus and Boethius.[67] There are excellent reasons to assign Milan as the place of his nativity.[68] So far as the medical acquirements of Elpideus are at issue, it is impossible to conjecture their excellence, inasmuch as no monument of especial worth in this respect has escaped to modern times.

Another physician and contemporary incumbent of the diaconate, Dionysius, is better known, who it has been alleged resided in the Italian capital during its siege by the Goths. An epitaph reproduced by Baronius,[69] fully commends the clerical practitioner for honesty, but fails to specify the particular eminence originating from his knowledge of medicine:

> "Hic Levita jacit Dionysius artis honestæ
> Functus et officio, quod medicina dedit."

Other ecclesiastics, during the period under notice, appear to have reached certain distinction, not for erudition in sacred and profane letters, but by reason of medical dexterity and successful treatment of maladies seemingly beyond recovery. Some of these, by their professional eminence, combined with substantial learning, attained the Episcopate.

The organization of that system, by which the pressing necessities of impoverished sick and incurably diseased were

---

65 Ennodius, Epistolar., Lib. VIII., Ep. 8; Lib. VII., Ep. 7, and Lib. IX. Ep. 14.

66 Procopius writes him: "Elpidio deinde medico." De Bello Gothico, Lib. I.

67 Ibid.

68 Tiraboschi, Storia della Litteratura, Tom. III., p. 64.

69 Baron., Annales, ap. an. 410; and Symmachus, Epistol., IX., Ep. 4.

attended through the benevolent aggregation and public disciplinary care, would seem to be due to Christian emperors who established such hospitals; although not necessarily a development of Christianity. These humane institutions were a well defined element in the Aztec civilization,[70] whose religion was celebrated amid priestly effusion of human blood.[71] It is, however, a matter susceptible of historical proof, that pagan emperors of imperial Rome had called into existence what evidently was the nucleus for hospital systems of a later period.

At the close of the first century, a Valetudinarium[72] for infirm soldiers, and a Veterinarium[73] for disabled horses were attached to the legionary camps as an indispensible feature when actually at war. Before this period, a sick or wounded warrior was subject to surgical attendance in his tent, or, the army changing its quarters, he was cared for in the neighboring houses.[74]

Previous to the incumbency of the imperial throne, Tiberius, and while yet heir apparent, exhibited the utmost interest in the welfare of his soldiers.[75] For the transportation of suffering sick, ambulances with the appliances of easy cushions, etc., were provided, and when the forces were regularly encamped, the construction of baths was ordered.[76] As late as the time of Germanicus, Trajan and Hadrian, these enlightened generals sought out their disabled soldiers in the tents or other quarters.[77]

In the second century, the first systematic aggregation of

---

70 Prescott, History of the Conquest of Mexico, Vol. I., p. 48.

71 Solis, Conquista de la Mexico, cap. 30.

72 Hecker, Geschichte der Heilkunde, Th. II., p. 270.

73 Ibid.

74 Sueton., in Vit. Tiber., cap. 11, records an order by which public edifices were placed in condition to receive the sick: "Jussique sunt omnes ægri in publicum porticum deferri, ac per valetudinum genera disponi."

75 "Quidquid ægrorum in civitate essit, visitare se velle: id a proximis aliter exceptum." Sueton., Vita Tiberii, cap. 11.

76 Vellius Paterculus, Hist. Rom., Lib., II., c. 114.

77 Spartian, Vita Hadriani, cap. 10.

the wounded and infirm appears in the Valetudinarium,[78] where, however, only such as were seriously afflicted by wounds or diseases received surgical attention, while those of a less aggravated type were treated in the usual Ægri contubernales.[79] The troubled condition of the times certainly hindered the full utility of those imperfect hospitals for the scientific treatment of diseases, established by Justinian in the middle of the sixth century.[80] Whether this institution as a strictly organized system of pathology be traceable to the terminal years of the fourth century, may remain an unsettled question, but that this establishment throughout the Roman empire, in its more humane and public character, was primarily due to other forms developed from the Christian church, admits of no controversy.

[78] Hecker, Geschichte der Heilkunde, Th. II., p. 284.

[79] Vegetius, De Re Milit., Lib. III., cap. 2.

[80] Procopius, De Ædificiis, Lib. I., cap. 2.

CHAPTER X.

Monastic Institutions—Beneficial Effects in Preserving Art, etc.—Rapid Degradation of Society in the Fifth Century—Monasteries Established under Protection of Civil Law—Various Convents Constructed in Gaul—Cultivate Medical Studies—Benedictine Monks—Conventual Infirmary—Saintly Cures Fostered by the Cloisters—Exorcism of Diseases by Saints—Miracles—Legends of Power of Martyrs.

NOTWITHSTANDING civil and religious society of the fourth century presented the external appearances of being christianized, and although sovereigns and people with great preponderance of numbers had embraced the new faith, they still remained paganized by force of custom, so far, indeed, that the laws, institutions and manners remained unaltered.[1]

Theodosius, one of the most pious monarchs of the empire, openly assumed the sacred and divine character of his imperial office. Valentinian, in essaying to excite decaying patriotic enthusiasm among the Romans against the Vandals, concluded the proclamation by declaring that it was signed by his divine hand.[2] Popular morals, under the pressure of direful governmental necessity, were so abhorrent and debased that fathers of families, according to Zozimus,[3] sold their daughters in prostitution at the Lupanaria in order to obtain money to liquidate taxes. The same author charged the Christians with the carefully-adhered-to policy of proselyting polytheists of his day, by promising them an entire remission of all crimes of whatever type, upon uniting with the dominant church.[4] At this epoch, according to the pithy utterance of Bossuet, everything

[1] Guizot, Histoire de la Civilization en France, Leç. 3.

[2] "Et manu divina propria." Novellæ, Tit. XX.

[3] Histor. Rom., Lib. II., cap. 38.

[4] Ibid., Lib. II., cap. 29.

was decaying in the East, and all things abandoned in the western empire.[5]

Contemporaneous writers draw a most deplorable picture of Rome. This great metropolis seemed in a moribund condition, deserted by its rulers and sacked by the Goths.[6] Certainly the marvellous development of the Latin monasteries was nurtured into hasty growth, by the propulsion of the frightful calamities threatening social dissolution, and in some localities, utterly destructive of human existence. These religious associations, to which, among other qualities, modern times owe the perpetuation of medical science, through monastic professors, and its revival at the close of the Middle Ages, appear to have originated in the Orient, where the more sensitive proselyted Christians were quickly driven to solitude for profound meditation upon divine things.

Provincial, isolated districts attracted in an unorganized form the increasing number of anchorites and recluses, who confidently believed uninterrupted and mental adoration to offer the surest progress towards Divinity. The sentiment among the Fathers was by no means unanimous, touching the utility of these organizations. In the year 390, by a rescript[7] of Valentinian II., these associated hermits were subjected to persecution. This law, evidently provoked by the opponents of Monachism, and perhaps the result of sound political economy, directed that all monks or professed anchorites, wheresoever domiciled upon the vast domains of the Roman empire, should forthwith depart the towns and cities, where they appear to have congregated in vast numbers from the time of Saint Basil, and the municipal authorities were required to enforce the decree which ordered them to seek deserted localities and waste solitutes as their habitations.[8]

---

[5] Histoire Universelle, 1ere P., Ep. XI.

[6] Sidonarius Apollonar., Carmen VII.

[7] "Quicunque sub professione monachi repperiuntur, deserta loca et vastos solitudines sequi, atque habitare jubeantur." XVI. Codex Theodosianus, Tit. III., De Monachis, Lex 1.

[8] XVI. Cod. Theod., Tit. III., Lex 1.

Theodosius, a few years later, abrogated this oppressive legislation.[9] In the year 340 Athenasius, fleeing the persecution of his orthodoxy by Arian enemies, arrived in Rome to implore the protection of the papal pontiff, Julius. While there, and during the prolonged session of an ecclesiastical council, which reaffirmed the boldly-asserted doctrines of the refugee, Athenasius industriously mingled with the religious element of the venerable metropolis, recounting the exploits so wonderful of Anthony and the Thebiade anchorites. These impressive statements appear to have produced almost the effect of a revolution.

Both sexes were incited to essay the establishment of cloisters.[10] Although the word monk was synonomous with ignominious infamy in vulgar prejudice, it quickly became a title of honor and sacred distinction.[11] After the death of the notorious Thebiade cenobite, Saint Athenasius wrote a biography of the deceased recluse, which was extensively circulated in Western Europe, and quickly attained the popularity of a legend and confession of faith. This simple narrative, after the lapse of time, was accepted as the foundation of occidental monastic superstitions, and out of it grew the rigid vitality of its laws, which endured for centuries.[12]

When the social debasement is considered, which prevailed among the Romans, it is by no means surprising that the suburbs of the city should be rapidly occupied by monasteries, filled with personages equally distinguished for illustrious birth, eminent science, and immense affluence, who preferred the surroundings of charity, sanctity and liberty,[13] to the companionship of degraded civilians of the Italian capital. During the latter part of the fourth century a tide of spiritual and pen-

---

[9] Ibid., Lex 2.

[10] On the signification of this word, vide IX. Cod. Theodos., Tit. III., De Custodia Reorum, Lex 3.

[11] Hieronymi, Vita S. Macari, cap. 4.

[12] Gregor. Nazien, Oratio 27.

[13] Hieronym. Epistolar., 66 ad Pammach.

itential life rose throughout the provinces, and swept before it the relics of ancient and glorious patrician families, which fled to these sanctuaries as a final refuge against the awful corruption of the age.

With characteristic boldness, Saint Jerome questioned alike the integrity of the Emperor Julian,[14] and denounced false monks and debased women who had procured access to the nunneries under the deceptive costume of widows or virgins, and secured a permanent abode, where with shameless hypocrisy they enjoyed the subsistence of these organized communities.[15] It is evident from the burning indignation of Jerome that already these beneficent institutions were thronged with disingenuous cenobites, who sought to combine the pompous splendor of the profane world with the humility of religion, or with mendacious presumption[16] captivated the confidence of affluent and exemplary noblemen, and as quickly abused it.[17]

To Saint Ambrose, whose pen has described the resistless march of isolated contemplation of divinity in a panegyric of unrivalled eloquence,[18] may be directly attributed, after Saint Augustine, much of that vitality which perpetuated monasteries throughout the middle ages, and with them the germs of science and the undying elements of art. The celebrated Regulæ, drafted by Augustine in the year 423, and originally intended to calm dissensions among the recluses of an African nunnery, were revived under Charlemagne, and furnished fundamental principles of mediæval monachism.

The institution of Saint Germain d'Auxerre has been traced to that period of the fifth century when the Teutons still derided the Christian faith in its most sacred recesses, and used the vestibules of its cloisters for stabling their horses, and pas-

---

[14] Ibid., ad Julian, Ep. VI., but partially excuses him for the reasons given.

[15] Ibid., ad Rustic., 225; and Ibid., ad Demetr., 140.

[16] Ibid., ad Rustic., Ep. 3.

[17] Ibid., ad Eustach., Ep. 18.

[18] Ambros., Hexameron., Lib. III., c. 5.

tured their migratory herds upon the herbage growing by the side of overthrown altars.[19] From these abbeys developed towns and villages, to which the effeminate Christian of the sixth century sought refuge from invading Gauls.[20]

From the vestments of dressed skins and common sandals or clogs, with which the earlier Gallic monk was attired in the penury of utter impoverishment, to more tolerable privations, the transition was accomplished by the modifying influences of years, although at an early age these provinces were remarked for their colonizing fecundity, and justly apostrophized as swarming bees abandoning their old for new hives.[21] Along the line of the Jura Alps, according to Sidonius Apollinarus, this form of religious development seems to have been carried on with great rapidity, and highly commended by him as a cherished aggrandizement.[22] The monastery of Saint Claude, so exposed to the incursions of the barbarous Alemanni that its prior was compelled to procure his supplies of salt across the Alps, signalized its superiority through Eugendius, abbot about the year 540, by an earnest and patient endeavor to inaugurate a taste for polite letters among his monkish subordinates. Greek and Latin were taught both clerics and laymen in this cloister, which attained high illustration in Gaul. The study of ancient authors[23] seems to have fascinated these monastic students, who also contributed to the preservation of such remnants of classical splendor in their custody by the transcription of manuscripts.[24]

However successful may have been the earliest expansion of an organization whose marvellous solidity was of incontestible and vital importance to medical economy during

[19] Sidonarius Apollonaris, Epistolar., Lib. VII., c. 6.

[20] Ibid., Lib. VII., c. 17.

[21] Vita St. Romani, cap 2, apud Acta S. S. Bol., Feb. 28.

[22] Epistolar., Lib. IV., c. 25.

[23] Too eager zeal for profane writers was expressly interdicted by Ambrose, especially if such fervor led to a neglect of sacred scriptures. De Officiis, Lib. I., c. 10.

[24] Vita S. Eugendi, cc. 2 and 3.

the Middle Ages, to the epoch when the treatment of the curative art was systematically pursued in the Universities of the fourteenth and fifteenth centuries, the services of Saint Benedict, exclusive of the extension of convents through the acceptance of his Regulæ, in founding the monastery of Monte Cassino, in the fifth century, of such signal benefit to medicine subsequently, must entitle him to unstinted admiration. Apparently influenced by the spontaneous impulse, hitherto mentioned, among eminent Romans, a youthful patrician seeking to flee the dispiriting influences of the age erected a refuge in solitude near Subjacio, whose locality, by the thunderbolt striking the shattered wine-cup from Nero's lip,[25] was thenceforth forever rendered safe from the footsteps of man.

This lad of fourteen years, of the highest susceptibility, in an age when the nervous organism of Christian devotees was abnormally quick, determined in the year 494 to renounce the attractions of science and mundane honors, in order to abide in that ecstatic grandeur, the outgrowth of profound meditative absorption, and abandoning the repressive presence of an old nurse, he sought the quietude essential to this existence amid the almost inaccessible routes of a locality[26] immortalized by Dante as the scene of the hermit life of Saint Franciscus.[27] On account of an infamous attempt by an associate priest to poison him,[28] the great precursor of modern monachism fled the companionship of such base machinations, and retired to Monte Cassino in the year 528.

Here, after the lapse of two centuries from the proclamation of Constantine the Great, still stood a venerable temple dedicated to Apollo and used for sacrificial rites by the pagan peasantry,[29] perhaps for the restoration to health. Persuading these polytheists to accept the new faith, Benedict constructed

---

[25] Tacitus, Annales, Lib. XIV., cap. 22.

[26] Gregor. Max., Dialog., Lib. II., cc. 1 and 8.

[27] Divina Commedia, Paridis. Can. XI.

[28] Greg. Max., op. cit., Lib. II., c. 8.

[29] Ibid. and Dante, op. cit., Can. XI.

two monasteries, of which one was placed under the patronage of Saint John, and the other dedicated to Saint Martin, whose medicinal potency had been essayed by Gregory, Bishop of Tours. After forty years of patient industry for the development of this powerful and munificent convent, to which the revival of medicine centuries afterwards may be accorded, its founder, the great legislator of the Benedictine monachism, died in the year 543, with the satisfaction of witnessing the rapid growth of that fabric which his religious meditations had doubtless suggested.

Up to this time the Latin Church followed with religious confidence the rules of monastic existence communicated through such eminent pontiffs as Augustine and Ambrose in the De Officiis. Benedict, in attempting successfully to reform the abuses of the Order whose doctrines he had embraced, by means of an economical and liturgical arrangement which collectively constituted the rule of conventual creed, also gave to the institution in western Europe a definitive and universal polity, from which developed the economy of medicine during the Middle Ages.

In his inflexible programme for daily action and labor, obedience was an essential principle. To banish indolence, which he declared to be a corroding element in the soul,[30] he regulated with exactitude the diurnal occupations of each monk, including divine service, and distinctively forbade singing amatory or libidinous songs when employed with secular artificers.[31] Under the Benedictine regulations, a monastery was regarded as a citadel unceasingly menaced by besieging foes, presumed to be demoniacal hosts arrayed in mortal combat against the church militant, of which the cloisters were an integral and important factor. It was, therefore, imperative in the internal organization of such establishments, to be possessed of a mill, bakery, various workshops, and a garden of greater or less extent, in order that none of the exigencies of

[30] Codex Regular., Pars. II., cap. 6, De Opere Monachorum, p. 560.

[31] Ibid.

existence should compel the external presence of their monkish garrison.[32]

A suitable cenobite was selected from the most eligible, and delegated under the name of cellarer,[33] or advocatus,[34] to supervise monastic goods and possessions, and especially to attend to such details as were required by the conventual infirmary.[35] This institution for proper treatment of maladies, in its essential features, the precursor of mediæval hospitals, was the enlargement of charity, as the dominant doctrine of abbeys and cloisters. We shall hereafter note the extensive use of the monastic infirmary, and scrutinize more closely its influence upon the enconomy of medicine. Through the practical application of the Benedictine regulations to the monasteries, the Western Empire was preserved from a profounder degradation of civilization and morals; while such fragments of ancient art and letters as escaped the destructive energy of the Teutonic races, were safely guarded by them. After the death of Benedict, the monastery of Monte Cassino was subjected to a temporary check in rapid progress, by the Longobards, who pillaged the edifices appurtenant, in the year 580.[36]

Notwithstanding these infelicitous events, this cloister maintained its advance towards that just celebrity ultimately obtained in contributing to the revival of medical science. In the year 718 Petroneas, a Brescian nobleman, at the instigation of Gregory II., reconstructed the monastery which afterward became so illustrious.[37] Towards the close of the sixth century Gregory himself assumed the direction of the convent of Saint Andrew at Rome. During his pontifical administra-

---

[32] "Hortos olerum vel apparatus ciborum propriis sibi manibus fratres exerceant." Ibid., p. 562.

[33] Du Cange, Gloss., sub v. Cellerar.

[34] Ibid., sub v. Advocatus.

[35] Ibid., sub v. Infirmarius; and Codex cit., cap. 48, col. 639.; vide Mabillon Ord. St. B. An., Tom. I., p. 56.

[36] Petrus Diaconus, Chronicon Casinense, sub an. 580.

[37] Mabillon, Ord. S. Bened. Annales, Tom. II., c. 32, p. 54.

tion of this abbey, an event occurred having direct reference to the history of medicine of the time.

One of the monks signalized himself as a dexterous physician; but, contrary to the stringent rules of the Benedictines, it appears he received three pieces of gold as compensation for skillful medical treatment of such diseased and infirm as sought the remedies at the Cloister Infirmary.[38] From this it is evident that as early as the period designated, this charitable apartment was frequented by those afflicted with bodily ills, in quest of medical curatives or the attendance of monastic surgeons, whose duty required gratuitous service. When the coins were discovered upon the body of the deceased cenobite, Saint Gregory peremptorily ordered them cast on the rigid cadaver, in presence of the brethren, who were directed to recite the terrible anathema: "Thy money be with thee in perdition!" but the complaisant humanity of the great Evangelist softened before this awful malediction.[39]

The extension of the Monastic order opened in the west of Europe scholastic institutions which propagated the orthodox creed and cultivated literature. In the city of Seville, a school was presided over by Leander, who directed the studies of his disciples by the supervision of sagacious masters.[40] Subsequent to the death of its abbot, this conventual organization was honored with the illustrious and erudite scholar, Isidore, who provided the people of the Western Church with the writings of Aristotle prior to the advent of the Saracens. In his Etymologaria many classical fragments are preserved, which, without this record, would have utterly perished. His compilation of the sciences of a more remote age and of a contemporaneous period, A. D. 636, equals in many respects

---

[38] Gregor. Maxim., Dialog., Lib. IV., c. 55.

[39] Unstinted admiration must be awarded this pope for his service to music, which he introduced on a scale of grandeur commensurate with the increasing pomp of the Romish ritualism. An amusing account of the attempted introduction of the pompous swell of the Gregorian chant to the harsh, guttural voices of the Franks, is given by the author of Vita Karoli Magni, p. 52.

[40] Montalembert, Les Moines d'Occident, Tom. II., p. 218.

the encyclopædical writings of the Alexandrine scholars, and entitles him to the profound esteem of modern scholarship. Among these are elaborate treatises on liberal arts and sciences,[41] law and philosophy, constituting an imperishable monument of curious erudition.

Isidore prepared an epitome of medicinal art and natural history, which, together with the works of Cassiodorus, were extensively used by the mediæval schools. In the Gallic provinces the Monastic system was permanently established as early as the time of Gregory of Tours, historian of the Frankish kings. The marvellous curative property of the Saints' relics, as attested by the personal test of the Turonese pontiff, have been alluded to; these remedies were rivalled by the living presence of St. Julian, a holy anchorite, the independence of whose solitude was soon interrupted by the indigent, and resonant with the despairing clamor of the sick, to whom he gave both alms and health.[42] How far the pontifical historian succumbed to the appearance of miraculous cures, it is impossible to determine; but the degradation of medicine may be presumed when he asserts that the diseases of the sick and infirm were banished upon the contact of a few drops of water drawn from a spring dug by Saint Martin's own hands.[43]

An additional event mentioned by this distinguished annalist will confirm the profound impression already made upon the popular mind, by remedial power attributed to personages of monastic habit and of extraordinary sanctity at the close of the sixth century. One day Aredius traversing Paris found Chilperic prostrate with a grievous fever. The royal sufferer besought the saint's prayers as an irresistible curative. Among the obnoxious measures charged against the Frankish King was a sweeping impost upon Gallic towns and municipalities.

---

[41] Isidore doubtless closely imitated the Opus of Martiani Capella, which divided art and science into Philologia, Grammatica, Dialectica, Rhetorica, Geometri, Arithmetica, Astronomica, and Musica.

[42] Gregor. Turoniens, De Miraculis S. Juliani, Lib. II., cc. 23–26.

[43] Gregor. Turon., De Miraculis S. Martini, Lib. II., cap. 24.

It should be mentioned as an honorable exception to the general drift of such legends, that although the saint had oftentimes interposed the immense puissance accorded him, it was not restricted to protecting religious houses and their consecrated sacerdoty, but freely exercised in favor of oppressed people. Disregarding the importunities of the diseased monarch, Aredius first demanded the absolute extinction of the assessment rolls, which were ultimately tendered him.

The abbot thereupon, surrounded by a great throng of persons, publicly fired the contribution registers, but before the fire had consumed them, announced the future health of the King.[44] Perhaps the most thorough attestation of the contempt into which physicians had fallen compared with saintly medicists, is the uncontroverted fact that such cures were invariably made after earthly medicine had been exhausted.[45] The establishment of such monasteries as Saint Gall, Luxeuil, and Fontanelle, should occupy the attention of the historian of medical economy of the early ages, inasmuch as these sacred organizations were the first to become solidly instituted through unequivocal marks of imperial favor from the Carlovingians, and as providing instructive information touching the venerable usages involved in curing the sick whose maladies were professedly demoniacal. After the departure of Saint Columban, the Irish evangelist, summoned to the Papal court, his authorized successor remained to consummate the ecclesiastical labors so auspiciously begun in the Gallic provinces.

Saint Gall, in whose honor the monastery was named, had occasion to vindicate the supernatural power of his master delegated to him, when the daughter of a Teutonic nobleman was brought before him seriously ill with an incurable disorder, presenting the livid appearance of an animated cadaver.[46] As an indication to what extent the doctrine of diabolical

---

[44] Ibid., Vita S. Aridii abbatis, c. 25.

[45] "Vero tradidit medicis." Gregor. Turonen., De Miraculis S. Martini, Lib. II., c. 24.

[46] Walafrid Strabo, Vita S. Galli., Lib. I., cap. 18.

causation of maladies had spread and entered into the faith as an integral portion at so remote a day as the period before us, the method applied for a remedy restoring health to the moribund princess is of great significance. Saint Gall approached the unconscious invalid as she reclined upon her mother's knees. Assuming the bended attitute of invocation by her side, the evangelist made a fervent prayer, and concluded by using the formal conjuration, evoking the demon producing the sickness to instantly depart.[47]

This species of exorcism, of more extended application at a later period of the Middle Ages, was oftentimes accompanied by an irresistible exorcism, by virtue of the unutterable name.[48]

The diabolical spirit quickly responded to the invocation of Saint Gall, that it was indeed he whom the exorcist had commanded to leave the virgin's body, and questioned not the resistless power of the abbot to cure the maiden's infirmity.[49] In the year 640, when this saint died, nearly the entire territory of Germany was Christianized, and around his cell were grouped the rudiments of a monastery, which became a celebrated school for the propagation of Christianity, a principal centre of intellectual brilliancy, from which radiated the mental culture of Mediæval Europe, and at an early period in the ninth century, drafted the plan of a perfect cloister, whose internal adjustments are of value to the subject of medicine at that distant epoch.

Of equal importance to the development of a system which exercised unlimited influence to retard the revival of medical science, although sharing with others its benefits for preserving

[47] "Domine Jesu Christe, etc., jube nunc immundissimum spiritum de puella hac pro tui gloria nominis exire. Impero tibi in nomine Domini nostri Jesu Christi, spiritus immunde, ut exeas et recedas ab hoc plasmate Dei." When the spirit conjured retreated, he passed across her lips in shape of a horrible black bird—"Avis nigerima et horrores terribilis." Ibid.

[48] "Per enarribile Nomen, per beloi hadonai," etc. Baluzius, Capitularia, Tom. II., col. 662, No. 10.

[49] Walafrid Strabo, Vita S. Galli., Lib. II., cap. 7.

art, was the erection of the monastic edifice at Luxeuil, in Western Gaul, and frequented in great numbers on account of the eminence of its schools.[50] Saint Vardrille, the founder of Fontanelle, in the year 648, exercised his remedial potency in healing the palsied arm of a forester, whose indiscreet zeal had induced him to transfix the sainted abbot with a lance.[51] Some of the monasteries engaged in the preparation of oil from whales, of which many appear to have entered the river Seine, and with this the gloom of their long winter evenings was brightened.[52]

A legend narrated by the chronicler of Saint Aichade's life, will attest the profound belief at this epoch, of that supernatural puissance which, it was devoutly accorded, manifested itself under specific circumstances, the development of which belief contributed to the prostration of medicine as a science, and established a practice of curing maladies, on the basis of an art, under the direction of angelic or divine forces.

This pious abbot, towards the conclusion of a long and eventful career, apprehending that his death might expose the Monastic brethren to the pitfalls of sin, earnestly invoked the Saviour to adjust the perplexing trouble. The following night he saw an angel gliding through the conventual dormitory. As the emissary of Deity, he touched one-half of the slumbering recluses, whose aggregate numbers reached nine hundred, with a staff, and at the same time promised the anxious prior, that when in a few days these four hundred and fifty monks ascended to heaven, they should advance to convoy him to the celestial sphere after his decease. Upon receiving notification of their approaching departure, the abbe prepared them for this grand journey with sacramental rites. Joining each other in the mystic celebration of the viaticum, they entered the chapel of the Monastery accompanied by the untouched recluses. Flanked by two confreres, the elect sounded with them

---

[50] Mabillon, Annales Ord. S. Bened., Tom. II., p. 603.

[51] Vita S. Ansberti, cap. 1; apud Mabillon, op. cit., Tom. II., p. 16.

[52] Vita S. Philiberti, cc. 1, 5, 6 and 32.

triumphal chants, and while the musical jubilee arose and swelled in harmonious echoes, the figures of those marked for ecstatic glory began to glow with unmistakable indications of coming transformation. Totally divested of suffering or pain, they passed away from their monastic associates, the first troop at the hour of terce,[53] the second at sextus,[54] the third at nones,[55] the fourth at vespers, and the last at completus.[56] For eight days their obsequies were celebrated by those whose passionate regrets broke forth into lamentations that they themselves were unworthy to thus ascend the resplendent pathway of divine bliss.[57]

Such traditions, while more firmly rooting the monastic system, and augmenting the numbers of those seeking the surroundings of a religious existence, developed without defiance in the popular mind, an unshaken belief touching the ocular exhibition of angelic power within the narrowed and secluded walls of cloisters, and accepted thus early in the sixth century the more ancient doctrines of ecclesiastical writers, who, as we have seen, asserted the interposition of Omnipotence in physical affairs, and adapted this faith to the curative art which preserved an existence throughout the Middle Ages.

The Irish, closely following the retreating footsteps of their Erse predecessors at this period, flocked to Rome in vast crowds, where they rendered the homage of an ardent devotion, and once, while progressing in their journey towards the Papal See, they thronged the xenodochium of a monastery in Gaul so densely as to cause a leper to lament outside the cloister gate, suffering from this horrible disease (which, as we shall hereafter discover, was perpetuated to modern times uninterruptedly), and recumbent on the ground, asking to be

---

53 Du Cange, Glossarium, sub v. Tertia.

54 Du Cange, sub v. Sexta.

55 Ibid., sub v. Nona.

56 Ibid., sub v. Completus.

57 Acta Sanctor., Bolland., Sep. I., Tom. V., p. 101; and Mabillon, Annales Ord. S. Bened., Saecul. 2, Tom. II., p. 930.

received within. The main entrance to the abbey was quickly swung open, and the diseased wanderer carried in upon the robust shoulders of the abbot himself, where he was provided a suitable place near the ruddy glow of the blazing fire. The prior then hastened to procure pure water with which to cleanse the leper, and linen to wipe his hands.

On his return the leprous stranger had disappeared, and as a convincing proof of his angelic presence, behind him was left an aroma so delightful that it penetrated the whole edifice, and could be compared alone to the perfumes of the Orient or the delicate distillations of springtime flowers.[58] Abbe Eustasius returning from Rome, whither a mission of Clothair II. had called him, was urgently summoned by the sorrowing parent of a Burgundian maiden, in the last agonies of a frightful malady, to appear and cure the moribund daughter. It appearing that his child had in her youth been consecrated by the vows of chastity, and shrunk from a marriage sanctioned by her parents, Eustasius reproached the father for his efforts to violate the solemn engagements of the virgin, and upon obtaining a formal renunciation of further attempts to coerce her into matrimony, the saint by personal intercession obtained a complete cure.[59]

From the preceding and rapid narration touching the organization and extension of the monastic system in Europe, from the time of Benedict to the eighth century, it is evident with their growth the doctrine that these cenobites, as persons of distinguished piety and exemplary lives, were endowed through superior sanctity with puissant forces, was accepted universally, uncontroverted and with absolute faith, and that these divine powers were oftentimes applied to cure such diseases as required miraculous treatment.

In unnumbered instances these convents were propagated by anchorites, whose adoring devotees frequently, upon exigent occasions, witnessed the actual operation of this resistless

[58] Vita S. Agilii, cc. 17 and 20; 4 ap., A. S. S. Boll., Tom. I., p. 14.

[59] Vita S. Eustasii, cc. 12 and 14; ap. Acta S. S. Bolland, Tom. II., p. 420.

potency, and when the monasteries attained to unqualified success and constituted an integral portion of the ecclesiastical and civil society, the reputation of unnatural cures, or the boldly-announced possession of wonder-working reliques, enlarged the number of monks and materially benefited the conventual finances.

CHAPTER XI.

Age of Charlemagne—His Enlightened Policy—Introduces Discipline in the Monasteries—Liberal Arts and Sciences Regulated by the Chartularies—The Emperor Adverse to Medical Attendance—His Israelitish Surgeon—Saracen Gift of Medicaments to the Gallic Ruler—Founding of the Celebrated Monte Cassino—Its Great Services to Medicine—Noted Medical Scholiasts of this Cloister—Nucleus of a Library of Medicine There—This Art Pursued in Italian Monasteries under the Carlovingians—Teutonic Laws on Surgical Evidence—Social Status of Surgeons Recognized by Edicts of Gothic Kings—Medicinal Art to be Taught in Monastic Schools—Phlebotomy or Conventual Blood-letting.

NEXT in importance to the progress of civilization in Western Europe, the reign of Charlemagne should be added to the establishment in France of the Monastic orders; and no ruler prior to the age of Frederick II. endeavored by the force of legislation more assiduously to provoke an interest in the study of medical art. The earlier years of this illustrious monarch having been almost exclusively occupied in strengthening his power among his own people and in subjugating the warlike Saxons after a conflict of thirty-three years,[1] in sixty mighty battles, with their unnumbered victims,[2] it was only towards the conclusion of prolonged and fruitful rule that he began to establish the practical details of uniform government, and to earnestly patronize intellectual culture.

After the successful termination of the colossal wars against the well-governed Saxons,[3] the most considerable illustration of his martial prowess was the complete overthrow of the Avares on the Danube, whose uncivilized forces at one period

[1] "Per continuos trigenta tres annos." Eiginhard, Vita Caroli Magni., cap. 7.

[2] Annales De Gestis Caroli Magni, Lib. II., Indic. 4, v. 95.

[3] Adam Brem., Gesta Ham. Pontific., Lib. I., c. 6.

threatened Constantinople,[4] and ventured to approach the delimitations of Frankish territory in the time of Charlemagne, and even at a more remote period.[5] In these unequalled conflicts, he fairly disrupted their military power, seized their treasures,[6] and utterly precluded their domination in Europe.[7] As the undaunted and martial evangelist of the Christian Church, this great monarch forced an unqualified acceptance of this new faith by the Saxons, of whom great numbers, yet devoted to the sanguinary rites and idolatrous worship of Thor, Odin and Frey, were baptized in one day.[8]

In the active pursuance of an enlightened policy, and incited by the ecclesiastical dignitaries of the empire, one of the first steps towards lasting dominion over the restless minds of his new converts was the subdivision of the conquered provinces into eight bishoprics, of which Mentz and Cologne were erected into the metropolitan see.[9] The utter extinction of Longobardic rule in Italy, under Desiderius, towards the end of the eighth century, established papal supremacy, and secured for Charlemagne the honors of imperial coronation.[10] From this era the whole weight of the Western Empire uniformly supported the pontifical dogmas, and with material and legislative force coöperated to their extension and maintenance.

To the expanding power of the monasteries throughout Gaul or France, as an integral element of the empire, the Frankish emperor added the active fruition of law, and sanctioned this increase by the influence of personal favor. Within a few years after the assumption of the imperial title, the vast

[4] Gibbon, Hist. of the Decline and Fall of Rome, Vol. IV., cc. 43 and 46.

[5] Aimonius, De Gestis Francor., Lib. III., c. 84; and Gregor. Turones., Histor. Francor., Lib. IV.

[6] Anom., Vita Caroli Magni, Tom. I., p. 55.

[7] Eiginhard., op. cit., cap. 13.

[8] Anom., Vita, cit., p. 52.

[9] Ad. Bremen, Gesta Ham. Pontif., Lib. I., cc. 12 and 13.

[10] Annal. De Gestis Caroli Magni, Lib. IV., Indic. 8.

district of domain extending from the Sicilian gulf to the extreme limits of Frisia, and from the Spanish peninsula to the Black sea,[11] began to exhibit architectural vitality, both sacred and profane,[12] while down to the date of his death, he appears to have contemplated the construction of a flotilla as a defence against the invasions of Norsemen.[13]

In addition to the dialects of his native country, the imperial Charles zealously aided in cultivating among his subjects a knowledge of both the Greek and Latin languages, with which he was familiar. The fundamental principles of art and science, such at least as survived the disasters of Gothic destruction, preserved by the Church at this period, and known according to the captious division of Martianus Capella[14] as the seven liberal arts and sciences, were most assiduously cultivated by the Frankish emperor, to that extent, indeed, which entitled him to the honorable distinction of Didasculus,[15] equivalent to master of learning. To the professors of the Trivium and Quadrium, which at a later date included medical art, marked honors were attributed, and valuable compensations awarded. During the active and bitter campaign in Italy, which terminated in the overthrow of the Longobardic dominion, Charlemagne was brought in contact with an erudite grammarian, in the city of Pavia,[16] whom Eiginhard designates as Peter Pisanum,[17] who obtained illustration on account of instructing the western ruler in the arts alluded to. Alcuin, a deacon of extended scholastic learning, was the tutor of this monarch in rhetoric, dialectics, and astronomy. As a fair attestation of astronomical knowledge, Charlemagne described the stellar movements in a metrical poem.

---

[11] Tiraboschi, Storia della Litteratura, Tom. III., p. 152.

[12] Eiginhard., Vita Caroli Magni, cap. 18.

[13] Ibid., cap. 17.

[14] Vide Supra, p. 155.

[15] Du Cange, Glossar., sub v. Didasculus.

[16] Tiraboschi, Storia della Litteratura, Tom. III., p. 155.

[17] Eiginhard, Vita Caroli Magni, cap. 25.

Before reverting to the private customs of the Emperor, which will justify a conclusion touching the status of medical practitioners and of this avocation at that period, the services rendered in aggregating the edicts of predecessors on the throne should be noted, especially as these collections were the laws by which the Monastic system was guided, and by which practical instruction in medicine was ordered to be given in conventual schools throughout the empire. Whatever may have been his intentions regarding the diversified laws among the different people subject to the government, he appears to have considered the necessity of adding to these such parts as were wanting, and of striking out portions, although of high antiquity, which demanded alteration in accordance with the changed order of religious affairs.[18] This design was thwarted, perhaps, by his death, as may be gathered from Eiginhard, who affirms that nothing was done in this direction, excepting the addition of a few capitularies, and those imperfect, to existing statutes.[19]

Nevertheless, the unwritten law of all his subjects was, by his order, reduced to writing. So far as those habits of dress and person are concerned, which tend to elucidate the condition of the curative art and sanitary notions in the Carlovingian age, it may be stated that this monarch, contrary to his descendant, Otho, wore the national costume, consisting of a linen camisa,[20] or underwear, next to the body, supplemented with short hose of similar stuff[21]—the disuse of which, in after ages, largely contributed to the propagation of epidemics and pestilential disorders.

Finely-dressed skins, more anciently adopted by the Romans,[22] and still used by the Huns,[23] completed the emperor's

---

[18] This expurgation was not so rigid as to exclude paganistic allusions. Lex Frision. Addit. Sap., Tit. XI., p. 37.

[19] Eiginhard, op. cit., cap. 29.

[20] Du Cange, Glossar., sub v. Casmia ; and Isidor., Etymologiar., Lib. XIX., cap. 22.

[21] Eiginhard, Vita Caroli Magni, cap. 22.

[22] Ammian. Marcellin., Gesta Roman., Lib. XXXI., cap. 2.

[23] Horatii, Satira, Lib. I., — 5.

external raiment. Although foreign vestments of most elegant texture were freely worn at the imperial court, Charlemagne invariably refused to invest himself with it, excepting at Rome, where in deference to the expressed wish of Hadrian, the Supreme Pontiff, and of Leo, his successor, he donned the Latin tunic, venerable chlamydis and sandals. In all his acts he powerfully aided in provoking a taste for the writings of the Christian Fathers, of which he preferred the treatise De Civitate[24] of Saint Augustin, otherwise surnamed the Pastoral.[25]

If it be possible to conclude upon the basis of sanitary economy, touching the advanced age reached by Charlemagne, perhaps such deduction may fail to vindicate a high estimation of the medical profession, but dignify the excellence of a temperate and frugal life, especially in the use of wine and food. With systematic regularity, after his nightly slumbers, all litigants were introduced before him, and their legal perplexities promptly adjudicated.[26] According to the reliable attestation of his biographer and son-in-law,[27] Imperial Chancellor, the Emperor preserved a robust vigor and firm step until towards the end of his career. For an interval of four years prior to his death he was troubled with frequent fevers, and lameness in one foot. In order to combat the encroachments of disease, which grievously afflicted him, he resorted to such medicaments as suit an arbitrary judgment, rather than follow the prescriptions and direction of physicians, for whom he professed great abhorrence.[28]

Notwithstanding the legislation and rescripts in the diverse codes sanctioned by the Gallic ruler, recognized the legality

---

24 Eiginhard, op. cit., cap. 24.

25 Thegani, De Gestis Ludovici, cap. 20.

26 Eiginhard, op. cit., cap. 24.

27 Vide Chronicon Laureshamensis, where the escapade of the emperor's daughter is detailed and concluded by marriage with Eiginhard.

28 "Et tunc quidem plura arbitratu suo, quam medicorum consilio faciebat, quos pene exosos habebat." Eiginhard, Vita Caroli Magni, cap. 22.

and functions of medical men in a limited signification, it is evident that throughout the colossal domains of the Frankish empire, such as pursued this art were of low attainments, though avowedly trained in the practice of medicine and surgery, or, exclusive of an Israelitish surgeon[29] and perhaps the distinguished Wintarius, who it is claimed was physician to the emperor,[30] in their use of remedies resembled the ambulatory professors of the pagan Teutons, and when exposed to the criticism of an unprofessional scrutiny become objects of suspicion and distrust. In the year 801, a Jewish ambassador to the Saracen court[31] at Bagdad, brought back with him as presents from the Caliph, among other gifts, a valuable selection of unguents, prized for their medicinal properties.[32]

One of the obnoxious regulations of his medical advisers, which seems to have provoked most unfavorably the great monarch, was a professional interdict laid upon the roasted flesh usually placed upon the royal table, and a somewhat compulsory persuasion to accommodate himself, instead, to broths or stewed meats.[33] As an additional preventative to declining health, the august patient gave himself to frequent equitation, in which he, with other Franks, was unrivalled. Recourse appears to have been had, in his day, to the medicinal benefits of bathing in the spray or steam of water naturally warm. For the purpose of diurnal natatory exercise in the tepid stream in the near vicinity of a royal domicil, he constructed a palace, where he resided at the time of his death.[34] In this sanitative habit, which he adopted at the instigation of his physicians, he was often accompanied by the

---

[29] Depping, Geschichte der Juden in Mittelalter, Th. I., p. 50.

[30] Lessing, Geschichte der Medezin, Th. I., p. 241.

[31] Anonom., Vita Caroli Magni, p. 58.

[32] Annalista Saxo., Histor. Francor., sub an. cit., p. 169.

[33] "Quod ei in cibis affa, quibus assuetus erat, dimittere, et elixis assuescere suadebant." Eiginhard, op. cit., cap. 22.

[34] "Delectabatur etiam vaporibus aquarum naturaliter calentium, frequenti natatu corpus exercens," etc. Eiginhard, Vita Caroli Magni, cap. 22.

princes and nobility, whose numbers sometimes aggregated more than a hundred.

Before proceeding to examine the condition of the healing art under the Carlovingian rulers, through their laws and the specific circumstances, either aiding to modify its scientific elements or retard its advancement and reduce it to the level of an empirical method, mingled with those supernatural auxiliaries provoked by demoniacal causes of maladies, which absorbed remedies into the hands of devotee monks, a sketch of the medical culture propagated by the monastery of Monte Cassino, will attest the vague and shadowy remnants of this science in its decadence, with sufficient vitality to prolong the fragile thread through two centuries, when it suddenly revived.[35]

If, at this epoch, amid so many revolutions to which society was subjected, the application of a higher type of medicine did not entirely succumb to the frightful catastrophes by which the most enlightened portions of Europe were clouded in the gloom of sanguinary violence, it was indebted, in conjunction with other arts, to the efforts of a few monasteries which preserved them from irretrievable destruction. The curative art, indeed, had receded from the higher altitudes of Galenic skill, and within the cloisters themselves was in perpetual conflict with the rapidly-expanding faith in the Satanic origin of sickness and diseases, making it quite impossible to trace these ills to natural causes, a difficulty aggravated as directly rivaling accepted dogmas of the Church; while among the people, Teutonic charlatans and impostors sadly supplemented the debasement of a science, provoked by ecclesiastical sanction at an early period of the Middle Ages.

To the monastery of Monte Cassino, in the ninth century, the impartial commendation should be made that in its incipient advance towards a more exact examination of ancient medical writers, a decided tendency manifested itself. It would no doubt be more in harmony with the facts relating to medical

[35] Tiraboschi, Storia della Litteratura Italiana, Tom. III., p. 263.

economy in this abbey, to record that the excellence of Saint Bertrarius in this art is rather individual than the culture of an entire monastery. Although thoroughly imbued with scholasticism, the writings of this monk reveal an unusual erudition for the age.

Of these, the most noted are his flattering biography of the founder of Western monachism, Saint Benedictus, and another treatise, in which he endeavored to harmonize conflicting passages of sacred Scripture, and bring them into chronological and historical concordance, an effort, for that period, worthy of the highest praise.[36]

Among such works, however, having direct reference to the matter under examination prepared by Bertrarius, the monastic chronicler relates the presentation, among other books, by him, to the conventual library, of two manuscript volumes.[37] In these, the erudite cleric had aggregrated great numbers of prescriptions and remedies for the cure of maladies, selected by personal labor from illustrious professors of the science in the past.[38] It would, doubtless, be elevating the medical services of Bertrarius to an unwarrantable height, if it were assumed that this industry partook of a scientific nature, when it is evident he was without more active incentive than the compilation of practical receipts.

The Carlovingian regulations stirred a zealous attention, among the monks of the empire, to the culture of medicine, denominated an art, and appear to have animated the convents of Italy and Gaul, during the progress of the ninth century; because, among other studies in which the monastic brethren were exercised, some attention was devoted to this as a branch of the liberal arts,[39] prescribed as fundamental in the monasteries, opened alike to ecclesiastical and lay students,

---

[36] Tiraboschi, Storia della Litteratura Italiana, Tom. III., p. 212 seq.

[37] "Duo codices medicinales, ejus utique industria de innumeris remediorum utilitatibus hinc inde collecti." Leo Ostiens, Chronicon Casinense, Lib. I., cap. 33.

[38] Leo Ostiens, Chronicon Casinense, Lib. I., cap. 33.

[39] Baluzius, Capitularia, Tom. I., col. 421.

and an extended aquaintanceship with these arts was made mandatory and a necessary prerequisite for the acceptance and conservation of postulants for church orders.[40]

In the venerable annals chronicling the events of the Torfa cloister for this period, it is stated the study of medicine was pursued at the convent, under the skilled direction of the abbot, Reoffred.[41] A disciple, studying cures and remedies for diseases under the personal tutelage of this prior, was a youth destined to monastic obligations, by the name of Campon. The progress of this stripling seems to have been rapid, and his tendency to vice and crime equally accelerated by an unholy ambition.[42] Having evidently acquired profound insight into the deleterious effects of certain poisons, this candidate for sacerdotal honors, instead of responding to the urbanity and paternal affection of his religious and medical preceptor, insiduously administered to him a mortal beverage, which quickly terminated the earthly career of the benevolent abbot.[43] As an attestation of the frightful depravity of the age succeeding Charlemagne, it may be stated here, that the monkish assassin intruded himself forcibly into the government of the Torfa cloister, and apparently before summary justice could prevent, he had dissipated the whole of its most valuable goods.[44]

That there were personages among the ancient Teutonic tribes who abandoned themselves to the practice of medicine in its varied and cognate branches, would seem to admit of no doubt. So far as the older Saxon races are concerned, who had attained a high civilization at the epoch of their utter subjection by Charlemagne, it has been asserted they possessed

---

[40] Capitular:, Aquisgran, cap. 70, An. 789; apud Baluz., op. cit., Tom. I., p. 237.

[41] Muratori, Scriptores Rer. Italico, Tom. II., pars. 2, p. 257.

[42] " Quorum unus Campo, ejus ab infantia alumnus et in arte medicinæ eruditus." Mabillon., Annales Ord. S. Benedict., Tom. III., p. 431.

[43] " Hausto letali poculo." Mabillon, Annales Ord. S. Benedict, Tom. III., p. 431.

[44] Ibid.

neither physicians nor surgeons.[45] If it be conceded that this people excluded practitioners of this art from their social organization, other less cultured nations appear to have departed from their example. For several centuries prior to the codification of laws governing the vanquished tribes of Gaul and Germany, subjected by the resistless forces of Charlemagne, the edicts and enactments of his predecessors, inspired with a desire to imitate the imperishible monuments of civil law,[46] distinctly affirm the existence among the Teutonic races of a professor of this avocation, alluded to and classified especially with the same formal phraseology as designated the learned physicians and surgeons of the Roman empire, viz: Medicus.

In all these statutory regulations this element is a well recognized one in the society of the German people, and appears to be as carefully defined and important as the judicial system, where this personage was required oftentimes to appear. One of the earliest records, so far as we know, which definely denominates among the Teutons practitioners of medicine, and distinctly recognizes them as personages of eminent social consideration and entitled to recognition for their profession, may be found in the laws of Dagobert, king of the Alemanni, which were drawn up and promulgated about the year 632.[47] In the Prœm or prefatory addition to the code, it is stated to have been agreed upon by the king, in the presence of princes and nobility, Christian pontiffs and populace, actually signifying their consent.[48]

The personal attendance of bishops when these enactments were decided upon might seem to warrant the inference that the medicus or medical man alluded to in these written laws, belonged to monasteries located in Gaul, subjected to pontifi-

[45] Heineccii, Antiquitates German., Tom. I., p. 606.

[46] Lex Alemannorum, cap. 98, sub fin. De Legibus; apud Goldast., Tom. II., p. 24.

[47] Goldastius, Antiquita. Aleman., Tom. II., p. 1.

[48] Ibid., Tom. II., p. 11.

cal control. We shall perhaps presently discover at this period and earlier, persons among the Germanic people who claimed to be endowed with a power to operate cures of maladies as marvellous as those performed by their scientific predecessors of the Roman Empire. Among other beneficial rescripts published by Dagobert for the better government of his subjects and the preservation of peace, it was solemnly declared,[49] if any person struck another on the head in anger so that a bony fragment should fall or fly from the wound, of size and density sufficient to be heard twenty-four feet when sounded upon a shield in the highway, such murderous assault should be compensated with a heavy fine. In case however the medicus or surgeon, to whose custody these evidences of an aggravated crime were entrusted, failed to produce them before the tribunal, he was privileged to swear that a bone had been removed from the head of the wounded person, and was lost.

If the wound opened a hole to the brain so that it appeared, or exuded, or permitted the medicus or surgeon to touch the same with an instrument in the nature of a probe, or with a napkin,[50] or in case the surgeon replaced it with medicaments or bandage, the convict should pay forty solidi.[51]

From the preceding statements it is clearly attested that so remote as the first half of the seventh century, the avocation of surgeon or medicus was recognized by the supreme code of the Alemanni and Langobards, which entitled him to be present in the courts in a professional character. Curiously enough, in an edict[52] of Rothar, monarch of the Italian Lango-

[49] "Si autem de capite os fractum tulerit de plaga, ita ut super publica via," etc. "Si autem ipsum medicus perdet," etc. "Si autem testa transcapulata fuerit, ita ut cervella appareant ut medicus cum pinna aut cum favone cervella tetigit," etc. Lex Alemannorum, cap. 58. For the character of the instruments mentioned in this citation, vide Du Cange, Glossarium Med. et Infim., Latinitas, sub. vv. Favone and Pinna.

[50] Lex Alemannorum, cap. 58.

[51] Leges Langobard., cap. 59; and Lex Alemannor., cap. 58.

[52] A. D. 643, Merkel, Geschichte der Langobardenrecht, p. 16.

bards, it was decreed that the loss of the fifth finger by violence should be assessed at two solidi, exclusive of the surgical charges for attendance.[53] It was also provided by the Langobardic jurisprudence, that whenever one person assaulted another with sufficient force to seriously wound him, he should at once seek the medicus or surgeon, and lay before him the condition of the wounded, in order that by the solemn sanction of the law medical service might be promptly at hand, to guard as far as possible the life and limb of the Lombards.

In case the party striking the blow failed to immediately notify a surgeon, then the aggrieved and injured person or his master was required to seek out and find a physician to whom the wounds were to be submitted for professional treatment.[54]

There is every reason to warrant the conclusion that the system of compensation for loss of a serf by death or debilitation through blundering medical practice, was adopted by other Teutonic tribes than the Wisigoths,[55] although this law of retaliation does not appear in the Roman codification, suffered to regulate civil and criminal procedure among the Germans vanquished by Charlemagne. The person striking the injurious blow was required by law to make good such loss as the wound entailed to servant or master, whether of the head or the body and its members, exclusive of charges for medical or surgical attendance, which compensation should be fixed by the judicious assessment of disinterested arbitrators.[56]

Professional skill thus provided, notwithstanding the long dominion of the Langobards in Italy, where the opportunities would appear to have aided in securing the services of a higher grade of physicians, must have emanated from those practitioners of the curative art whose status was carefully

---

[53] "Si quintum digitum de manu excusserit componat solidos II.: excepto operas et mercedis medici." Edictum Rotharis Regis., cap. 118.

[54] Edictum, Rotharis Regis., cap. 118.

[55] Lex Wisigothorum, Lib. XI., Titulus I., Lex. 4; apud Canciani, Leg. Barbar., Tom. IV., p. 180.

[56] "Qui plagas fecerit ipse querat medici," etc. "Et ille qui caput rumpit, et operas reddat et mercedis medici persolvat." Edictum, Roth., cit., cap. 128.

determined by the Teutonic statutes of a more remote epoch. Wherever indeed among the earlier German races reference is made by contemporaneous history to the enforcement of the penalties against an ignorant physician or unskillful surgeon, for the indemnification of a nobleman's life or a slave's loss through his blundering, or by edicts this class is prominently alluded to, such personages without doubt were ambulatory medical advisers, who followed these nations in their migratory movements whither the desire of conquest or lust of gain led them. As the immediate predecessors of the Carlovingians, to whom European civilization is largely indebted, the Salic legislation is of equal interest as a historical thread by which the condition or existence of practical medicine, in the custody of persons exclusively devoted to this avocation, can be traced anterior to the imperial rescripts of Charlemagne which prescribed its study in the monastic schools of the Empire.

About a quarter of a century subsequent to the formal promulgation of the Rotharic edicts, recognizing the social status and certain privileges of the medicus or surgeon, in a convocation of the Salic nation, it was enacted when a blow or stab within the ribs or abdomen should expose the viscera, and become an incurable wound, the convict should pay a heavy fine as a punishment, exclusive of the medicaments or such charges as were demanded by the surgeon into whose care the disabled person was delivered.[57] Upon the accession of Charlemagne to the imperial dignity, a steady and unswerving zeal seems to have characterized all the efforts of this illustrious monarch to so solidly establish the varied interests of his vast empire, under the sanction of civil and canonical authority, as would admit of a perpetual existence.

With enlightened judgment, imitating the munificence of the great Theodosius and Justinian, his predecessors in the Latin empire, the Teutonic ruler attempted through the mediation of legislation to inspire into the partially civilized minds of his subjects an enthusiasm for polite arts, and to preserve them

---

[57] Pactus, Legis Salic., Titulus XX., cap. 6.

from the iconoclastic movement of the age, by the protective influence of ecclesiastical canons.[58] In the year 804, by a decree granting valuable forest lands, with immunities and perquisites, to the bishopric of Osnaberg, it was expressly stipulated to be for the maintenance of a school in which the Greek and Latin languages should be taught in perpetuity, according to the tenor of the grant, in order that such persons intending to assume clerical orders might not be deficient in a knowledge of these, or, at least, might have the opportunity of acquiring them.[59]

The schools of the empire, by a law of Ludowig the Pious, issued in the year 823, were made to partake more of the character of a public institution, accessible to such as desired educational facilities, and especially was it directed that these scholastic establishments should be conveniently located in suitable places.[60] By the sanction of the Church authorities the pupils were to be instructed in liberal arts, which were particularly specified as psalmody, notation, chanting, computation,[61] grammar or reading, and transcribing Catholic books.[62] It was doubtless an unequivocal advance, and of the highest importance for the future of medical culture in the monasteries, whither this art had fled and preserved a fragile vitality, oppressed by the gloom of increasing superstition, when Charlemagne in the year 805, by a chartulary entitled De Causis Ecclesiasticis, enacted that in addition to the science of calculation, the medicinal art must thenceforth be taught the pupils of the monastic schools of the empire as a portion of the prescribed studies, receiving the active sanction of the sacerdotal authorities.[63]

---

[58] Baluzius, Capitularia, Tom. I., p. 645.

[59] Baluzius, Cartularia, Tom. I., p. 419.

[60] Ibid., pp. 634, 737.

[61] "Psalmos, notas, cantas, computum, grammaticam per singula monasteria vel episcopia discant." Carulor, anno 789, cap. 70; ap. Baluz., op. cit., Tom. I., p. 237.

[62] Ibid.

[63] "De compoto ut veraciter discant omnes. De medicinali arte ut infantes

Previous to this year, instruction in the curative art was apparently abandoned to the discretion of abbots, who doubtless heeded the urgent admonition of Cassiodorus touching the necessity of a careful study of the writings of medical sages, but these priors as chief of the cloister schools, evidently through personal ignorance, neglected the counsels of the Benedictine anchorite, or inculcated such notions of remedies as were an absolute necessity for emergencies, without the spirit of scientific investigation which vitalized the theme.

Too high commendation cannot be awarded the illustrious Carlovingian for this rescript, which thenceforth made a study of medicine an element in all the imperial monastic schools, for by the virtue of this law forcible attention was devoted to the writings of Galen, Hippocrates, Celsus, and Dioscorides, which not only tended to their preservation, but, it may be confidently asserted, prepared the way for the revival of this science during the Middle Ages. The Frankish emperor, following the custom of the period, in regulating the compensation for wounds, declared that just charges for medicaments were to be allowed, independent of the penalty for violating the law.[64]

A further regulation of the Church as a sanitary measure, may be mentioned here, sanctioned by the Church under Lewis the Pious, who left the use of the bath among the conventual brethren entirely to the prior's arbitration. From the same edict it can be gathered that certain monks subjected themselves at stated intervals to cupping or phlebotomy, so that they might procure in the infirmary a more delicate diet than was usually allowed robust cenobites, and as a preventative the canon established the rule that no blood-letting should be performed at fixed periods—only according to necessity.[65]

---

hanc discere mittantur." Capitular., Teotan., cap. 5; Baluz., op. cit., Tom. I., col. 421; and Lex Salica., Tit. I., cap. 5, Ed. Eccardi, p. 178.

[64] Lex Salica, Tit. XIX., cap. 6; and Baluzius, Cartular, Tom. I., col. 294.

[65] "Ut certum phlebotomiæ tempus non observent, sed unicuique secundum necessitus expostulat concedatur." Capitular., Aquisgranense, anno 817, cap. 11.

Notwithstanding the manifest debasement of medicine to the level of the charlatan and empiric among the Teutonic nations, and the fanatical practitioners within the monasteries of this age, occasional allusions indicate an experimental spirit with the use of remedies in curing diseases, under the expansive rule, "different ills demand different treatment,"[66] that "where the wound is closed medicaments must be introduced within to insure a cure."[67] Minute and specific directions were given in an ordinance by Charlemagne in the year 800, touching the planting and raising of herbs and vegetables in all the gardens appurtenant to the royal domain. The concluding paragraph of this statute is of the highest utility in tracing the progress of horticulture.[68]

---

66 Baluzius, Cartularia, Tom. I., p. 1191.

67 "Ubi autem vulnus infixum est, medicina adhibenda est." Capitular., Aquisgran., an. 803, cap. 4; ap. Baluz., op. cit., Tom. I., 380; and Tom. II., p. 158.

68 Capitulare, De Villis, cap. 70; apud Baluz., op. cit., Tom. I., p. 342.

CHAPTER XII.

Nature of Medical Culture among Ancient Germans — Controlled by Sacerdoty—Healing Virtues Attributed to the Mandragora—Used with Runic Characters—Publicly Sold at Fairs—Magic Power of these Effigies—Magic Ligations, Potions, etc., for Herds and Men—Teutonic Women Skilled in Medicine—Curative Virtue of the Runes—Toxicology—Storm-Evokers or Tempestarii—Profession of Curative Art Recognized at an Early Age—Pagan Word for Surgeon—Ambulatory Physicians—Archaism of Germanic Medical Derivatives—Formulas for Cure, of Ancient Magicians—Virgins Specially Adapted to the Healing Art—Cure of Luxations.

MEDICAL knowledge among the ancient Germans prior to the Carlovingian dynasty was no doubt confined to practical use of simple medicaments, and such skill in surgery as the emergencies of individual accidents admitted. The Teutonic surgeon, whose status was clearly defined by the several edicts of a martial and sanguinary race, was of either sex indifferently, and, without the union being susceptible of demonstration, identical with its more remote usage in the temples of Apollo, medicine remained in the custody of a sacerdoty who performed ritualistic ceremonies before Norse divinities. So far as a similarity may be instituted between the system of cures accepted by these hardy warriors for themselves and families, and that pursued as a science to its decline amid the general crash of arts, it would seem that the Germanic medicus or physician also assumed the endowment of magical properties whose skilled operation perfected cures. How far indeed the secrets of medicine may have been transmitted to these races or their priesthood, by the Greeks and Latins,[1] at a period beyond exact research, there is no doubt that the people of Gaul, through the convenient centre of civilization at Marseilles, procured varied methods for palliating serious dis-

[1] Rothii, Disquisitio de Vocabulo Artzt., cap. 1, § 19, p. 38.

eases, especially when it is considered that the Gallic nobles frequently attended studies in the lyceum of this city, among which was taught the science of medicine.[2]

One of the principal herbal medicines to which magical potency was universally ascribed, and which survived the downfall of northern temple-worship through the introduction of Christianity, was the mandragora, or alraun plant.[3] To this unusual power was attributed, and in diversified forms it appears to have been used for the provocation and irresistible cure of maladies.[4] It was eagerly sought for by sterile women, and for obstetrical labors.[5]

In its most ancient adaptation, this alraun, or its cognate, the Runes either carved or shaped like an image, was regarded as arcane, or possessed of secret inherent forces, which were transmitted under the profoundest mystery.[6] This root, after having been gathered amid impressive and solemn ceremonies,[7] was carved into the rude effigy of a Norse deity, three of whom, represented by gilded images, still stood in a heathen temple in the time of Columban in Germany.[8] Thus prepared, these mandragora figures were sold or traded to Teutonic purchasers, as endowed with magic curative forces. From their attributes of peculiar efficiency to prevent evils to herds, and other mishaps against life and property, similar to the Latin tutelary divinities, they were oftentimes carried around enclosures in solemn procession.[9] To this custom without

---

[2] Strabo, De Situ Orbis., Lib. IV.; and Cæsar, De Bello Gallico, Lib. VI., cap. 14. Apollo of the Gauls, patron of the sick. Ib., Lib. VI., cap. 17.

[3] Grimm, Ueber die Deutsche Runen., p. 68.

[4] According to Arætaeos, De Causis et Signis, Lib. I., c. 6, p. 78. This herb, when mingled with food, produced insanity.

[5] "Opem enim, quæ credulorum persuasio est, mulieribus, sterilitas vitio et partus onere laborantibus, ferunt." Rothii, De Imagunculis Germanor., Alraunicis, p. 10.

[6] Grimm, op. cit., pp. 71, 207.

[7] Rothii, op. cit., § 3, p. 6 seq.

[8] Walafrid Strabo, Vita S. Galli., Lib. I., cap. 4, p. 144.

[9] Rothii, De Imagunc., p. 19.

doubt, so deeply rooted as a part of these paganistic rites against which Christian pontiffs combated by canons and civil law, should be attributed the cause of an interdict by Charlemange at Lepinta, setting forth that such *simulacra* or figures were borne with heathen celebration through fields and groves as a propitiatory scheme under the invocation of Norse gods, and peremptorily forbidding such practices under the heaviest penalties.[10]

These images endowed with curative powers survived to Christianity as an element of saintly remedies. In nearly all the diversified nationalities of the Germanic race, similar properties were attributed to the effigies of their divinities, prior and subsequent to the adoption of a new faith. Among the Norsemen, in the regions of Scandinavia, where the worship of Thor was preëminent, carved types of this battle-god were assumed to possess unlimited puissance as a horoscope and talisman—the basis for which was almost invariably the alraun or mandragora. Thus, for instance, when it is stated such images were borne about by Halfred, a poet, and Helogren in a bag, although sculptured from a whale's tooth, and charged with the subtle essence of vaticination, it is to be understood they assimilated with the Runic Lares of the ancient Germans.[11] Scandinavians carried metal effigies carved out of gold or silver, or incised upon tiles, perpetually as amulets and safeguards against diseases and physical infirmities.

An early Christian Synod convoked in the year 690, in Burgundy, a century subsequent to the formal introduction of this religion by Clothair's edict,[12] interdicted communicants and proselytes offering oblations in their own abodes, pervigils in the festivities of saints, or on the highways, to sacred trees, and forbade them pledging vows to fountains; but decreed when a convert had a vow to consecrate it should be performed

---

[10] Indiculus Superstit. et Paganiar., cap. 1, 26, 27; apud Balazius, Cartular., Tom. I., col. 150; and Sulpicius Sever., Vita S. Martini, cap. 9.

[11] Rothii, De Imagune, Germ. Alrunis., p. 24.

[12] Baluzius, op. cit., Tom. I., p. 6 seq.

by vigils in a church, and the compensation involved in this act should be tendered the matriculæ or poor.[13] This provincial council concluded its ordinance by forbidding proselytes manufacturing carved or sculptured effigies with a foot, or linen male figures.[14]

The sculptilia pede facta[15] placed under ecclesiastical ban, were images of human feet, which the humbler Teutons erected at cross-roads, in order to secure restoration to health and a cure for maladies.[16] An early evangelical pontiff, whose Episcopate extended over the converted Germans, ordered a great number of these curious remedies for sickness and disease to be burned, some of which were composed of wood, linen, and other materials.

Touching effigies fabricated of linen texture, whose use was equally sanitary, and of greater magical efficiency than the carved foot, these appear to be identical with the simulacra de pannis facta, or cloth images, specified in the Indiculus above quoted, and were disposed of to paganistic and proselyte purchasers, as sanitative amulets, by perambulatory physicians, who trafficked extensively upon the credulity of the suffering sick and infirm. The remedial potency of these Norse cures was assumed to be intensified, when the mandragora, mystically prepared, was steeped in liquids. Thus, for instance, after soaking this potential effigy in water, wine or beer, it communicated a curative energy to the fluid, claimed to be an infallible and prompt remedy for the most aggravated disorders. In Charlemagne's age, headache was frequently cured by saintly recommendation to shape a figure of the head and place it on a cross.[17]

The water in which these images were steeped, was oftentimes given to domesticated herds, as a certain remedy for the

---

[13] Labbe, Collec. Concil., Canon: III., Tom. V., p. 958.

[14] Du Cange, Glossarium, sub v. Compensum.

[15] Rothii, De Imagunculis Germ. Alraunic., p. 25.

[16] Du Cange, op. cit., sub v. Sculptel.

[17] Vita Idæ Duchessæ, cap. 19; apud Leibnitz, Tom. I., p. 176.

disorders of cattle and horses. As a preventative this fluid was copiously sprinkled in the sheds where the animals herded.[18] Added to these sanitary forces, this renowned plant was accorded talismanic powers which repelled noxious elements; ills of whatever nature, whether superinduced by incantations or magic arts, upon man or animals. In their domestic application these Runic effigies were wide-spread and as piously adored as the lares of fleeing Priam,[19] constituting an effective palladium against the encroachments of sickness, aiding a restoration to health, expelling anxious inquietude, and were especially relied on to prevent sorrowful misfortunes from breaking the integrity of the home circle. Nor was this vast efficacy limited to such desirable results, but it descended to preserving the exhilarating wine and beer against loss of its intoxicating property, rendered successful commercial negotiations, and infallibly promoted rapid and enormous affluence.

Other virtues of a surprising character were awarded the omnipotent mandragora. It conciliated affection and maintained friendship, preserved congugal fealty and developed benevolence.[20] The immensity of worth inherent in this mystical medicament, its vital essence, was by no means confined to sustaining health and providing certain remedies for infirmities; its power manipulated tribunals[21] and secured judicial favor at court; and when this resistless amulet was held under the arm by a suitor at law, however unjust his cause, the vegetable Rune controlled the forum and obtained the verdict.

Evidently this puissant plant was before the mind of the Langobardic monarch, who enacted that in the doubtful struggle of a juridical duel neither of the combatants should carry

---

[18] Rothii, De Imag. Ger. Alraun., p. 10.

[19] Virgil, Æneid, Lib. V.

[20] Rothii, op. cit., p. 11.

[21] "In foro patroni dissertissimi vicem obit imagunculo alrunica. Favorem enim judicis, litiganti certissimum comparat, atque sub brachio amuleti instar, recondita, efficit." Rothii, op. cit., cap. 1, § 6.

a talisman which should render the conflict unequal.[22] To the usage among the ancient Teutonic races, of women devoting their time to the practice of medicine and surgery, may be traced the perpetuation of this custom at a later period of the Middle Ages, by their female successors. As early indeed as the age of Tacitus, the wives and mothers of German families were celebrated for the skillful use of medicaments and the dexterous manipulation of wounds received by their husbands or sons in sanguinary battle.[23] It is a matter susceptible of historical proof that the feminine Vates of the Druids and consorts of Northern princes had at a remote epoch obtained a just renown for medical skill. At a short distance from the mainland, in the Senna Isles or Heiligland, scene of the mystical cult of Norse deities,[24] the priestesses were reputed to possess such medicinal knowledge as permitted them to speedily cure those diseases universally regarded elsewhere as utterly incurable.[25]

This unequivocal acknowledgment of the ability of Teutonic women in the practice of medicine, has especial adaptation to the Scandinavian females, whose prowess in this valuable art seems to have become so celebrated during their earthly career that monumental honors were erected after death to such notables as Eyra, Tyrfa, and Groa Volva.[26] To the sepulchures which concealed the decaying remains of these famous women, pilgrimages were made from distant provinces and remote cities by the incurably diseased, in the earnest hope that the essential virtue of that puissance so notably manifested in

---

22 "Nullus camphio præsumat, quando ad pugnando contra alio vadit, herbas quod ad malificias pertinet super se habere," etc. Edictum Rotharis Regis, cap. 368; and Concilium Bavaricum, A. D. 772, cap. 3.

23 "Ad matres, ad conjuges vulnera ferunt; nec illæ numerare aut exigere plagas pavent," etc. Germania, cap. 7.

24 Cluverius, Antiquitat. Germanic., Lib. III., cc. 23–34.

25 "Sanare, quæ apud alios insanabilia sunt scire," etc. Pomponii Melae., De Situ Orbis., Lib. III., cap. 6.

26 Rothii, De Imagunc. German. Alraun., pp. 20, 35.

life might still surround the sombre portals of the tomb, and perform a miraculous cure.[27]

In the presence of these memorial obelisks, flowers, herbs, and fruits, rudely reproduced on stone tablets, were delineated as symbols of the materials from which the remedial restorers had been extracted. Germanic matrons were long distinguished in those arts appertaining to obstetrical gestation, or the cure of sterility. In such physical infirmities recourse was had to simple medications and the forcible energies of magical curatives.[28] These excellent endowments were applied to remedy the disorders of herds with the same alacrity as the ills of humanity, and the potency of magic, as well as chemical forces of vegetable productions, were applied indifferently to heal wounds and luxations.[29] At a period considerably remote from the Carlovingian age, veterinary surgery seems to have been practiced with success by women, by the potential means of a mirror placed in a window, especially the cure of fractured bones.[30]

More anciently, the care of herds and flocks naturally devolved upon this sex in the absence of their warlike husbands.[31] The earliest and most practical legislation touching paganistic rites and customs of the converted Germans, and conjointly promulgated by pontifical and imperial authority, attests the vigorous existence of a power accorded Teutonic matrons to render men blind, enervated, or insane, through magical medicines. Acts superinducing imbecility[32] were particularly the

[27] "Vata pro salute et corporis incolummitate a popularibus æque ac pereginis facta sint et soluta." Ibid., p. 36.

[28] Eccardi, Comment. Rer. Orient. Franc., Tom. I., p. 840.

[29] "Ut noverint magicas artes incantationesque quibuslibet infirmitatibus hominium nihil posse remedii conferre." Baluz., Cartular., Addit. Tert., cap. 93, p. 1174.

[30] "Mulier quædam est hic in vicino, quæ per incantationes et demonum invocationes, homines et animalia, præcipue equos, defectum in membris habentes, curare consuevit." Buschius, De Reformat. Monaster., cap. 51.

[31] Tacitus, Germania, cc. 5 and 15.

[32] "Qui dicitur portasse strias cocinant," etc. Pactus Legis. Salic., Tit. LXVII., cap. 1. Also, Lex Aleman., cap. 22.

object of canonical and civil animadversion, and that rite also by which utter destruction might be invoked upon a hated personage,[33] was interdicted under severest penalties.

Such ills of body or of mind, to which man or animal was subjected through enmity of dexterous female magicians, were invariably assigned to women physicians for remedies, in which their excellence was unquestioned. Magic and soothsaying entered largely into the curative art, applied by means of formal murmured words, which promptly expelled maladies from the sick and infirm sufferers.[34] According to the marvellous properties attributed to the Runes, their vast medicinal potency constituted an inherent essence and liberally used by the Norse women, of whom Eir, as the surgical deëss of Asgard, appears to have been the patroness.[35] A remedy professedly of great virtue, has survived to modern times, in the shape of an adage: "The hair of a dog is good for its bite."[36]

Although the narrative of Tacitus seems to conclude the question touching the knowledge among the Germans of his time of the secrets of letters,[37] the subsequent advent of foreigners doubtless persuaded their cultivation fcr poses, introduced certain immoral customs, which early Wisigothic rescripts severely censured. Archæologists, with unrestricted avowal, have sought to portray a golden age of innocence among Teutonic families in their paganistic era,[38] but the historian must with impartial justice proclaim that in the short period of a few centuries, this primeval civilization, utterly unconscious of shame, with its total absence of vice to provoke a blush upon the brow of a fair-haired Saxon, had so completely vanished, as to demand the stringent repressive

---

[33] Lex Salic., cit.; and Baluz., Cartular., De Partibus Sax., cc. 6 and 9, Tom. I., p. 294 seq.

[34] Snorro Sturlon., Heimskringla, Lib. I., cc. 4 and 8. Sigfridrîfumâl, str. 9 and 11.

[35] Gylfag., str. 35.

[36] Lordfafmrs., str. 138.

[37] Tacitus, op. cit., cc. 18 and 19.

[38] Cluverius, Antiquitat. German., Lib. I., c. 16, p. 115.

power of criminal law and ecclesiastical authority to guard against national debasement.

Thus, for instance, the Gothic and Salic maidens and their lovers, unrestricted by modesty, invented amatory arts to conciliate affection, collected herbs whose medicinal qualities served for convenient poison to translate an indiscreet husband, or when united with alraunic characters, were used as amulets and talismans, disclosing the secrets of incantations and magic letters, and recommended immodest decoctions to pervert nature.[39]

In toxicology or poisons, Scandinavian females excelled German matrons. Heuta, a Danish lady of high rank, was so erudite in the preparation of such drugs, that she compounded a philter by which the Norweigian ruler Hringwen was fascinated, and remained her lover for many years.[40] Teutonic maidens, dexterous in this art, appear to have confined the practical application of this science to the strict limits of medical economy, at times, indeed, exercising supernatural power to soften the minds of men to benevolence and mercy, over which they glorified the control.[41] In addition to this knowledge, they were accorded the power of raising storms and tempests, and were generally classified as Tempestarii.[42] These destructive disturbances, it was claimed, originated in the Runic effigies,[43] as personifying an evil spirit, controlled by the material type, and in its general signification corroborated popular belief among Christian converts of demoniacal creation of natural phenomena.

Priestesses consecrated to the gloomy rites of Norse divini-

---

[39] Lex Wisigothorum, Lib. III., Tit. IV., Lex 3. "Si quis mulieri herbas dederit, ut infantes habere non possit." Lex Salica, Tit. XXI., c. 4; and Lex Bojuvarior., Tit. I., cap. 18.

[40] Rothii, De Imagunc. Germ. Alraun., p. 43.

[41] "Si aliqua femina sit quæ per quædam maleficia et incantationes mentes hominum se emmutare posse dicit, id est, ut de lodis in amorem aut de amore in odium convertat." Regino, De Disciplino Ecclesiastic., Lib. II., cap. 5, n. 45.

[42] Du Cangius, Glossarium, sub v. Tempestiarii.

[43] Rothii, De Imagunc. Germ. Alraun., p. 46.

ties were assumed to possess the prerogative of provoking violent rain or hail storms, hurricanes and whirlwinds, by the delusive mediation of murmured chants, and when thus suddenly evoked by these divine servants, the same potency might instantly end them. At least such is the unequivocal attestation of Pomponius Mela, who affirmed the female sacerdoty in Heligoland were able by magic songs to stir up storms by sea and land.[44] Honors similar to those rendered the gods of Asgard, were paid the mandragora images, the chief curative method of the ancient Teutons, with identical ceremonies and equal idolatry.

When ambulatory physicians sold these effigies to credulous sick, they distinctly declared, to frequent change of vestments, ablutions usual in those ages[45] should be added in order that the divinized types might not be infested with insects or attacked by moths.[46] How profoundly the idolatry of these medical talismans had descended among converted pagans prior to and during the reign of Charlemagne, may be gathered from the dauntless struggle of the people for those customs, alluding to their extinct temple worship and the uncompromising attitude of canonical and secular power against them. Unsubdued Saxons, in valiant defiance of imperial rescripts, placed banqueting boards before these divine effigies, and with gay festivities by day and night honored the curative power of their divinities through symbols. A portion of animal food was abandoned reverently to these deities, which was consumed by the celebrants of sacrificial rites, in joyous conviviality.[47]

---

[44] De Situ Orbis., Lib. III., cap. 6.

[45] Tacitus, Germania, cc. 17 and 22.

[46] "Cautio, qui propterea illas aqua saepius ablui jubent, ne carie infestentur atque tineisque in esum cedant, aut mucescant divinæ illæ effiges." Rothii, op. cit., p. 55. Vagrant medicastres in the fifth century, Rog. Wendor., Flor. Histor., sub an. 497, Tom. I., p. 51.

[47] Baluz., Cartular. De Partibus Saxon., cap. 21, Tom. I., p. 254; and Gregor. Turones., De Gloria Confessor., cap. 2.

That nation which devoutly believed the gods oftentimes assumed a corporeal human form, and directly operated earthly events, nor disdained tempting feasts,[48] coöperated to perpetuate those myths which, in the Middle Ages, to great degree underlay the system of medicine. At the period under examination, vagrant medici or physicians,[49] on foot and on horseback, from Italy, Spain, and the Gallic provinces, seem to have found a ready sale in Germany for their mandragora images, where they arrived in troops among a rude and partially Christianized people, who eagerly sought these wandering medicine vendors, and purchased their curative wares for genuine figures of the Alraun spirit.

Frequently other materials, such as lustral water, consecrated wax, and fragments of the cross, of unquestioned medicinal potency, helped to dispose of the pharmaceutical stock the more readily. While thus captivating the superstitious fancy of the uncultivated populace, these migratory physicians, in addition to harmless medicaments with magical attributes, plied a nefarious industry at fairs and public marts in larger towns and municipalities of the newly-vanquished country, where they were aggregated in crowds to sell noxious drugs and poisons, whose terrible efficacy was presumed to be increased by the resonant and elongated names given the vendible goods.[50]

In the year 822, when Waldger sought to enter into the presence of Ludwig, Emperor of Germany, he arrayed himself in the foreign costume of a physician, and under this attire the monarch regarded him as a vagrant medicus or surgeon, and ordered him admitted,[51] a convincing proof of the roving and doubtless degraded character of the drug and medicine vendors of that age. According to the usual system of living

---

48 Tacitus, Germania, cap. 40.

49 Rothii, De Imagunculis Germanor. Alraunic., p. 68.

50 Rothii, De Imagunc. Germ. Alraun., p. 69.

51 "Sub habitù peregrino." Herman. Corner. Chronicon, sub an. 822, Eccard. II., col. 448.

among the earlier Germans, which involved the simplest diet and most vigorous physical exercises, it is evident this uniformity must in a measure guard against the approach of maladies incident to the more luxurious refinement of civilized society.

Mêdicinal art, under these surroundings, necessarily failed in developing great curative properties, and was doubtless restricted to the cultivation of remedies appropriate to wounds, fractures and luxations. The cure of bodily infirmities resulting from a martial life, necessitated the neophyte in medicine becoming familiar with strange powers of runic herbs to heal serious wounds.[52] In order to procure certain remedies, the leaves, flowers, and fruit of fructiferous trees were gathered with scrupulous selection, a duty devolving upon Druidesses. Before the thorough Christianization of their race, the Germans themselves recognized a medical avocation, the practitioners of which were in a greater or less constant demand. At the close of the eighth or commencement of the ninth century, this profession was specifically designated in native vernacular as ercetere or medicus,[53] and is to be accepted to signify the medicasters so frequently referred to in the semi-barbarous rescripts of the earlier Teutons from the sixth to the close of the eighth century.

In a metrical poem of Conrad of Wissenburg, a versifier of the ninth century, this word is written "arzat," almost identical with the modern name, and clearly designates the ancient physician or surgeon.[54] In the next age arzat and arzater[55] occur, and signify a physician and medicaments, or the primative pigmenteria,[56] or apothecary, and attest a practical sys-

---

[52] "Runas arboreas nosse debes, si egregii medici nomen sustinere velis vulneraque ex arte curare." Olans Magni., in Specimen. Lexici Runici, p. 109.

[53] Sigfrîdfumâl, Str. 11.

[54] "Thoh ni was gevvisse er arzat niheiner." Lib. III., c. 14, v. 19; ap. Schilter., Thesaur. Antiq. Teuton., I., p. 184.

[55] Pezii, Thesaur. Anecdot., Tom. I., p. 384.

[56] Du Cange, Glossarium, sub v. Pigmentarius.

tem of medicine, doubtless transmitted from paganism to Christian converts, after the period of Clothair. As a cognate word the Gallic arzan, in its archaic interpretation, had the sense of healing or curing from sickness or wounds.[57] In this signification is to be understood the formal interdict of the early ages: wine should not be medicated with chalk or the white of an egg.[58] Ancient paraphrases of Scripture use the word as a healer or one who cures diseases, fairly interpreted by its Latin vocable medicus.[59] A curious confirmation of this allegation may be found in Anglo-Saxon versions of Biblical writings,[60] which quaintly affirm: "De Arstedye Kumpt vom derne Allerhögesten; de Here leth de Arsedye uth der Erden wassen," that is, "The Lord is creator of medicine, and the Master lets medicaments be produced by the earth." Arzt, meaning surgeon, has been traced to these ancient Germanic roots as incorporating the idea of curing and healing diseases, with its possible origin in the medicinal properties of mandragora effigies.[61]

From these statements it appears in a remote antiquity, among these people, there existed a profession pursuing a certain system of medical economy.

Eccard, however, distinctly asserts the philological derivation of this word as coeval with the epoch at which medical art was recognized as an element of scholastic culture, in the monasteries of the Latin Church, and prescribed to be taught as medicinalis arte,[62] which the erudite commentator claims is the lineal precursor of Arzt, or surgeon.[63] Through its trans-

[57] Wachter, Glossar., Voce Gerzan., p. 22. In the twelfth century pharmaceutical Latin was translated into German vernacular. Macer., De Virtutibus Herbarum, Anzeig. Blatt., No. 39, an. 1827, p. 19 seq.

[58] "Win arzen mit kolk, oder eyer-klar." Schilter, op. cit., v. arzat., p. 65.

[59] "Wenke ik bin de Here dyn arste." Exod. XV., cap. 26.

[60] Rothii, De Vocab. Arzt., p. 15.

[61] Ibid., p. 18 seq.

[62] Lex Salica, Capitular. De Causis Ecclesiast., cap. 5, p. 178.

[63] "Sed medicina jam olim ars dicta est, et medicus artista. Use vetus arzat et nostrum ars medicus derivandum." Scholium, ap. Leg. Salic., op. cit., p. 178.

formations and linguistic changes, the original meaning of the word Arzat, as implying the preparation or growing of herbs for medicinal purposes, reappears with reasonable lucidity.[64] Under this sweeping classification, the older Germanic medici, of pagan and early Christian times, were distinguished as personages whose lives were passed in rural districts, wanderers of the fields, where they gather herbs for cures of sickness and wounds.[65] Their avocation closely identified with meadows, glades and woodland, they traversed these gloomy groves in troops, and with anxious sagacity cut the sanitative vegetation, or eradicated it with magic rites and ceremonies.[66] Frequent reference is made in the historical writings of northern authors, to the dexterous compounding of medicines by both sexes, who were sufficiently fortunate to preserve the inestimable lives of royalty. A youthful monk, by the name of Johannes, native of a contiguous province, whose knowledge of this art had reached the grievously stricken Waldemer, a Scandivavian king, was summoned to the palace, where by an adroit mixture of powders with his patron's food, he managed to prolong the monarch's life for a limited period only.[67] The monastic attire, as we have seen at an early age, appears to have added force to the professional vagrancy of the mediæval physician. Another, a rustic, uniting extensive information upon the properties of medicinal herbs with agriculture, was enabled to save the life of Harald, brother of Saint Olave, king of Norway, suffering with a malady provoked by seven wounds.[68]

---

[64] Lex Bojar., Tit. XII., c. 8; and the Aranmûnmoth of Charlemagne, Eiginhardi, Vita Caroli Magni, cap. 29.

[65] "Germanorum medici, quippe qui, ut herbas, usui sibi in medendo futuras, colligerent, silvos ac saltus discurrebant," etc., "immo vero superstitiosa diligentia varii generis ritus, plures herbas abscisuri ac radices evulsuri per artis suæ et religionis præcepta, observare debeant." Rothii, De Vocabulo Arzt., p. 74.

[66] Plinii, Hist. Nat., Lib. XXV., cap. 9.

[67] "E scania accersitus," Saxo Grammaticus, Historiæ Danicæ, Lib. XV., p. 581. Touching the skill of Northern people in herbal medicines, vide Olaus Magnus, Hist. Septent., Lib. V., cap. 16, cc. 50-52.

[68] Rothii, De Vocabul. Arzt., p. 76.

Archaic words in use among the Gauls and Germans as early as the eighth century, having a signification exactly corresponding to the medicus or physician, and pigmentum or medicaments of the imperial codes, further attest the presence of a vocation identical with the medical profession. In Tatian's paraphrase of the Evangelists, drawn up for use in proselyting the worshipers of Norse idols, about the middle of the period before us, the vulgate medicus or physician is translated into the vernacular by Lachs, or in its plural form Lachin.[69] A like vocable among the Franks currently expressed the act of healing or curing maladies. Laec or Lec of the Anglo-Saxon, attested by the Old Testament, signified this: while laecman or laecdom stood for medicine in its abstract sense.[70]

Older versions by Ulphilas in the fifth century, contained words expressing systematic healing of bodily ills, by a person practising the craft professionally,[71] and the more recent Eddaic songs, distinctly individualize an avocation of practical medicine as a well-defined element in Norse society. In the Scandinavian province Laekner accurately reproduced the Salic medicus or physician, and by the nomenclature of laekning, a system of curing is affirmed.[72] It is doubtful whether the Teutonic professors were more careful in avoidance of unjust exactions for medical services than their predecessors under Theodoric, the Gothic ruler, and his illustrious secretary, Cassiodorus, or the Wisigoth kings, whose codifications regulated, as we have stated, their salary and basis of compensation.[73]

From this legislation, and the various codes cited hitherto, it is manifest when the medicus was summoned to attest certain physical mishaps, he was entitled to demand and receive such wages as were fixed by disinterested parties. In the

---

69 Rothii, Disquisit. Nominum, p. 79.

70 Psalm L., Com. III.

71 Ulphili, Versio Evangel. IX. Matth., c. 12.

72 Rothii, Disquisit. Nomin., p. 85; and Edda Snorii, Mytholog., 30.

73 Lex Wisigothorum, Lib. XI., Tit. I., Leg. 1–5.

Middle Ages wealthy patients obtained double attention and additional drugs from the peripatetic apothecaries, while the impoverished and indigent sick on the contrary received just one-half the attention, and medicines strictly necessary. A celebrated mediæval practitioner of the curative art urgently instructed his disciples against curing diseases or administering remedies to affluent valetudinarians without first receiving payment.[74] It is doubtful indeed, whether among the earlier Germanic physicians at the period of Christianization a schedule of charges for medical treatment was extant, excepting perhaps the ambulatory surgeons, who certainly procured heavy compensation for their wares, while the practitioners along fixed routes, doubtless were largely rewarded by gratitude.

In the economy of poison cures, the suction principle of the Teutonic Leck was continued to a later epoch of the Middle Ages, when the favorite of a king purged a poisoned wound by this method. Whenever anciently surgical instruments appropriate for prompt and thorough cleansing of aggravated wounds were not procurable, or perhaps yet in use, practical purgation was accomplished by lip-suction, after which sanitative herbs were applied.[75]

According to Kero's Teutonic Glossary, prepared by a monk of Saint Gall, under Pepin, the Carlovingian king, the Latin vocable medicamina or medicine, is translated by Lahchida, which in this word signifies a system of cures;[76] and the Lexicon of Hraban Maur, of the ninth century, interpreted by Vursari,[77] by the literal sense of pharmacy, indicating the existence of a class in society occupied in gathering herbal remedies; meaning the early surgeon or medicus. Groa Volva, celebrated by the Norse in written and sculptured monuments,

---

[74] Freind, Historia Medicinæ, p. 551.

[75] Rothii, Disquisitio Nomin., p. 102.

[76] Goldastius, Aleman. Antiquit., Tom. II., pars. 1, p. 81. Vide Du Cange, Glossarium, sub v. Lecator, who demonstrates social debasement of mediæval Europe in the propagation of this name from its surgical origin.

[77] Rothii, De Nom. Wursari, p. 119.

13

as presenting curatives drawn from Asgard to Thor,[78] gave the nomenclature to a system of curing by herbal medicaments, and may be taken to attest the close relationship supposed to exist, by the early converts to Christianity, between the practitioners of medicine and the Norse divinities.

The vestments in which the Norsemen arrayed their sanitary deès were imitated by the professional raiment of physicians, composed of a linen mantlet, clinging to the figure, and succinctly girded by a band of like texture.[79] This was likewise the dress of Druidesses, whose dexterous curative knowledge has been alluded to.[80] The corrugated face and silvered hair of this Deity may be assumed to represent the advanced age and inspiring experience of the physician. In the right hand the image grasps an urn filled with health-giving plants and fruits, and doubtless reproduces a more ancient Æsculapian symbol. The left hand, holding a plow wheel, typifies not only care and patronage over rural affairs, but prosperity and health of the devotees of this cult. In many German provinces where pagan customs survived to Christianity under other forms, the people were accustomed amid varied rites and ceremonials to fasten the wheel emblem above their doorways, or over the forum of principal houses, on Saint John's day, fully persuaded such types would protect the inmates during the year from maladies and bodily harm.[81]

The name common to the Teutonic races, by which the followers of the curative art appear best known to that portion of the Middle Ages when the doctorates were issued from medical colleges, was the word helari, corresponding to medici or physicians of the codes. Metrical versifiers, so early as the eighth and ninth centuries,[82] use it in this sense, and a similar signification is conveyed in the fragmentary romance of Charlemagne's struggle with the Saracens, written in the

---

[78] Rothii, Eplic. Vocab. Græd., p. 123.

[79] Ibid., p. 122.

[80] Pompon., Mela. De Situ. Orbis., Lib. III., cap. 6.

[81] Rothii, Eplic. Voc. Græd., p. 125.

[82] Othfried, Liber. Evangelica, Lib. II., c. 14, v. 242; and Lib. III., c. 12, v. 35.

thirteenth century by an anonymous author.[83] This poem aptly compares the Saviour to a healer or medicus, in the same phraseology with which classical Apollo might be thus denominated. Belgic conservatism,[84] and English pertinacity, in defiance to dialectic corruption through Norman French, maintained the Heelmester of ancient Frisia, and the healer of the Anglo-Saxons, to that period of the Middle Ages when these were substituted by medicus, Doctor physicus of the university vellum. Before concluding this somewhat detailed inquiry into the external condition of medicine among the ancient Germans, it should be added that in the Beeta of the Runic Chapter, a direct recognition appears of a necessity to combine magic as a potential element in the economy of medicine.[85] The circumstances under which these pagan nations accepted Christian dogmas, without rudimentary alteration of social habits and usages descended from Norse temple worship, contributed to vitalize the doctrine of sickness and disease as the direct outgrowth and emanation of evil spirits, so thoroughly believed by the evangelists, and actually survived, as a part of their own mythology, to these semi-civilized proselytes, and passed with them into the new faith.

At the period of this transmission, the art of curing, whether practised by men or women in the provinces of Germany, had descended the degrading slope of imposition; and in the uncertain amalgamation of Norse polytheism with Christian ritualism, that portion of the healing methods classified as Boeter, involving the use of magic, evidently obtained the ascendency; inasmuch as reiterated Carlovingian legislation was impotent to hinder oft-recurring practice of incantations, soothsaying and prognostications, credulously sought as sure means to health, or prevention of infirmities. Each disease and sickness, afflict-

---

[83] Apollo ther mare,
Unde andere Hailari,
Apollo the renowned,
And other celebrated physicians.

Apud Schilter, Antiq., Teutonic, Tom. II., p. 45.

[84] Rothii, Eplic. Voc. Heilari, p. 128.

[85] "That kann eg beeta, brätt." Runa Capitale, Str. 9.

ing a suffering invalid, the Germanic soothsaying physician asserted could be quickly cured or expelled by the magical insufflation of a murmured word, or by means of enchanted herbs and vitalized stones,[86] a system exactly described in the Boeter.

The prolonged obstinacy which these people exhibited in preserving faith in the efficacy of curious medicinal modes, provoked the ponderous repressive power of the Carlovingian edicts, which categorically interdicted to the populace superstitious usages, and imperatively directed the sacerdoty themselves to desist from propagating these injurious customs, through imprudent indifference or actual acquiescence.[87] Medical formulas of older magicians for centuries survived to their mediæval successors, the rural medical charlatans, who professed prompt cures of ophthalmic disorders by the recitation of ritualistic words, accompanied with suitable gestures of the arms and fingers over the diseased eyes, thrice touched amid guttural murmur as a necessary adjunct to the operation. The following scheme sets forth substantially the curative potency of established methods used by three maiden surgeons, and is an evident perpetuation of that singular remedy for maladies designated by the nomenclature Boeter or Invocation:

"Et gingen ens dre Mäge,
Up enen greunen Wege:
De ene waste wat vorn Bley.
De aure waste wat vorn starr,
De drûdde vôr de hidd vorwar:
Un bôdden dat alle enerley.
Im Namen + Vaders + Sohnes und + Heiligen Geistes. Amen."[88]

---

86 "Nullus morbus, valetudo nulla nullumque infortunium est, quæ non certo oris murmure, attactu, spurcio adflatu, atque fatuis herbarum, ossium, lapidum aliorumque rerum," etc. Rothii, Vocabul. Bœter., p. 139.

87 Baluzius, Cartular. De Partibus Saxonum, cap. 21, Tom. I., col. 254.

88 "Three maidens once going
On a verdant highway;
One could cure blindness,
Another cured cataract,
Third cured inflammation;
But all cured by one means."
In the name of the Father, Son, etc. Rothii, De Vocabulo Bœter, p. 141.

In this venerable conjuration, announcing the prowess of ambulatory female medicists to cure a suffusion and spotted discoloration of the eyes, the essential remedial energy inheres and appears in the bödden, or invocating formula, anciently deduced from a system of incantations accompanied by muttered phrases and geometric figures. We have hitherto narrated the important element of the alraun or mandragora effigies in medical economy, even so late as the age of Charlemagne.

With these and the enchantments, by which cures should be obtained, the runics also figured as a conspicuous factor in the problem. Inasmuch as German virgins,[89] in more remote times, notably essayed the expulsion of diseases, as attested by the preceding spell, they also sought to vanquish by means of curious letters, the spiritual essence of evil, causing bodily infirmities, and combined them with the resistless force of alraun figures.[90] With these images Salic herders distinctly marked their cattle and flocks as an amulet, to paint or brand which upon stolen herds was subject to heavy penalties.[91] The Frisian code, possibly reduced to a written form as early as the time of Charles Martel,[92] and certainly sanctioned by Charlemagne, permitted the use of runic marks in the solemn investigation of assassinations, and thus proclaimed their potency to aid in the detection of crime.[93]

Luxations were cured with speed and certainty when the injured member was brought under the influence of such magic rites. Thus, for instance, beneath the puissant force of Odinic charms, the broken bones of man or beast were readily reunited in perfect health.[94] It may be added here, as indicating

89 Ammianus Marcellinus, Gesta Rom., Lib. XXXI., cap. 2.

90 Grimm, Ueber die Deutsche Runen, p. 296 seq.

91 Lex Salica, Titulus X., cap. 1.

92 Introductio ad Leg. Frision., p. 21.

93 Lex Frision., Tit. XIV., cap. 1.

94 Grimm, Ueber drei Entdeckten Gedichte. Soranus cured maniacs by incantations. Hieron., Mercurialis, De Arte Gymnastic., Lib. VI., c. 5.

the progress of such medicinal methods, after the extinction of the sombre celebration of Norse religion, and its survival under new names to Christianity, that magical rhythms of equally potent surgical properties passed from the sagacious Phol and Odin to the sainted evangelists and their divine Masters.[95] A knowledge of runic remedies appears to have prevailed wherever the Teutonic races were dispersed. So far as the application of these letters to prognostics and auguries may be traced, it is probable the concurrent usage of mandragora cures was equally extensive.[96]

From the previous statements touching the veritable condition of medicine among the people of Western Europe down to the Carlovingian period, and including such nomenclature as aptly expressed the vocation, it is evident that so early as the seventh century the Latin distinctive term of the professors of this art had begun to diminish the frequent use of the native word. A gradual change from the medicus of that epoch, and a total exclusion of vernacular terminology during succeeding ages, elevated the vocable physicus[97] to signify the person, and physicia the occupation, and incorporated the notion of an art practised with thorough cognizance of the recondite secrets and mysteries of natural sciences.

Indeed, from the twelfth century to the close of the Middle Ages the denomination of physicus, or physician, was an equivalent for the vernacular terms above enumerated and explained, as designating a personage abandoned to the curative and medical art, and in no other signification is it used in the mediæval records. In modern times a bold separation of the originally aggregated words, physicus and chirurgicus—physician and surgeon, has divided these to mean prescriptive skill and manual dexterity, although during the Middle Ages they were nearly synonymous.[98] The causes provoking an

---

95 Thorpe, Northern Mythology, Vol. I., p. 23.

96 Beda, Historia Ecclesiastica, Lib. V., c. 11.

97 Du Cange, Glossarium, sub voc. Physicus.

98 Ibid., sub v. Chirurgicus.

ultimate division of a profession formerly uniting both branches of the Æsculapian science, may be gathered from a subsequent portion of this work; and it will suffice to add here, in the literary monuments towards the end of the fifteenth century the words are invariably conjoined, thus: physici chirurgii.[99]

This disjunction, at an earlier period of the Middle Ages, may have been aided by the potential example of Saracen professors of medicine, to whom, throughout this era till the fourteenth century, students of Germany, France and England, and indeed other European countries, faithfully subjected themselves as an obedient soldiery. Moslem scientists, in abandoning almost with contempt the practice of surgery, and confining their erudite investigations to the chemical development of medical science, doubtless largely influenced the debasement of a valuable art.

Other causes forced surgical operations into a most disreputable class of medicastres, to which reference will be made hereafter. Toward the conclusion of the period noted, the vocable physicus or physician, in addition to its curative signification, including surgery, came to receive a more enlarged sense. Popular belief, industriously nurtured by professors of medicine, elevated them to the highest point of scientific knowledge of natural phenomena relating to the human body, and involved mirific puissance to heal present diseases, together with a species of augury and divination for future maladies.[100]

As this word, in its primary meaning, was equivalent among the vulgar and lowly to a penetrating cognizance of natural science, consequently physiculatus, derived from the above, was used from an early period as expressing the skilfullness of a prophet and horuspice.[101] These physici or physicians of

---

[99] Rothii, De Vocabulo Physic., p. 152.

[100] Ibid., p. 154 seq.

[101] "Vox augurum, et aruspicium." Du Cange, Gloss., sub v. Physiculatus; and "Physiculator, augur, naturas in extis aminantium quærens." Martianus Capella, De Nuptiis Philolog. et Mercur., Lib. I.

so remote an age assimilated to their more ancient precursors, in claiming to be illuminated by the divine afflatus of Apollo, and as a sequence asserted their endowment with miraculous abilities to exactly comprehend present diseases, boasting supernal virtues touching possible vicissitudes of fluctuating health and convalescence, even to the fortuitous death of men.[102]

When such high and mighty attributes, arrogated by the mediæval physici, are considered, it will excite no surprise when the tendencies of the times accepted a knowledge of corrupt Latinity as a colossal acquisition favored in University, hall and court, that the vernacular classification of the healing art should recede before this transcendent dialect, and from physicus and chirurgicus, even in smaller provincial towns, arose the modern physician and surgeon.[103]

---

102 Rothii, De Vocab., Physic., p. 154.

103 Du Cange, Glossar., sub v. Chirurgius.

CHAPTER XIII.

Survival of Paganism in Christianity Affects Medical Economy—Abjuration Formulas Recognize Supernatural Forces—Norse Deities of Avowed Personality—Index of Pagan Superstitions as Proscribed—Includes a System of Curatives—Effigies for Medicinal Usage—Sortilege to Evoke Pestilence—Such Remedies Characterized by the Ecclesiastics as "Execrabile"—Sanitary Amulets—Ligatures, or Charmed Remedial Surgery—Preternatural Virtue Recognized by the Chartularies of the Eighth Century—Progress of Saintly Cures—Great Faith in Reliquaries—Trade of Venetians in Reliques—Theft of—Source of Wealth to Cloisters—Their Medical Properties.

THE introduction of Christianity among the Teutonic races offered no hindrance to a perpetuation, under new forms, of those social observances with which Norse temple idolatry was so intimately associated. Offering to proselytes an unlimited number of demoniacal æons, similar in individuality and prowess to those peopling the invisible universe, Northern mythology readily united with the Christian demonology.

This belief, as accelerating the downfall and maintaining the utter prostration of medical science, preserved its primitive vigor by means of the splendid and imposing ceremonies of baptismal rites. During the celebration involved in this solemn service the satanic hosts, as originators of sin, vice, and maladies, were expelled the human body by exorcism,[1] insufflation of the officiating cleric, sign of the cross, and invocation of the Triune Deity. Earlier formulas for such expulsion directed a double exhalation of the priest.[2] Close upon abjurations followed consecration of baptismal fluids, in which the catechumen was placed entirely nude.[3] As early as the fifth century, the formal portion of the abjuration phrases subsequently

[1] Formulæ Exorcismorum; apud Baluz., Cartular., Tom. II., col. 639 seq.

[2] Gregor. Nazien., Orat. De Sec., Adv. —.

[3] Ambros., De Initiat., cap. 11.

adopted by the Latin Church were in vogue, according to the following, reproduced from Salvianus, of Marseilles: "Quid est in baptismo salutori Christianorum prima confessio? Quæ scilicet nisi est renunciare se diabolo ac pompiis ejus, atque spectaculis et operibus protestentur? Abrenuncio enim, inquis, diabolo, pompis, spectaculis et operibus ejus. Et quod postea? Credo, inquis, in deum patrem omnipotentum, et in Jesum Christum, filium ejus.[4]" The synod held at Lepinta in Germany, in the year 743, established by the perfunctory force of civil and canonical law, articles of faith which in future should be received as ecclesiastical dogmas by converted pagans, and in addition to these, promulgated, apparently, a written renunciation of Norse worship.

How far the more venerable abjuration formulas were adhered to may admit of doubtful solution, although it as a manifest portion of ancient rituals become incorporated with the new, particularly the expulsion clause of insufflation.[5] In accordance with an unswerving pontifical and secular policy, the three principal divinities of Asgard, whose original seat of worship was in Upsala,[6] at the period before us, had receded from their exalted eminence as patrons of those virtues so dear and so closely interwoven with the texture of social existence and become distinctly classified as forbidding and repulsive demons, whose ancient puissance to charm away sickness vanished, and was now claimed to create it. The necessity of preparing renunciatory formulas attests the prolongation of a creed in this diabolical essence, and actually accredited by an erudite sacerdoty. These forms, yet extant, are monuments among the oldest of German letters, and of priceless worth as a memorial of an extinct civilization.

Catechumens standing before the sacred font as early as

---

[4] Gubernatione Dei, Lib. VI., cap. 6.

[5] "Deinde exsufflas in Faciem ejusdem et dices; Exi ab spiritus immunde, et redde honorem," etc. "Et dices tribus vicibus." Massman, Abschwöworungs Förmeln, p. 68, No. 2.

[6] Olaus Magnus, Histor. Septentr., Lib. III., cap. 6.

the first half of the eighth century, preceding a formal baptism and acceptance into the Christian Church, were severally interrogated:

"Forsachistu diabolæ?
Et resp. Ec forsacha diabolæ,
End allem diabol geldz?
Respoñ. End ec forsacho allum diabol geldæ.
End altu diaboles vvercum?
Resp. End ec forsacho allum diaboles vvercum and wordum thunaer ende vvoden ende saxnote ende allem them unholdum the hira genotas sind."[7]

It is made imperative, in this confession, to forsake or renounce the culture of other subordinate deities, so numerous in Norse mytholygy, and here referred to under the general denomination of unholden or proscribed demons and their associates.

Another equally important formulary, republished by Massmann, under the caption of Interrogatio fidei,[8] was propounded to the neophyte before entering into full communion:

"Forsachistu unholdun?
Ih forsacho, etc.,
Forsachistu indiwillon?
Ih, etc..
Forsachistu allem dem bluotstrom them heidine man hym Zablustrom in dizageldon habent?
Ih forsacho," etc.

The triple divinities specified in the first abjuration, had a temple, previously alluded to as standing on the shores of Lake Constance in the year 612, which enclosed three gilded effigies—tres deauratas imagines—and was destroyed by Saint Colomban.[9]

Carlovingian rescripts required the church regulation that these formularies be memorized, to be rigidly enforced,[10] and

[7] Massmann, Abschwörungs Förmeln, p. 67, No. 1.

[8] Ibid., fol. 68, No. 2.

[9] Walafrid Strabo, Vita Sancti Galli., Lib. I., cap. 6.

[10] Massmann, Abschwörungs Förmeln, p. 6; and Baluz., Cartular., Tom. I., p. 579.

enacted at Lepinta, that whoever should be convicted of heathen practices, and contrary to the Roman law, including magic remedies for diseases, must liquidate the misdemeanor by a fine of fifteen solidi.[11] The latter chartulary, and the second promulgated in Carloman's reign for the better government of the Latin Church, will fully attest the vitality of paganistic customs, in defiance of an evangelical zeal of nearly two centuries; and to crush out these this edict was especially framed.

The Indiculus Superstitionum et Pagianorum, appended to the rescript, summarizes heathen observances, and categorically forbids them. In their general tendency these interdicted customs involved superstitious recognition of invisible forces, open to possible control for nefarious or benevolent purposes, some of which were directly germane to the curative art. Consequently we reproduce them here:

"I. De sacrilegio ad sepulchra mortuorum. II. De sacrilegio super defunctos, id est, dadsisas. III. De spurcalibus in Februaris. IV. De casulis, id est fanis. V. De sacrilegiis per ecclesias. VI. De sacris silviarum, quæ nimidas vocant. VII. De his quæ faciunt super petras. VIII. De sacriis Mercurii vel Jovis. IX. De sacrificio quod fit alicui sanctorum. X. De phylacteriis et ligaturiis. XI. De fontibus sacrificiorum. XII. De incantationibus. XIII. De auguriis, vel avium vel equorum vel bovum stercore, vel sternutatione. XIV. De divinis vel sortilegis. XV. De igne fricato de ligno, id est, nodfyr. XVI. De cerebro animalium. XVII. De observatione pagana in foco vel in inchoatione rei alicujus. XVIII. De incertis locis quæ colunt pro sacris. XIX. De petendo quod boni vocant Sanctæ Mariæ. XX. De feriis quæ faciunt Jovi vel Mercurii. XXI. De lunæ defectione, quod dicunt Vinceluna. XXII. De tempestatibus et cornibus et calceis. XXIII. De Dulcis circa villas. XXIV. De pagano cursu, quem Yrias nominant, scissis pannis vel calceis. XXV. De eo quod sibi sanctos fingunt quoslibet mortuos. XXVI. De simulacro de consparso farina. XXVII. De simulacris de

[11] Baluzius, Cartularia, cap. 4, Tom. I., p. 150.

pannis factis. XXXVIII. De simulacro quod per campos portant. XXIX. De ligneis pedibus vel manibus pagano ritu. XXX. De eo quod credunt quia feminæ lunam commendent, quod possint corda hominum tollere juxta paganos."[12]

This canonical interdict of these usages, closely identified with the polytheistic celebration of Thor and Odin, designated by the names of Roman prototypes, placed under the ban, sacrifices to these divinities, either upon stones—supra petras;[13] or in shady groves;[14] festivities to the dead—super defunctos—celebrating military prowess of those resting forever beneath a monumental sepulchre, or awaiting the funeral torch to fire the consuming fagots, around which an impatient multitude awaited a generous distribution of dadsisas[15] or death food, partaken at the convivium,[16] or banquet, following the funeral service. The chapter on the sacrifices performed in churches, indicates the prompt amalgamation of not merely ideas touching the puissance and sanctity of Christian martyrs, an exact reproduction of supernatural attributes of Norse deities, but the rapid subrogation of that external pomp which added imposing splendor to the Northern temple worship, and was boldly adapted to the Romish ritual.

Included in the forbidden practices was the preparation of inartistic effigies, carved in imitation of the Upsala deities, sold at trifling cost, and extensively used in sacrificial offerings. The purchase or consumption of these figures was endowed with that marvellous curative and talismanic property which illustrated the mandragora runes, and consequently, was interdicted to Christian proselytes. As a substitute for the effigy of Thor, in the processional circumambulation around the circuit of

---

[12] Baluz., Cartular., A. D. 743, Tom. I., p. 150.

[13] Indiculus Superstit. et Paganiar., cap. 7; ap. Baluz. Cartular., Tom. I., p. 150.

[14] Cluverius, Antiquitat. German., Lib. I., cap. 24.

[15] This food, in the nature of witzelbrod, appears to have been eaten at the tomb. Du Cange, Glossarium, sub v. Dadsisas.

[16] Ibid., sub voc. Convivium.

tillable lands, a statuette of the Holy Virgin was produced, and accorded omnipotent powers to protect future crops and health of herds.[17]

Reference has been hitherto made touching the assumed power of medical women among the pagans, to provoke tenderness and weaken the courage of the boldest into timorous apprehension, by means of irresistible magic spells. The exercise of a potency so dangerous to martial society and the religious fabric of this era, quickly received vigilant attention from ecclesiastical authority, and was promptly forbidden. Identical with the belief of their older Christian precursors, the power of incantation was fully admitted as an essential factor in the causation and cure of sickness; and as an outgrowth of this puissance, prognostications touching the future, whether of health or infirmities, were faithfully accredited.[18]

Sortilege by the brain or other animal matter of man, bird or beast;[19] evoking destructive storms, whether of wind, rain or hail; or auguries from ascending smoke, and the first animal fortuitously met, were solemnly denounced.[20] Of all recited paganistic usages, the practice of which was subjected to pecuniary punishment, those involving the suspension of wooden limbs at the intersection of highways for remedying diseases,[21] and the use of ligatures and phylacteries, are of greatest importance in their connection with the medical economy of the early ages.

So far as the imitated effigies of Northern divinities are concerned, in close relation with the curative property of mandragora runes, we have previously examined this interesting branch of Teutonic medicine. Ligatures, similar to the earlier amulets, whose efficacy was accepted by some medical writers

---

[17] Indiculus, Superstit. et Paganiar, cap. 30.

[18] Rothii, De Vocabulo Physico., p. 54; and Martianus Capella, De Nuptiis Philolog., etc., Lib. I.

[19] Indiculus Superstit., etc., cc. 13, 14 and 16.

[20] Ibid., cc. 17 and 22.

[21] Ibid., c. 29.

and rejected by others[22] as remote as the time of Isidore, appear to have been freely applied to the prevention and cure of maladies.

This erudite encyclopædist, stirred with burning indignation at the successful introduction of a system of cures apostrophized by him as the "most execrable of remedies," proceeds to describe the method of their preparation. After the imposing invocations and addition of mystic characters, these medicinal charms were presumed to be of the greatest efficacy and ready for suspension to the neck. While the Spanish scholastic does not deny the remedial qualities of these ligatures, he expressly charges that they were known and used in Hippocrates' day; and the production of the most pestiferous society of men and malevolent angels, and concludes, "Since they have so diabolical origin, all good Christians should avoid and execrate them."[23]

It will explain the extensive use of the medical curatives by proselytes, when it is stated that the authority of pontifical and secular power, for ages prior to the Carloman chartulary, was indispensable, not alone to hold popular tendencies to such talismans in subjection, but the priesthood itself, a little more enlightened perhaps than the people, was addicted to fastening these ligatures about the necks of men and beasts, and justified the practice on the ground that they contained extracts from sacred scriptures. The pontiffs distinctly asserted that these, instead of constituting a Christian remedy, were the very venom of the Devil.[24]

Oftentimes these sanitary amulets among the Northern converts were prepared with the most pompous incantations and sortileges.[25] As a tribute to the saintly character of a devotee

---

[22] Du Cange, Glossar., sub v. Ligaturæ. The adhesion of Villanova to their effectiveness is doubtful, De Physicis Ligaturis, p. 619; Phylactery talismans in the year 1016. Annalista Saxo., sub an., cit.; ap. Eccard. I., p. 442.

[23] "Salisatores, etc. Ligaturæ execrabilium remedium quæ ars medicinum condemnat." Isidor., Hispal. Etymologior., Lib. VIII., c. 9.

[24] Du Cange, Glossar., sub v. Ligaturæ.

[25] Gregor., Turones. De Miraculis S. Martini, Lib. II., c. 45; and Lib. IV., c. 36.

in the time of Martin, the Frankish saint, it is recited that visiting a sick woman, found with these ligatures upon her, and after removing this evidence of pagan futility, the diseased person was instantly restored to perfect sanity by pouring into her mouth the oil of a holy sepulchre.[26] Down to the age of Boniface, bishop of the Mayence episcopate, these remnants of paganistic medicinal remedies appear to have survived all the the enactments of canon and civil law, inasmuch as this pontiff expressly charges[27] that some of the women of his day were seen with ligatures and phylacteries on their arms and legs as infallible protectors against maladies. Bede states that the Anglo-Saxons made zealous use of such medicinal curatives.[28]

From the text of the rescript decreed by a council of bishops, under the sanction of Charlemagne, in the year 787, at his imperial residence, the followers of this avocation were classified by law as obligatores, who arrange these medical amulets designed to expel demoniacal sickness from the human body.[29] The chapter of the Indiculus above quoted as No. XV., De igne fricato de ligno, id est Nodfyr, seems to have been a usage adopted to a variety of purposes,[30] among which was preservation against diseases by the assumed sanitative power of fire produced by prolonged friction of two twigs.[31]

The apparent singularity of the customs cited recedes before a demonstrable fact, that all these observances and methods, so universally adopted in the interest of good health and indemnity from disease, which indeed, with aged pagans, was equivalent to assassination,[32] were based upon the doctrine of controlling the invisible deities of Asgard and their subordi-

[26] Ibid., op. cit., Lib. II., cap. 32.

[27] "Dicunt quopue se vidisse ibi mulieres pagano ritu phylacteria et ligaturas, et in brachiis, et cruribus ligatas habere." Du Cange, op. cit., v. Ligaturæ.

[28] Beda, Vita S. Guthberti, cap. 16; Ibid., Histor. Ecclesias., Lib. IV., c. 27. On their more ancient use, Eutropius, Hist. Breviar., Rom. Lib. III.

[29] Capitular., Aquisgran, cap. 63.

[30] Du Cange, Glossar., sub v. Nodfyr.

[31] Roskoff, Geschichte des Teufels, Th. I., p. 295.

[32] Simrock, Deutsche Mythologie, p. 232.

nate divinities, the incorporeal but visible beings of Nifelhel. The duration of such faith facilitated the introduction and rapid amalgamation of prior teachings of the Christian Fathers, with the crude yet well defined mythology or demonology of Northern converts. The colossal dimensions of this notion may be inferred from the abjuration formulas reproduced above; and how profoundly the popular mind was impressed with the vast resources of demoniacal hosts, can be gathered from the creeds and confessions prescribed in the eighth century[33]—where the forces of idolatry, poisonings, conjurings, sortilege, and belief in were-wolves,[34] are distinctly incorporate together with diabolical prerogatives.

The cautionary counsels of the Church authorities against the use of phylacteries and the ligatures, were finally, after useless appeals to the clergy and people had been issued, formally interdicted,[35] together with such mystic formulas and prognostications as foolish men hazarded under the very shadow of sacred edifices redolent with paganism, in the name of Holy Martyrs or Saints of God, thus provoking them to wrath, including sacrilegious fires commonly called Nedfratre.[36] Observances of this nature were subject to the prohibitory penalty of reasonable fines, but this practice by the Saxon proselytes was punishable with death.[37]

Substantially the same heathen usages were pressed upon the attention of the clergy by a decree of Charlemagne, in the year 769, with positive instructions to prevent their repetition.[38] To the clergy were committed the grave functions of enforcing varied ecclesiastical statutes enacted to eradicate the vital growth of paganistic rites, among which was the preparation and sale of amulets, ligatures and talismanic phylacteries for

---

33 Massmann, Abschwörungs Förmeln, p. 121, No. 20.

34 Roskoff, Geschichte des Teufels, Th. I., p. 298.

35 Cartular., Carolimanni, an. 742, cap. 5; Baluz. I., col. 148.

36 Du Cange, Glossarium, sub v. Nedfratres.

37 Cartular., De Partibus Saxon., cap. 8; Baluz. I., col. 250.

38 Baluz., Cartular., Tom. I., col. 191.

the prevention or cure of fever and pestilence. While, however, these enlightened edicts added the ponderous force of penal law to this task, the subject-matter of each rescript frankly admitted the abstract existence of those demoniacal powers whose potential elements were only checked by Christian faith and the full exercise of martyrology.

The ordinance of 789 recites the arch-demon as an actual being, and admits the Satanic domination, in declaring: "If any one, deceived by the devil, believes, after the manner of Pagans, that a certain man or woman is a witch and devours men, and shall therefore burn the one so charged, or give the decedent's flesh to be eaten, or eat it himself, he shall be punished with death."[39]

In a cartulary of the same date, the potential invocation of supernatural forces is clearly set forth in an interdiction laid upon the conjuration of hail storms, by means of charts affixed to beams;[40] and it likewise forbade the baptism of bells, presuming, perhaps, the concession of a sacred rite against the mighty bolt of Thor or thunder, might vitalize a venerable heathen superstition. Canonical laws, combined with Carlovingian edicts, were alike impotent to eradicate effectually the supernal force and virtues accorded the ligatures, phylacteries, runic effigies, and other medicinal symbols of the northern proselytes; and in defiance to such legislation they survived as unquestioned curatives to a late period of the Middle Ages.[41]

The politic introduction of idolatry of sainted relics at this period, divided the vulgar mind between a gradually increasing apathy to more ancient rites, and the transmission of medical puissance of older ceremonials to visible remains of divinized martyrs and saints. The attractive elements of this culture involved both financial and spiritual gain to the chapels and monasteries possessing such holy fragments, as

---

[39] Baluz., Cartular., cap. 6, Tom. I., col. 252.

[40] "Nec chartas per perticas appendant propter grandinem." Capitulare Tertium, cap. 18; Baluz., op. cit., p. 244; and Du Cange, Glossar., sub v. Pertica.

[41] Delrio, Disquisition, Magicar., Lib. I., II. and III.

they not only provided a certain remedy for all maladies and criminalities, but as talismans, preserved the devotee against the terrible afflictions of famine in food or water, pestilence, battle and sudden death.[42]

Charlemagne materially enlarged the scope of their possible energies, by an edict requiring all oaths[43] and other civil obligations to be attested upon them by actual contact. Wherever, indeed, these holy remains of martyrs and saints, dead in the odor of superior purity, were exposed to excited impulse of vulgar superstition, whether in cloister or cathedral, a knowledge of their miraculous puissance quickly extended throughout contiguous provinces, and oftentimes into foreign countries.

The chief object in those remote ages appears to have been the possession of desirable reliques, not alone for intrinsic worth, but for the steady and uninterrupted revenues derived from their exposure to suffering sick and infirm, by which means streams of wealth and affluence flowed into monastic and chapter treasuries. In more ancient times these inert objects only obtained simple adoration from zealous Christians, as typical representatives of those who had suffered martyrdom for the new faith, which rapidly increased into a credulity of their supernal powers, at first in the Eastern Empire,[44] and with the introduction of the monastic system in the West the potential efficiency of this cult was quickly recognized.[45]

As early as the ninth century in Western Europe, translation of sainted bones was attended with elaborate and formal ceremonies. When a final depository had been selected, either within the perpetual enclosure of a stone sarcophagus, or exposed to external examination, a sacred edifice of imposing

---

[42] Roskoff, Geschichte des Teufels, Th. II., p. 55.

[43] "Omne sacramentum in Ecclesia aut Supra reliquias juraretur." Cartular., Quartum., an. 803, cap. 57; Baluz., Tom. I., col. 398.

[44] Beausobre, Histoire du Manicheisme, Tom. II., pp. 638–642, 652.

[45] Gregor., Turones. Vita S. Martini, Lib. II., c. 32; and Lib. IV., c. 36; and Beda, Histor. Eccles., Lib. I., cc. 18 and 21.

proportions was erected over them, and thenceforth the affluence of their religious custodians was assured. It is related when the body of Saint Sebastian, legitimately procured from Rome, together with the purloined remains of Saint Gregory, arrived at the cloister of Soissons, so great was the spontaneous aggregation of invalids who sought the medicinal virtues of these relics, that they came in troops, weighted with bodily ills, but departed wholly healed and thoroughly robust.[46] The influx of gold from grateful donors was so vast that the monks actually counted eighty measures of money, and a hundred pounds in coin.[47] The immense value of such objects may be readily calculated when it is stated in the year 1056 Berengar pledged securities to the amount of ten thousand solidi, for the production of the reliques of SS. Just and Pastor, upon the legal decision of ownership between him and a Narbonnese Archbishop.[48]

Among the first to realize the unbounded commercial worth of these adored and medicinal materials were Venetian merchants, whose resources, developed by the fortuitous circumstances of their illustrious metropolis, enabled them to undertake this lucrative traffic in oriental ports, where naturally these revered remains were most plentiful. Notwithstanding the government of Venice delayed instituting public marts or fairs until the eleventh century, there were in the cities of Rome and Pavia such enterprises a long time anterior, for commercial exchange.[49]

In order to swell the concourse of pilgrims frequenting these displays, originally suggested by pious and infirm wanderers to the sacred relics of an enshrined martyr, especial indulgences were granted by the pontiffs, together with important

---

[46] Acta SS. Boland., Jan. 20, Tom. II., p. 259.

[47] Roth., Beneficienwesen, Th. I., p. 255.

[48] "Et volui ei dare obsides per decem millia solidos, ut si ullus homo vel femina ullam vim ei faceret de ipsorum corpora sanctorem," etc. Baluz., Concilia Narbonn., p. 15.

[49] Du Cange, Gloss., sub v. Foras.

immunities and franchises. Meanwhile nothing was neglected which could augment the patron saint's celebrity, under whose tutelary protection the fair was solemnly placed, and each opportunity was eagerly seized of procuring relics already celebrated for their miraculous powers.[50]

As a suitable guarantee for the institution of a public mart in Germany, the Reichsberg annals[51] state that the emperor demanded certain hostages, or the holy arm of Saint George. The Venetians, not satisfied with establishing a fair in honor of Saint Mark, their tutelary protector, and others, purchased famous relics wherever they were procurable. It is, indeed, stated by way of accusation that a negotiation for an exchange of a well-preserved body of Saint Tairise, ancient patriarch of Byzantium, having terminated unsuccessfully, because the Greek monks who possessed it refused absolutely to sell or barter, these enterprising traders quietly stole the desired skeleton.[52]

Mediæval bishops used these saintly fragments to obtain contributions for the construction or repair of sacred edifices. For this purpose these venerated objects were circulated among the people of the episcopate under priestly surveillance, and formally presented with urgent request for pecuniary gifts;[53] and as a consideration for liberal advances, these bones were as freely applied to the cure of obstinate diseases, as the rifled contents of the Wisigothic tombs.[54]

Official sanction, given at an early age to the Agnus Dei, excited a deep and devoted interest in their medical economy.[55] These pellets of paschal wax, distributed to the people after the impressive ceremonies of Sabbatic consecration, were care-

---

50 Daru., Histoire du Venise, cap. 33, Tom. I., p. 30 seq.

51 Chronicon Reichensperb, p. 263.

52 Daru., Histoire de Venise, Tom. I., cap. 34. In the year 1175 the Venitian merchants stole such sanctified bones from Alexandria, in Egypt. Arnoldi, Chronic. Slavorum, Lib. VII., cap. 8.

53 Du Cange, sub v. Reliquæ.

54 Lex Wisig., Lib. IX., Tit. II., Lex. 2.

55 Walafrid Strabo, De Rebus Eccles., cap. 22.

fully preserved in humble domiciles as a resistless amulet against disease, or set up within the circumscribed precincts of vineyards and arable fields, became a talisman against demoniacal prestige, and the crushing force of thunder.[56]

---

[56] Du Cange, op. cit., sub v. Agnus Dei.

CHAPTER XIV.

Rise and Progress of Saint Gall—Its Influence on Art and Medical Culture—Lazaretto for Lepers Early in the Ninth Century at this Cloister—Gardens for Botanicaland Pharmaceutical Purposes—Hraban Maur Digests in the Ninth Century a Glossary of Physiology in the Native Idiom for Teutonic Students—Collection of Medical MSS. by this Monastery in the Early Ages—Noted Professor of this Art—His Knowledge of Chemistry—Miracle Cures—Curious Means of Preserving Infant Life—Precious Relics—Sources of Monastic Affluence.

FROM the middle of the eighth century until the early part of the ninth, the cloister of Saint Gall advanced slowly, if at all, along the splendid pathway predicted by its founder.[1] Exposed from its very origin to unmeasured exactions and impositions of the bishops of the Constance Episcopacy, its progress in the development of those arts and sciences receiving close and faithful attention, was hindered for nearly a century. In the year 816, abbot Gozpert having secured a ratification of the ancient conventual franchises, and the concession of priceless immunities, upon the abbey subjecting itself to a scrutinizing inquisition,[2] he was at liberty to construct an edifice of suitable proportions for monkish abodes, and in harmony with the monastery's great name.

From the plan of this prospective structure in its architectural details, indications sufficiently attest a decided advance in this art, under the cultivated attention of an expert draughtsman, evidently the illustrious scholar, Raban Maurus.[3] Among essential apartments sketched out as the draft of the new cloister, was the school-room for conventual pupils, and an infirmary or hospital for the sick and infirm, and a sort of Lazaretto for those suffering from contagious diseases.

[1] Otte, Geschichte der Bankunst, p. 101.

[2] Ratpert., Monach. De Origene et Diversis Casib. S. Galli., cap. 5.

[3] Otte, Geschichte der Bankunst, p. 96.

This erudite scholastic, in accordance with whose plan, still preserved on parchment, the monastery was constructed, also drew out private chambers for a chief physician—medici ipsius. These were composed of three communicating apartments contiguous to the Lazaretto. To these in close union was added a room where medicaments were stored and classified under the denomination of pharmacy. Equally significant for the possible progress of medicine within the abbeys of this age, was a botanical garden attached to this convent, and whose productions of vegetables, plants, roots, etc., were gathered especially for medicinal purposes.[4] Raban Maurus, to whom the above described vellum plan of the medical and pharmaceutical apartments has been justly ascribed, was tutor of Walafrid Strabo, the celebrated historian of Saint Gall, and as chief of the Fuldane school, was evidently selected for his artistic abilities and sincere piety. That Maurus evinced a deep and enduring interest in the substantial advance of medicine, and therefore drafted suitable chambers for the monastic medicus or physician, rests upon other and more positive information touching his skillful knowledge of the human frame.

Whether prior or subsequent to the year 820, when the plan alluded to was traced, this scholastic priest, afterwards bishop of Mayence,[5] carefully collated and translated the names of minutest portions of human physiology from their Latin terminology in the Teutonic language.[6] Such translations were evidently rendered essential to the tuition of convent scholars, who by the law of Charlemagne at this epoch, were required to be instructed in medicinal art. For the German youth a glossary of this description was an indispensable necessity for a correct understanding of the subject.

It should be added that the German language of that date appears to have readily provided proper names to the several

---

[4] Ibid., p. 101.

[5] Goldastius, Rerum Alemannic., Tom. I., p. 140.

[6] De Partibus Humani Corporis; ap. Goldast., Tom. II., p. 64 seq.

hundred technical Latin terms descriptive of human anatomy.[7] The formal consecration of a part of the newly-erected edifice and its outlying grounds to medical habitation and pharmacy, attests unequivocally that as early as the ninth century the Carlovingian rescript was effectually followed by instruction in the art and preparation of medicines, and administering remedies thus prepared to the inmates and distressed strangers applying for succor.[8] About the middle of this century, Grimold, who had successfully conducted the priory of Saint Gall for many years, influenced by the infirmities of an advanced age, surrendered the practical administration of this rapidly increasing cloister into the hands of his colleague Hartmuth. With the sagacious supervision of this illustrious monk, the new edifice advanced to completion, rendered additionally attractive by the embellishments and decorations of foreign and conventual artificers. Hartmuth's especial claim to illustration was justly due to an aggregation of manuscript volumes, which for that period, and at so remote a distance from the centers of such traffic, where books were multiplied by copyists and sold for enormous prices, may be characterized as extraordinary.

Great zeal was manifested by Charlemagne to propagate this interesting branch of industry, who sought by personal example,[9] and by an edict, to render the multiplication of copies an uninterrupted portion of the monastic system.[10] To the manuscripts already at hand, collected by the enlightened efforts of his predecessors, especially by the renowned Gozpert, Hartmuth, during the lifetime of his inferior associate, added a

---

[7] A curious exemplar of such translation may be found in Nithardi, Historia de Dissent., Filior., etc.; Lib. III., sub an. 843, at which time the imperial contestants obligated themselves with vernacular oath. Correct construction of this formula in Massmann, Abschwörungs Förmeln, p. 180 seq.

[8] "Fuere autem qui medicinem et herbariam profiterentur, tanta facilitata, ut externos etiam et peregrie profectos ad curationem admitterent." Vadian, De Colleg. Monast. Veterib., Lib. I., p. 23.

[9] Eiginhard, Vita Caroli Magni, cap. 25.

[10] Cartulare, an. 789, cap. 70; ap. Baluz., Tom. I., pp. 237 and 714.

great quantity of original treatises, or as the chronist modestly states it, "he assembled no small lot of books."[11] Among this commendable selection, as may be supposed, such works relating to ecclesiastical history, dogmas and monastic regulations, naturally exceeded the books on other subjects.

The writings of Josephus and the encyclopedia of Isidore were collected by the enthusiastic scholastic, and placed with others in the conventual library.[12] Upon the accession of this monk to an undivided prelatial dignity in the year 872, he further enlarged the library by an addition of the biographies of the founders of the abbey Saint Gall; Martin, the Gallic martyr, and Saint Othmer, together with one volume of the polyhistor Solinus.

This collection was afterwards increased by a donation of other books which he had prepared for personal use and in the most pleasing style.[13] The writings of Bœthius, De Consolatione, so highly prized during the Middle Ages, and frequently translated into vernacular dialects,[14] and the treatises of Orosius Martianus,[15] De Nuptiis Mercuri et Philologiae, otherwise the Seven Liberal Arts, at a later period of his life were added to the abbey collection. It seems the abbot possessed a duplicate copy of the Consolatio by Bœthius, in five volumes, and also executed with his own skilled hand a map of the world in the most subtle and accurate style.[16]

Included in the aggregation of books made by Hartmuth, and presented to the abbey library, were two volumes of the Etymologies of Isidore, one of which was exclusively confined to the subject of medicinal art.[17] Whether this monastery

---

[11] "Librorum etiam non parvam capiam sub eodem abbate Hartmatus Composuit," Ratperti, De Origen. et Divers. Casib. S. Galli., cap. 9.

[12] Ibid., cap. 9.

[13] Ratpert, De Orig. et Diver. Casib., cap. 10.

[14] Jo. Crofti, Chronicon, sub an. 1401.

[15] Usually written with Capella, Orosius suppressed.

[16] "Inter hos unam mappam mundi subtili opere patravit." Ratperti, op. cit., cap. 10.

[17] Nec non et Homiliæ Caesarii in Vol. I.; Etymologiorum Isidori, Vol. II.; "Medicinalis liber unus." Ibid.

possessed the writings of other medical authorities besides Isidore and Hippocrates, is uncertain, although it is by no means improbable that outside of the cloister of Monte Cassino, where this art was treated as a system, such treatises by pagan scholars and scientists were exposed to suspicion at this early age. Among the scholastic magnates domiciled in Saint Gall under the priorate of Cralo, four were especially famous: Geraldus, on account of his solid erudition in the liberal arts and sciences, was master of the convent school from early youth to advanced age; Burkhard, from his singular wealth of scientific and religious endowments, was deemed a suitable personage for the sacerdotal robes; and Notker, alike distinguished for the severity of discipline which secured for him the cognomen of Pipergrannus,[18] or bitterly severe, and his high excellence as doctor and painter. Of those gifts, however, which elevated him above his associates, a rare acquaintanceship with the practice of medical art signalized him in the early part of the tenth century.[19]

The monastic chronicler distinctly asserts that the contributions of Notker, the Doctor, to both the arts of painting and medicine, would amply furnish materials for a great volume.[20] Of the former, many specimens were yet visible in the time of Ekkehard, his biographer, preserved in elegant ornamentation of the portals and mural decorations of the church of Saint Gall, and in the attractive illuminations of numerous manuscripts in the convent library. At a comparatively early period of his habitation in the monastery, under the administration of Solomon, abbot, he was celebrated for a profound knowledge of musical science.

Whether it was the figures of the notes, with their heavy sombre colors, or a supposed intimacy with demoniacal spirits, during the last years of the ninth century this illustrious

---

[18] Du Cange, Glossar., sub v. Pipergrannus.

[19] Ekkehardi, jun., De Casibus Monast. S. Galli., cap. 9.

[20] "De Notkero vero doctore, pictore et medico, cum materiam grandis voluminis habeanus." Ibid., cap. 13.

scholastic and physician was accused of unnatural arts, attested by the actual presence of black books of the Devil,[21] an inculpation urged against him by a monastic inmate—the master of conventual builders—decanus operis.[22] In the curative art, however, his knowledge and successful cures were so great that he was distinguished from a predecessor of like name, by the nomenclature of physicus or physician.[23] From the close of the ninth to the third decade of the tenth century,[24] the reputation of Notker was continually ascending, on account of remarkable cures performed by his medical treatment of maladies universally regarded as incurable. In addition to the medicinal etymology of Isidore, which the monastic library possessed since the time of Hartmuth, this illustrious monk had profoundly imbued his mind with the medical aphorisms, specific antidotes, and prognostics or diagnosis of Hippocrates;[25] so that his acquaintanceship, and, indeed, a remarkable one for that period of medicine, was procured from the writings of the sage of Chios, and, doubtless, involved familiarity with the abstract principles of this art.

Notker's evident readiness in detecting the trick of Duke Henry, by substituting human fluids in order to test the knowledge of the Saint Gall physician, attests both a high proficiency in the essential elements of chemistry, since he not only discovered the crafty substitution, but predicted events based on this inspection, which ultimately occured,[26] and dem-

---

[21] "Ne miremini, inquit, si Diaboli, à quo nigros libros noctibus discunt, falcinatorum suorum," etc. Ibid., cap. 3,

[22] Du Cange, Glossarium, sub v. Decanno Operis.

[23] "Unus dicebatur Notkerus Physicus, vir multæ scientiæ," etc. Ekkehardi, Minim., De Vita Notkeri Balbuli, cap. 4.

[24] Vadiani, Chronologia Abbat. S. Galli., sub an. 942.

[25] "Medendo autem mira et stupenda frequenter fecerat, quoque, quoniam et in Aphorismis medicinalibus, speciebus quoque et Antidotis, et Prognosticis Hippocraticis erat instructus." Ekkehardi jun., De Casibus et Eventibus, etc., S. Galli., cap. 13.

[26] "Ut in urina Hienrici Ducis versute se decipere temptantis apparuit." Ibid. Urinal inspection in Cassiodorus' day as part of medical practice. Edicta Reg., Ostrogothor., c. 19.

onstrates further the undoubted application of strangers to the conventual pharmacy for medical treatment.

When, moreover, the diocesan bishop was produced before this renowned physician for medicinal attendance in a pustular malady, he unhesitatingly asserted his ability to repress the eruptions, but declined, and attributed the refusal to a disinclination to become incriminated with the prelate's death, which would surely ensue if such treatment were adopted. He also predicted an entire cure for the pontiff without the disorder leaving the slightest trace visible.[27] According to the phraseology used by Ekkehard, the annalist of Saint Gall, in portraying the closing scenes of the venerable Keroldo's life, resembling the imposing death of the Anglo-Saxon Beda,[28] when the dying monk, whose eminent abilities and many virtues entitled him to exalted praise, asked for Notker, it is parenthetically stated he was then "in the royal hall, selecting remedies."[29]

During the audience with Otho, emperor of Germany, to whom a delegation of monastic electors officially announced the death of his predecessor and the elevation of Notker to the vacant priorate of Saint Gall, he was referred to as a medicus, in terms indicating a celebrity even in the imperial court.[30] In alluding to certain conventual brethren of this renowned abbey, who were regarded as pillars of the church by their utterances and example, a venerable chronicler praises the clerical surgeon for his mathematical skill.[31] The curious means resorted to for the preservation of the infant existence of Burkard, subsequently prior of Saint Gall, as a sample of surgery towards the close of the ninth century, will attest the anxiety to prolong human life in those remote ages. When it became an unquestioned fact that the mother was rapidly

---

[27] Ekkehard, jun., De Casib. et Eventib., etc., cap. 18.

[28] Simon. Dun., Histor. Ecçlesiæ, Lib. I., cap. 15.

[29] "Erat enim ille tunc pro remediis in aula regia." Ibid., cap. 14.

[30] Ibid., cap 16.

[31] Cunrad. Fabar., De Casib., Monast. S. Galli, cap. 3.

declining in health before the entire fruition, preparations were made to save the offspring.

Fourteen days prior to full maturity the parent died, whereupon, according to this startling legend, the child was removed by excision, yet alive, and carefully wrapt in the skin of a swine just slaughtered.[32] During the priorate of Thieton, in the first part of the tenth century,[33] the cloister chapel was almost totally destroyed by fire. Pending this sad fatality, which, however, attested the notable puissance of saintly relics, great numbers of the books in the abbey library were stolen by irresponsible persons summoned thither under the ostensible purpose of aiding to save the edifices adjoining the burning church. Most strenuous efforts were made by the conventual brethren and their lay assistants, to preserve the holy bones of Saint Othmer from combustion.[34]

However singular it may appear, the facts confronting us even simultaneously with the undisputed excellence of Notker's medical skill, require an unreserved admission that, notwithstanding the possession of treatises on medicine by Isidore and the illustrious sage of Chios, permitting the application of this art to diseases in the infirmary of Saint Gall, the anomaly of the Middle Ages exists, of an increasing confidence in miraculous cures by consecrated wax, or contact with idolized relics. Before the middle of the ninth century, an event occurred in this cloister, which offers the exact prototype of a saintly pathological remedy in the twelfth century at Monte Cassino, where scientific curatives had been exhausted, and as a last resort St. Bernard, of Clairvaux, was called to operate a restoration to health.[35] A certain monk of Saint Gall, as the annalist alleges, "possessed of no slight instruction in medical science,[36]

---

[32] "Infans excisus et aruinæ porci recens erucæ ubi incutescere et involutus." Ekkehard, op. cit., cap. 10.

[33] Vadiani, Chronologia, sub an. 923.

[34] Ekkehard, jun., De Casib. Monaster. S. Galli, cap. 6.

[35] Fleury, Histoire Ecclesiastique, Tom. XIV., p. 509.

[36] "Frater quidam ejusdem congregationis medicinali scientia non ignobiliter instructus." Walafrid Strabo, Vita B. Galli, Lib. II., cap 37.

at a time prescribed for such operations by canon and imperial law,[37] attempted the regulation blood-letting or phlebotomy by incising a vein; but owing to the haste with which the surgery was performed, not only the arm actually lanced, but his entire body, swelled up as a vast tumor. His condition became quickly moribund, especially after the application of the highest skillfulness known to medical art had proved nugatory. The ensuing evening he beheld a personage of candid and venerable appearance approach him in a dream, who inquired touching the mortal infirmity. Upon being informed of the fruitless attempts of science to restore health, the old man directed him to repair at morning twilight to the crypt, where a flaming light blazed in perpetual flame before an altar within which reposed the bones of Saint Gall, and that of the oil which furnished the material for such holy combustion, he should anoint his wounds, which act would instantly heal the suffering invalid. Following the advice of the nocturnal visitant, and applying the remedy, he was immediately cured.[38] In the year 811, Wolflems having resigned the direction of this cloister upon his accession to the Constance episcopate, he dedicated a church to the patron Saint of the monastery and the Holy Mother. The relics, or body of Saint Gall, being translated to their final domicil—an altar especially constructed for this purpose—proved to be a standing and effective remedy for the cure of gout.[39]

Fragments of the true cross suspended to a tree, in addition to sanitary powers, were of sufficient potency to evoke divine manifestation for the proper location of sacred edifices. Saint Magnus,[40] who appears to have carried these puissant objects around with him, completely vanquished demons who fre-

---

37 By a cartulary of Charlemagne in the year 789, the nuns were forbid resorting to this operation in order to provoke an unnatural fairness of face: "Et de pallore earum propter sanguinis minuationem." Capitulare Tertium, cap. 3.

38 Walafrid Strabo, Vita B. Galli, Lib. II., cap. 37.

39 "Curatus à podagra per ipsius merita." Vadiani, Chronologia, sub an. 811.

40 Theodor. Eremit., De Vita S. Magni Confessoris, Lib. II., cap. 6.

quented a locality selected for a chapel, through the terrible name of Adonai.

When the omnipotent relics of Saint Blasius were translated from Rome to the monastery of Saint Gall, the specified spot for the altar which contained them was designated by a miracle as strange as the supposed talismanic powers of its patron's mouldering bones.[41] Among other wonderful attributes conceded to the celebrated Isone, a monk inhabiting this cloister, was the preparation of an ointment of such resistless curative virtue, that oftentimes lepers, paralytics, and the sightless, were instantly restored to perfect sanity by anointing the affected parts.

The supremacy of the founder of this abbey over the foul demon vexing, as we have narrated, the ducal daughter of Burgundy, was revealed in a miraculous cure of the suffering girl; and as usual in such cases, the grateful prince caused the construction of an imposing edifice for a perpetual monument of the demoniacal exorcism and of parental gratitude.[43] The chronicler of this saint's life, as a fitting testimonial of his divine prowess in posthumous remedies for the sick and infirm, states that wax from tapers illuminating the ends of the altar enclosing Saint Gall's mortal remains, was an instantaneous cure in violent toothache, diseased eyes, and total deafness.[44]

Eyesight was restored to the blinded orbs of a humble merchant, seeking the blood-stained marks upon the chapel of Saint Magnus, under the inspiration of a divine impulse, and feeling his uncertain way by a staff to the place where these discolorations reappeared more distinctly after each washing

---

[41] Anonym. Script., De Vita S. Findiani, cap. 6.

[42] Ekkehard, jun., De Casib. Monast., cap. 2.

[43] Walafrid Strabo, De Vita B. Galli, Lib. I., cc. 16 and 19.

[44] "Nam quicunque dentium fatigatii doloribus vel oculorum latitudine vel aurium præclusione laborantes de eisdem cerus quippiam ceræ tulerunt," etc. Ibid., Lib. I., c. 34. Dental surgery was carefully prescribed in the 11th century by Constans Afer., Liber de Chirurgia, cap. 35, p. 339.

with heavy layers of lime.[45] A vase used by the martyred Willabrod for bathing thrice a year, still holding its partially solidified water by divine invocation after her death, was of great medicinal energy in diverse ailments.[46] How profoundly this system of ready recurrence to saintly curatives was impressed upon early mediæval medical economy, appears from the hasty recourse to the restorative forces of this virgin, by an artificer wounded in elevating, with his confréres, an enormous quadrate stone to an elevated point in a side wall. This block, through incautious handling, glided and fell upon a workman's foot and crushed it. He was immediately carried to the diversorium or infirmary, and the mangled member carefully anointed with wax. Insisting upon being borne to the sepulchre of Willabrod, it is asserted he obtained so quickly the gracious attention of the entombed saintess, that the following day at dawn, entirely restored to primitive vigor, he went to work with the operatives.[47]

It will sufficiently appear from the summary touching medicinal puissance of sainted relics, how vast, of necessity, the affluence of wealth must have been to a conventual treasury, where fragments of martyred dead were endowed with miraculous remedies. Further reference to this usage will be made hereafter, as an index of that abiding faith of the Middle Ages touching demoniacal causation of sickness, whose prompt and efficacious expulsion was submissivly conceded to be inherent in adored types of Omnipotent force, which vanquished diabolical and vexatious maladies.

Therefore, the possession of valued relics was an unfailing source of riches to a cloister, and oftentimes the unremitting exertions of these religious bodies to procure them provoked an interference of authority to divide contested acquisitions.[48]

---

45 Hepidani Cœnob., De Miraculis Wibordiæ Virginis, Lib. I., c. 35.

46 "Sed etiam post martyrium pro diversis languoribus medicabile fuit, et est." Hepidani, Cœnob., De Miraculis Wibord. Virgin., Lib. I., c. 20.

47 Ibid., Lib. II., cap. 16.

48 Wolteri, Chronica Bremensis, sub an. 888.

Not unfrequently documentary evidence of authenticity accompanied a gift of relics, and furnished legal proof of ownership, as early as the ninth century.[49] Such donations were regarded as the most precious presents, and chronicled in the conventual annals as events of high importance.[50] The procuration of Saint Peter's knife by a German monastery in the twelfth century was deemed the most illustrious act of a benevolent abbot.[51]

In the same age a certain nobleman, on a pious pilgrimage to Jerusalem, after long and patient importunity, succeeded in obtaining at enormous cost trifling particles of the relics of Abraham, Isaac, and Jacob, which, enclosed in a priceless box, he donated to the monastery of Saint Gall. This gift was regarded so inestimable that it is the single event of the year; but when it is considered, wherever these sainted fragments were deposited, throughout that vicinity there was uninterrupted peace, unstinted plenty, and salubrious air, the suppression of other matters is amply explained.[52] Amid the sacking of Constantinople by the Frankish forces in the beginning of the next century, the principal object of their ferocious cruelties and vigilant searches was the acquisition of precious relics.[53]

Among these were drops of the Saviour's blood, large pieces of the true cross, bones of Saints John the Baptist and James, and parts of the body of Saint George. Many of these it seems were obtained by a Cistercian monk by the name of Martin, through whom portions were distributed throughout Alsace and Germany.[54]

---

[49] Ibid.

[50] Chronicon Rastedense, sub an. 1121.

[51] "Et hic gladium sive cultrum Sancti Petri," Ibid., sub an 1190.

[52] "Ubicumque autem reliquæ fuerint, ut illi testati sunt illic pax, et augmentum, et lenitas æris semper erit." Hepid. Cœnob., Annales, sub an. 1180.

[53] "Spe lucri . . . reliquiis sanctorum innumerabilium, quibus hæc civitas præstabat omni Orienti." Otto Fris. Chr. Cont. Sanblas, cap. 49.

[54] Otto Frising. Chronicon, Continuat Sanblas, cap. 49.

These relics, captured in Constantinople, were divided by the troops under Marquis de Montfort, with the same justice as prevailed in the division of other booty. In this way the Venetians were enabled to enrich their metropolis with a piece of the sainted cross, an arm of Saint George, part of the head of Saint John the Baptist, the entire skeleton of Saint Luke, that of the prophet Saint Simeon, and a small bottle of Jesus Christ's blood.[55] The Greek capital from the remotest times appears to have monopolized this traffic in sacred wares, claiming to possess a fragment of the stone on which Jacob slept, and the staff transformed into a serpent by Moses.

Here also were guarded the Holy Virgin's vestments, her spindle, drops of her milk, the cradle in which the Saviour had lain, a tooth from his adolescent jaw, a hair of his beard, a particle of bread used in the Last Supper, and a portion of the royal purple worn by him before Pilate.[56] Naturally clerical adventurers among the occidental Crusaders, pending the sacking of the Byzantine city, sought out most zealously these valuable remnants of pristine glory, and in obtaining them were by no means scrupulous with menaces and violence.[57] When scattered through Western Europe, in the monasteries and other religious places, their curative properties increased the pilgrimages thither of the sick and diseased.

---

[55] Daru., Histoire de Venise, Tom. I., p. 64 seq.

[56] Roskoff, Geschichte des Teufels, Th. II., p. 54.

[57] Daru., op. cit., Tom. I., p. 64.

CHAPTER XV.

Monastery of Salerno—Celebrated for its Medical School in the Ninth Century—Contest of Duplicity and Poison between a Bishop and a Salernite Professor—MSS. of Hippocrates and Galen Carried in Journeys by Monks—A Youthful Cleric and Medical Student—Monkish Professor of this Art—Progress of the Celebrity of Salerno in the Tenth and Eleventh Centuries—Doubtful Methods of Increasing this Fame—A Monopoly of Curatives Established by Force—Imperial Sufferers seek Remedies There—Metrical Version of Hygienic Advice to an English King—Archbishop as Skilled Surgeon—Professional Writers of this Age—Avocation of Medicine Exclusively in Hands of Clergy—Its Great Lucrativeness—Synods Interdict its Practice by Ecclesiastics for Compensation.

THAT Carlovingian legislation, touching the medical education of youth aggregated in monastic schools, manifested beneficial results from an early period, independent of the high powers attributed to relics as curatives, admits of historical proof, although to what extent such instruction was based on the writings of Hippocrates and Galen is uncertain. Before the close of the ninth century, under the reign of Carloman, king of Bavaria, Wigbert, ordained as bishop of Mayence, appears to have attained, prior to the year 880, when he died, a high distinction for profound knowledge of medicine.[1]

In addition to this justly acquired celebrity, the illustrious pontiff obtained grateful recognition from his monastery by the gift of books which he had accumulated and adorned entirely by personal embellishment.[2] It may be fairly inferred that a portion of these numerous volumes included treatises on the practice of that science which had aided in his illustration. In the year 946, a species of contest for medical supremacy

[1] "Qui suo tempore medicinæ artis peritissimus fuit." Annalista Saxo, sub anno 880.

[2] Catalog., Episcop. Hildes, ap. Leibnit., Tom. I., pp. 743 and 772.

occurred between bishop Deroldus and a Salernite physician, in the presence of Otho, emperor of Germany.[3]

This incident vindicates the assumption that early in the tenth century, the subsequently renowned school of Salerno was already reputed for its comparatively elevated standard of the curative art. This struggle, attesting an expansion of a system beyond the crude remedies of holy shrines, is worthy of reproduction. Deroldus, for whom the king entertained a passionate attachment, had the fame of profound medical skill. It is narrated of him by a contemporary annalist, that being deceived by a Salernite medicus or physician, he succeeded in duping the scholastic of the celebrated college.

Notwithstanding the rivals were equally versed in a knowledge of medical secrets, the royal preference leaned towards the skillfulness of bishop Derold, while the queen consort especially patronized the Salernite. A discussion arose between them touching individual profundity in the nature of things confessedly within the boundaries of this art.[4] To propositions upon such subjects hazarded by the king in their mutual presence, answers were made with the best possible effect. It is stated that the ecclesiastic, from his thorough acquaintanceship with letters, responded with greater lucidity; while, indeed, the Salernite, unskilled in polite literature, was impartially awarded superior natural endowments, and a more correct experience in the disputed subject.

One day, occupying the regal table, where they dined together, a heated argument originated as to the relative remedial properties of pharmacy, surgery and botany.[5] It will be observed that at the remote period under notice a clear distinction appears to have been obtained touching the technical denomination of these branches of medicine; and strange to relate, the Salernite medicus or physician, ignorant

---

[3] Richerius, Historiarum, Lib. II., cap. 59.

[4] Richerius, Historiar., Lib. II., cap. 59.

[5] "Tractatumque uberius, quid efficiat farmaceutica, quid vero cirurgica, quid etiam butanica." Ibid.

of the foreign names given to these divisions, blushed and was silent.[6] So highly incensed was the Italian medicastre that he dexterously infused a deadly poison into the pontiff's food, which caused him to fall. Upon removal, he administered an andidote—teriaca—which as promptly expelled the destructive principle of the noxious drug. Three days afterwards he returned to the royal court, and, on answer to inquiry, responded that his infirmity "was a severe cold,"[7] in order to quiet the defiance of the Salernite, and render him incautious.

The crafty bishop, thoroughly skilled it appears in toxicants, with the utmost dexterity concealed a powder between his fingers, and while his medical antagonist raised a portion of food to eat, slyly scattered the deadly granules over it unperceived.[8]

Upon the king's most imperative request, and the suffering Italian's vehement prayer, the bishop administered antidotes, but carefully desisted from entirely curing his penitent rival; as a consequence, the left foot was permanently affected.[9] The response made by the Salernite physician, touching his infirmity, is abundant evidence of the degraded condition of medicine at that epoch. He asserted "the poison had been driven by the antidotes through the veins into the disabled limb." Finally the epidermis seems to have been attacked by the venomous drug, sickness ensued, and, to save his life, the foot, amid great agony, was amputated by surgeons.[10] In those distant ages it was by no means an infrequent occurrence for a cleric, devotedly inclined to a practical culture of the Æsculapian art, to carry with him a well-worn manuscript copy of Hippocrates or Galen, in order to study the rudiments of cures

[6] "Et Salernitanus, peregrina nomina non advertens, ab eorum interpretatione erubescens quiebit." Ibid.

[7] "Fleumatis frigdore se levitur tactum respondit." Ibid.

[8] "Deroldus toxicam inter auricularem ac salutarem, occultatem ejus cibo sumend respersit." Richer., Historiar, Lib. II., cap. 59.

[9] "Nam sumpta teriaca, vis veneri in pedem sinistrum penitus dilapsa est." Ibid.

[10] "Factoque morbo, post a cirurgis miserabiliter absciditur." Ibid.

commented upon by these venerable writers of medical science.

In the year 991, a monk traveling from the city of Rheims to Carnotum or Chartres, utilized with avidity the time consumed in the journey by pondering the logic of Hippocrates on liberal studies.[11] The monastic student, having accomplished the object of the voyage alluded to, and being relieved of all solicitude, proceeded with the study of the Hippocratian aphorisms, under the direction of Herbrand, a person of eminent celebrity and science.

When at length the youthful cleric had familiarized himself with the prognostication of diseases, and recognized that a simple acquaintanceship with maladies would not suffice a person desiring thorough information, he besought his patron to permit him the perusal of a work evidently digested by Herbrand, which was inscribed: Concordance of Hippocrates, Galen and Soranus.[12] This he obtained, and it was deemed a treatise equally erudite in dinamidia—perhaps dynamical forces—pharmacy, botany and surgery.[13] His master, the compiler of the volume, used by the scholastic youth with excellent fruits, was a Carnotum ecclesiastic. From an incident which happened to Richerius, the medical student designated, when arriving at the entrance of this municipality, it is clear Herbrand was widely famed for skillful pharmacy and surgery.

The clerical historian, the disciple of this monkish professor, states upon reaching the city of Carnotum, he was met by a

---

[11] "Cum aviditate discendi logicam Yppocratis Choi de studiis liberalibus sæpe et multum cogitarem, quadam die equitem Carnotinum in urbe Remorum positus offendi." Ibid., Lib. IV., cap. 50.

[12] "In quibus cum tantum prognostica morborum accessissem, et simplex egritudinum cognitio cupienti non sufficieret, petii etiam ab ea—Herbrando—lectionem ejuslibri, qui inscribitur de Concordia Yppocratis Galieni et Surani," Richer. Histor., Lib. IV., c. 50. Vide Fabricius, Biblioth. Græca, Tom. XI., p. 714, touching Soranus.

[13] "Quod et obtenui, cum eum in arte peritissimum dinainidia, farmaceutica, butanica atque cirurgica non laterent." Ibid.

lad who apparently, like Richerius, was proceeding to the domicile of Herbrand for the expressed purpose of procuring proper instruction in the study of medicine. At all events, the production by this juvenile scholar of an advisory letter touching the readings of Hippocrates' Aphorisms,[14] warrants the conclusion that in this town, not far from Rheims, a clerical professor was engaged in the systematic tuition of several disciples of the curative art, and had attained to considerable eminence.[15]

Similar to the irregular movements, in a progressive form, of philosophy and mathematics, after having been neglected for several ages, medical studies began to revive in those parts of Italy, enlightened by the careful policy of foreign or native dominion, and radiated a certain beneficence to other quarters of Western Europe. By direct influences of such Italian professors of the curative art, as had obtained celebrity, the fame of localities chiefly monasteries, under Teutonic subjection, expanded with increasing attraction in the North and occidental Europe, and secured most favorable consideration and substantial rewards to these educational institutions from sovereign potentates, whether papal or imperial.

The Salernite school, whose ranking distinction among the later medical scientists of the Middle Ages was everywhere avowed, should receive the highest eulogies on account of its early elevation of a rational standard of remedies, at an epoch when flimsy pretexts of such a system were equivalent to ecclesiastical censure. We have seen, at a compatively early period of the tenth cenutury, a physician of Salerno justly distinguished for his knowledge of medicine and its cognate filiations of surgery and pharmacy, at the Othonian court, contesting publicly with a more eminent surgeon, bishop of Amiens.[16]

Gervaise, of Tilbury,[17] in sketching out the original rise of

[14] "Epistolam protulit ille hortatoriam ad Aphorismorum lectionem." Ibid.

[15] Richerius, Historiarum, Lib. IV., cap. 50.

[16] Ibid., Lib. II., cap. 59.

[17] Otia Imperialia, Divis. III., cap. 15.

this science at Salerno, makes the singular accusation against the medical students and professors, that when its celebrity was established and success assured, they resorted to a disreputable artifice in order to obtain exclusive control of the patronage seeking the monastery and vicinity for a cure of vexatious maladies. He alleges that in the Neapolitan city, otherwise Civitas Putoleum, the wizard Virgil had constructed baths of perpetual utility to the people, with admirable art, and to be exclusively devoted to healing internal and external diseases.

In order to render so valuable a gift practicable for stricken sufferers for whom it was designed, certain shells were inscribed with the particular curative property attributed to these waters, together with a full description of the malady. Afterwards, however, when the study of medicine vigorously flourished at Salerno, the scholastics, influenced by envy, destroyed the notices affixed to the neighboring baths, apprehensive lest the knowledge of their sanitary powers might divert or diminish their lucrative profession among invalids. The gossipping abbot adds that the baths were for the most part intact in his day—A. D., 1211[18]—and a certain remedy for diverse diseases; but sagaciously concludes, those should be suspected which lacked a proper notice, because the medicinal forces of the one might provoke the very disorder it was intended to cure.[19]

Notwithstanding this sweeping diatribe against the medical scholars of Salerno, there are indications that this city was already, at the end of the tenth century, extensively known for the renowned excellence of its physicians, both at home and among foreigners. In the year 984, Adalberane, occupant of the Vendome Episcopate, in France, was transported thither in quest of such curatives for his infirmities as it would appear were not procurable elsewhere.[20] About the same period,

---

18 Leibnitz, Rer. Bruns., Tom. I., p. 995.

19 "Ipsa tamen balnea pro maxima parte intacta, diversis morborum generibus medelam tribuunt." Gervasii Tilburnensis, Otia Imperialia, Divis. III., cap. 15. Other mechanical marvels constructed by Virgil are described in cc. 13 and 16.

20 Tiraboschi, Storia della Litteratura Italiana, Tom. III., p. 394.

Desiderus, abbot of Monte Cassino, afterwards pope under the name of Victor III., seeking a remedy for an aggravated malady with which he was afflicted, had recourse to Salernite physicians.[21]

Almost simultaneously with the pilgrimage of the religious head of Monte Cassino, searching for medicaments in supreme Salerno, to cure an infirmity caused by unremitting labor, an emperor of Germany, Henry, son of Otho the Great, in the year 1002, ascended the heights where Saint Benedict, ages before, had founded the great monastery of Cassino, eagerly pursuing the hope of a permanent cure from a distressing disorder. From the details of the operation to which the emperor was subjected, it is evident lithotomy was successfully practiced in the infirmary or hospital of this cloister, in the tenth century.

After the extraordinary campaign in Italy, which resulted in restoring Apulia to the Roman crown, on his return from these ancient Greek provinces he was attacked with most painful calculus, and although suffering great agony, endured it with patience. Ascending Monte Cassino, through adjurations to Saint Benedict and the Holy Virgin, he craved a restoration to health. Slumbering in the conventual hospitium, he saw the sainted founder approach, who after addressing consoling words opened that portion of his body where the disease was seated with a "medicinal iron," and the distressing object gently removed, at the same time instantly healing the incision.[22] When the imperial patient beheld the stone in his hand, he manifested unlimited gratitude, by rich donations to the abbey.

Great diversity of opinion exists touching the antiquity of the Salernite medical school in its collegiate form,[23] although there

---

21 "Medendi gratia Salernum perrexit." Leo Ostiens, Chronicon Casinense, Lib. III., cap. 7.

22 "Cum ferro medicinali partem illam corporis ubi habitabat calculus." Chronica S. Ægidii, sub an. 1002.

23 Savigny, Geschichte Rœmischen Rechts, Th. III., p. 156.

certainly seem to be reasonable probabilities of the advanced qualities of its medical institutions, which so early as the first half of the tenth century, as we have seen, had obtained honorable recognition.[24] There can be no doubt, however, that at the close of this age these establishments were extensively known.

About the middle of the ensuing century, an annalist, speaking of the erudition of Rodolphus, a monk of this convent, affirms, "among other learning, such as grammar, dialectics, astronomy, and music, he was as deeply versed in medicine as the Salernites, whose school of the curative art had existed from ancient times, and where none equalled him in this science, excepting a skilled matron."[25] Odericus Vitalis, the chronicler cited, carried down his annual record to the middle of the twelfth century, at which period he died. Two centuries prior to this era would be fairly within the annalist's meaning, and vindicates the statement of Richerius, touching the Salernite physician of his own time.[26]

A metrical version of the curative properties of certain materials, addressed to Robert of England in the twelfth century, has been assigned to earlier writers, in order to extend the origin of this medical school to an immediate institution by Charlemagne in the eighth or ninth century. Doubtless, the significance of this would be simply tracing, as other monastic medical schools, these establishments to the Carlovingian cartulary prescribing the study as a part of conventual education.

Whether the excellence of Salerno, prior to the advent of Constans Afer in the eleventh century,[27] in medicinal culture was unique, or transcended the eminence of other institutions, a positive beneficial influence arrived with the famous African scientist, or according to the rational conjecture of Tiraboschi, through Saracen residents of Sicily, introducing Arabic science,

---

[24] Richerius, Historiar., Lib. II., cap. 59.

[25] Odericus Vitalis, Historia Ecclesiast., sub an. 1059, Lib. III. c. xi.

[26] Historiarum, Lib. II., cap. 59.

[27] Petrus Diaconus, De Viribus Illustratibus Casinens., cap. 23.

who, domiciled under Christian domination, furnished medical as well as other books[28]—an event rendered quite certain by the sagacious system of legislation adopted by Robert Guiscard at the epoch before us, which promoted a free interchange of Moslem knowledge.[29]

The conquest of Spain by the Arabs, and their rule for centuries, constituted the principal source from which emanated the energizing forces whose operation modified at length the crude medical systems of Europe, and gave them a stricter scientific tendency. The rythmical prescriptions offered the English king by the school of Salerno, assisted in extending the fame of this great monastery to the most distant countries of Europe. These receipts, in alternative hexameter and pentameter, are known differently as Medicina Salernitana, De Conservanda bona Valetudine, Regimen Sanitatis Salerni, and Flos Medicinæ.[30]

Whether other versions of this curious sanitary poem exist is uncertain, although with the usual prolixity of mediæval versifiers, some of these reach beyond a thousand lines,[31] while abbreviated ones are limited to less than four hundred. The main purpose of this hygienic poem appears to have been the procuration of royal favor from an adventurer then sojourning in Salerno, perhaps Robert, Duke of Normandy, son of William the Conqueror. It is, indeed, possible to have been written at the expressed wish of the king himself.

Popular legends so frequently repeated in the Middle Ages, touching a poisoned wound received by this prince at the siege of Jerusalem, and his probable application to Salernite surgery for medical advice, may have suggested the poem, which prior to his departure for England was prepared in the

[28] Tiraboschi, Storia della Litteratura, Tom. III., p. 396.

[29] Bazancourt, Histoire de la Sicilie sous la Domination des Normands, Tom. II., p. 79.

[30] Villannova, Proemium in Lib. Regim. Salutatis Salernit., col. 1874.

[31] Vossius, De Natura Artium, Lib. V., cc. 11 and 12; and Regimen Salernit. Scholæ, p. 50, § 7.

nature of detailed hygiene for the preservation of health, by the physicians attending.[32] Doubtless the vivid recommendations of this versified prescription added to the increasing celebrity of Salerno, maintained it for many ages in great repute, until it became the subject of frequent commentaries in many languages, by those interested in propagating the system of this medical school among other nations.[33] The authorship of this celebrated sanitary treatise has been attributed to John of Milan,[34] who it is urged compiled it while a student of medicine at Salerno, and which obtained the concurrence of the medical professors[35]—an allegation most unequivocally denied by the erudite historian of Italian letters.[36]

As further proof that the masters of the great school were consulted for a remedy in an incurable disorder, it is vehemently urged that these scientists after careful study, declared the poison could be extracted through suction, which it will be remembered was an important element of surgery, and that there was no remaining cure for this fistular malady.[37] The king refused to submit to such operation, which, however, was successfully performed during his slumbers, by the devoted sacrifice of Isabella, the royal consort.[38] How fragile and unreliable such popular traditions may be, though propagated by written records, readily appears from the metrical rescript itself, as the production and utterances of the united Salernite professors, touching an accepted cure of this identical ailment:

"Auri pigmentum, sulphur miscere memento:
His decet apponi calcem: conjunge saponi:

---

[32] Regimen Salernit. Sanit., Prœm.

[33] An English metrical version of the Regimen was published in London in 1607 for practical use.

[34] "Io. Mediol. inscriptor totum collegium Salernitatum." Zac. Silvii, Præfat. ad Scholam Salernitat., cap. 3.

[35] "Anglorum Regi scripsit schola tota Salerni." Reg. Sanitat., v. 1.

[36] Tiraboschi, Storia della Litteratura, Tom. III., p. 402 seq.

[37] Freind, Historia Medicinæ, p. 530 seq.

[38] Oderic., Vital., Histor. Eccles. Lib. x., c. xi., sub an. 1100, does not mention such event.

Quator hæc misce, commixtis quator istis
Fistula curatur, quator ex his si repleatur."[39]

In this quotation nothing appears to assume a possible cure from suction alone. These hygenic verses, if designed exclusively for a sanitary guide to the wounded ruler of England, embodied excellent hints for the preservation of health, in the nature of dietary considerations, which at the time were, indeed, but little regarded. In its essential advice, this venerable regimen might be followed still most advantageously.

The Norman prince is urged, if earnestly desiring robust, uninterrupted health, to avoid the oppressive weight of grave cares, flee unjust anger as profane and especially injurious to a sanitary condition; while a parsimonious use of wine and frugal meals would produce a strong and vigorous physical system; that it was desirable to arise and exercise after dining, to the utter exclusion of post-prandial slumbers. Such hygenic attentions, with others, it was claimed, would procure a long and comfortable life.[40]

Expanding celebrity rapidly followed the fame obtained by this production of Salernite medical professors; so much so, indeed, that in the middle of the next century, Romoaldus, archbishop of Salerno, asserted the city to have been preeminent and illustrious for centuries, on account of its studies in medicine and other arts.[41]

William, King of Sicily, summoned the archbishop to his court as expert and skilled in medical culture, according to a confession which he makes himself.[42] Here his profound acquaintance with this art provided suitable remedies—a rose syrup, etc.—for an aggravated disease with which the monarch was suffering.[43] Towards this epoch an erudite Israelitish trav-

---

39 Regimen, Sanitatis Salernit., v. 83.

40 "Surgere post epulas, somnium fuge meridianum." Ib., v. 15; and "Hæc bene si serves, tu longo tempore vives." Ibid., v. 17.

41 "Civitatem medicinæ utrique artis diu famosam." Muratori, Scriptor. Rerum Ital., Tom. VII., p. 172.

42 "Qui in arte medicina erat valde peritus." Ibid., Tom. VII., p. 206.

43 "Nam siruppum rosatum simplicem fuisse quem dederat." Ibid., op. cit., Tom. VII., p. 320.

eler by the name of Benjamin, whose writings have been published, having journeyed to Salerno, about the year 1170, bestowed upon this city the cognomen, Schola medicinorum Idumeorum—which he intended to signify as a school of medicine designed for occidental Christians. He adds further, what is of interest at this time, that there were over six hundred Hebrew students of this science at Salerno, and of these he mentions some as already famous.[44]

At Amalfi he found about twenty Jews, of whom Hananæl, a physician, was a principal man of the city.[45] From the mention hitherto made, touching the presence in France in the tenth century of a Salernite medical professor, it attests that at so early a period in the Gallic kingdom, it was an advantageous recommendation for a practitioner, if his studies in medicine were pursued at Salerno. In the year 1140, Roger I., the Sicilian monarch, promulgated an ordinance, prescribing that none should presume to practice medicine in his kingdom without first obtaining the consent of magistrate or judges, and in case of failure to comply with the conditions of the law, the delinquent should be pnnished with forfeiture of his goods and chattels.[46]

When it is considered that the edict referred to is the precursor of more elaborate regulations of the Hohenstaufen emperors upon this subject, and published for guidance in the monarchy of Sicily, where medical research had become famous prior to the twelfth century, it should excite little surprise that both in Salerno and its neighboring cloisters, many writers devoted their energies to elucidate the practical details of medicine. Of these Matthew Platearus, a Salernite physician, toward the termination of the age under notice, compiled a treatise on Antidotal Selections, and a work on the virtues of Simple Medicines.[47]

---

[44] "Salernum devectus sum, urbem medicinorum scholis illustrem." Benjam. Tudelensis, Itinerarium, p. 22 seq.

[45] Ibid., p. 23.

[46] Constitutiones Regni Siculi, Titul. XXXIV., De Probabile Experentia Medicorum, p. 367.

[47] Fabricius, Bibliotheca Latinit. et Infim., Tom. V., p. 52.

In the year 1163, Saladin of Ascoli, physician to the prince of Sorrento, prepared a compendium on the nature of aromatics.[48] Erotus and Garioneponte, likewise of Salerno, obtained distinction in this age, the former as author of a valuable treatise on the maladies of women, the latter as writer of eight books on different diseases.[49] With rare exceptions, students of medicine of this and preceding centuries acquired a practical familiarity of the curative art as a means to procure ecclesiastical eminence within the range of monastic and social existence, or as a fruitful source of gain, although few of these monkish scholars illustrated their knowledge of remedies by erudite compilations. One of the disciples of Constans Afer, Otho, evidently a German, and chaplain to the Empress Agnes, translated into the Roman or vulgar idiom of Italy those works on the healing art, which his master had reproduced from Greek, Arabic, and other oriental languages, into mediæval Latinity.[50]

Another scholar of the Carthaginian Constans, named John, subsequent to the death of his master, wrote a work of erudite importance on medical aphorisms,[51] which was particularly acceptable and essential to physicians of that age.[52] This writer closed his earthly career at Naples, to which city he bequeathed the entire medical books of Constans, his tutor.[53] Other monasteries in Italy cultivated to a high degree the art of medicine at this epoch and earlier, since, about the middle of the eleventh century, Dominicus, abbot of the Pescara

---

48 "Compendium Aromatorum," Ibid., Tom. VI., p. 142.

49 Tiraboschi, Storia della Litteratura, Tom. III., p. 404.

50 "Capellanus Agnetis Imperatricis, ea quæ Constantinus de diversis linguis transtulerat, cothurnato sermone in Romanam Linguam descripsit." Paulus Diaconus, De Virib. Illustr. Casinensis, cap. 24.

51 "Joannes medicus, supradicti Constantini discipulus et Casinensis monachus vir in physica arte dissertissimus Aphorisimum edidit.," Paul. Diac., op. cit., cap. 35.

52 "Physicis satis necessarium." Ibid.

53 "Ubi omnes libros Constantini sui magistri reliquit." Ibid.

cloister, received especial distinction from Henry III. of Germany, on account of medical knowledge.[54]

Bernard, a Ravennate monk, in 1028, through skillful use of medicaments, obtained specific mention in the annals of his time.[55] Endowed with superior culture, both in letters and a rudimentary science, closely associated with the healing art, Italian monks, in its broadest signification, possessed enlarged educational facilities over their confréres of more distant European countries. In consequence of such beneficial endowments, other nations gladly welcomed their culture and skill, and advanced them to positions of clerical honor.[56] Thus, for instance, a Tuscan early in the twelfth century, having performed for many years the abbatial functions of an Aberdeen cloister, with distinguished abilities, was a formidable competitor for the Canterbury archbishopric,[57] but national prejudice against the "Langobard," as he was denominated, prevented his election. Great eulogy is awarded the Italian prelate, for the indomitable energy of his character, and the notable achievements performed by him at his abbey in Aberdeen, which signalized the administration of the monastic property and hierarchial annals, at the period of Robert, Duke of Gloucester's adventurous landing in England.[58]

Of his medical acquisitions, the ancient records speak in panegyrical terms, and William of Malmsburg, in a summary of Foricius' attainments, asserts in laudatory language his distinguished eminence in the art of medicine.[59] The zealous devotion of ecclesiastics, pontifical[60] and cleric, to the practice of this science, especially in Italy, had caused such grave

[54] "Et eruditus arte medicinali, pro qua multi placuit imperatori." A. D. 1046, Muratori, Script. Rer. Ital., Tom. II., Pars. 2, p. 854.

[55] "Bernardus quidam, Ravenna monachus medicinæ artis peritus." Mabillon, Annales Or. S. B., sub an. 1028, Tom. IV., Lib. LVI., p. 345.

[56] Wm. Malmsb., De Gestis Pontific. Angliæ, Lib. II., p. 253.

[57] Wm. Malmsb., De Gestis Pontif. Angl., Lib. II., p. 230.

[58] Gesta Stephan., p. 56.

[59] Wm. Malmsb., op. cit., p. 230.

[60] Dithmar., Chronicon, Lib. VII., an. 1017.

irregularities that several Church councils endeavored to suppress this ardor under the punitive power of canonical law, with indifferent success. Although it was admitted at the first synod where this matter was inquired into, that the enthusiasm for the culture of medicine, when confined within proper limits, might be highly laudable, it had after the lapse of time, and as early as the year 1136, degenerated into abuse.

Many monks upon acquiring skill in this art used it as a pretext to remain at inconvenient distances from the cloister, and as ambulatory medici or physicians, wandered between large towns and princely courts. Like inculpation was urged against clerical students of civil and ecclesiastical law.[61] Therefore, in the twelfth century, a general council, held by Innocent II., enacted and promulgated certain laws as a remedy against this infraction of ecclesiastical rules. It was charged that great numbers of regular and canonical monks, after having assumed vestments and made monastic profession, abandoned the Regula of the cloisters, urged on by a desire of lucre, and devoted themselves to the theory of law and medicine. Such illicit use of secular knowledge was peremptorily forbidden, and bishops, abbots and priors, were threatened with heavy penalties if they culpably permitted these abuses.[62]

In the year 1179, similar ordinances were reënacted by the Turonese synod under Alexander III., which further enlarged the scope of the older canon, so as to interdict the regular clergy from teaching either law or medicine in schools.[63] Subsequent general and provincial councils reaffirmed these prohibitory canons.[64]

---

[61] Labbe, Concilia Lateran, II^s, Can. IX., Tom. XXI.

[62] "Spreta beatorum magistrorum Benedicti et Augustini regula leges temporales et medicinam gratia lucri temporalis addiscunt." Labbe, Concilia Lateran, II^s, Can. IX., Tom. XXI.

[63] Wm. Neubrig., Historia Anglicana, Lib. III., cap. 3.

[64] In the year 1195 the following was ordered at Montpelier: "Prohibuit prætera sub omni severitate ecclesiasticæ disciplinæ ne quis monachus vel canonicus regularis aut alius religiosus ad seculares leges vel physicam legendas accedat." Concil., Narbonens: XV.; apud Baluz., Concilia, Tom. I., p. 35.

Notwithstanding the vast number of practitioners devoting time and abilities to the culture of medicine, it made little progress towards an exact science, and was enriched with no new discoveries. Students and professors of the art, in its universal signification, were apparently occupied exclusively either in translating or compiling the works of ancient medical writers. Doubtless, these efforts ultimately aided an advance towards a more perfect system in the next century, at which period the full benefactions arising from the scrutinizing spirit of Arabic scientists, had so abundantly prepared the way for the immense progress of medicine towards the close of the Middle Ages.

Frequent and uninterrupted intercourse with these scientific enthusiasts was maintained at this epoch, and no doubt the European mind was abundantly prepared to receive and act upon a transmission of chemical and medical culture from the Spanish Arabs through such Christian students as attended the great schools of Cordova.

The diminutive advance of curative art to a more elevated standard subsequent to the advent of Constans Afer, who, as we shall presently discover, was deeply learned in the lore at the time, the exclusive property of Mahometan scholars and Oriental Israelites. unequivocally attests that the imposing movement of those ages, provoked by philosophers and skeptical inquirers after realities in the West, opened the entire range of Arabic science, and adopted it when the disintegrating elements of slothful ignorance began to recede before profounder knowledge of mathematics, astronomy, philosophy, and medicine. In the tenth century, the studies of Gerbert among the Saracens were apparently in an age when his contributions to the European stock of learning were lost in the dense gloom of superstition.

CHAPTER XVI.

Arabic Influence on Medical Art in Europe—Rapid Rise of Mahometanism—Caused by Justice to Subjects and Conquered Provinces—Their Swift Attainment to Science—Saracens Welcome Christian Scholars—Latter Sect Selected as Tutors by Haroun al Raschid—Translations into Arabic by These—Galen's Medical Books Rendered in the Saracen Tongue—Hippocrates' Treatises Preserved at Bagdad—Scholastic and Scientific Culture Arise in Arab-Spain—Sanitary Arrangements of Abderaham—Early Writers on Medicine—Students Flock Thither from other Nations in Europe, Asia, etc.—Moslem Ruler by a Rescript Organizes the Professors of the Curative Art—His Interdict against Charlatans—Hospitals—Possible Early Knowledge of the Use of *Aqua Vitæ.*

FROM whatever causes Mussulman power ascended so swiftly to dazzling greatness, and by the rapid extension of its conquests obtained the most cultured portions of the Orient and Western Europe within two centuries of its organization by Mahomet, is not germane to this treatise. In the seventh century the Arabians had overrun Syria, Egypt, Persia, and Africa, and subjugated these nations under lasting dominion; while in the next era Spain received these invincible conquerors, whose rule was to continue for many centuries. The resolute opposition with which they were confronted on Gallic soil, near Tours, by the Frankish forces under Charles Martel,[1] doubtless preserved the whole of Europe from permanent Moslem empire. In its earliest efforts, this power was exercised in rigid and inflexible vindication of Mahometan faith, uncompromising exaltation of the law, and as a development of this, the highest attributes of justice.[2] Wherever the

[1] Mariana, Historia de España, Lib. VII., cap. 3.

[2] The appeal of dissatisfied Christian subjects of Roderick, inviting a Saracen ruler from Africa to Spain in the eighth century, was based on this notion. Conde, Historia de la Dominacion de los Arabes en España, p. 13.

Arabs appeared, and elevated the standard of their fanatical armies, the literature of the Greeks, their pompous and turbulent hierarchy, unprincipled civilization, and religious polemics, receded before the fiery zeal of these fervid warriors.

Everywhere in their triumphal march, to the very portals of Tours, these Oriental invaders appear to have acted upon practical notions of steady and lasting conquest; and as rapidly as the subjugated territory opened, helplessly in advance of the martial tread of resistless forces, the Arabs immediately domiciled themselves in abandoned towns and deserted villages, in order that the faith of Mahomet might, by their presence, stand as an imperishable monument for all time. Early in the eighth century, actuated by this principle of permanent occupancy of conquered provinces, great numbers of them, with their families, entered into Aquitania,[3] where they certainly remained to the time of Charlemagne.[4]

When the Mahometans first issued in vast hordes from the Arabian deserts, they possessed a slender knowledge of astronomy, combined with Oriental poesy vivid with the burning imagery of their uncultivated minds. Under the Ommiades, immediate successors of the prophet, the study of the Mahometans seems to have been confined to native poetry and the interpretation of the Koran;[5] but the trifling culture of this people, upon first emerging from their fiery sands, was swept away before the great whirlwind of fanaticism for that religious fabric which blinded the quickened devotion of its adherents and eloquent orators to the cultivated excellence of strange letters, which, indeed, were scattered by the destructive march of these uncivilized devotees, or, amid lurid flames, vanished as a holocaust to Mahometan law.

Persian incursions into the literary city of Alexandria in the

---

[3] Regino, Chronicon, sub an. 655—where they entered: "Quasi in ea habitaturi."

[4] Anon., De Gest. Carolimagni, an. 797, Lib. III., c. 4, v. 327 seq; and Mariana, op. cit., Tom. I., p. 328.

[5] Gibbon, History of the Decline and Fall of the Roman Empire, Vol. V., p. 300.

year 616, under Chosroes II., spared the intellectual accumulations of ages,[6] but the first expedition of the Arabs in 640 was as disastrous to Christian zealots as to the literature of Greece. One of their own historians of the twelfth century distinctly states the conflagration of the great Alexandrine library by his ancient compatriots; while another chronicler of Arabic nationality and historical events as unequivocally asserts, in the ensuing century, that an incendiary fire destroyed the last famous aggregation of books upon the command of Omru, commander of the invading armies.[7]

The seductive pen of the skeptical Gibbon,[8] raised objections against the accuracy of these narratives, although more recent researches would seem to conclude further controversy upon this act. Inasmuch as it is agreed on all hands that the earliest followers of the prophet were actuated by a devotion for propagating the law, and that Grecian letters were the especial object of their hatred, the elucidation by Matter,[9] led to the conclusion, as stated, touching the Moslem destruction of the great library of Alexandria; but as late as the year 1175, the gymnasium still stood outside the city, and appears to have been used at that time by numerous schools for the purpose of teaching Aristotelian philosophy.[10] For a century or more subsequent to the death of their religious head, the Saracens were totally illiterate, and divested of all scientific culture; and while extending the energizing forces of Mahometan faith, were apparently content to remain so.

Notwithstanding the burning animosity of the fervid doctrines of the Moslems, they were not entirely indifferent to the comparative quietude in religious matters so earnestly desired by their conquered subjects; and under the influence of an undeviating principle of justice, allowed the Christians of the ac-

[6] Matter, École d'Alexandrie, Tom. I., p. 333.

[7] Abulfagus, Historia Moslem., p. 114.

[8] Gibbon, op. cit., Vol. V., p. 343.

[9] École d'Alexandrie, Tom. I., p. 332.

[10] Benjam. Tudelensis, Itinerarium, p. 101.

quired country to maintain, in accordance with the binding force of treaties, the practice of their faith, and prosecute the imposing ceremonies of their worship.[11] In the eastern habitations of the Arabs, thus disposed by an equitable inspiration towards the devotees of other dogmas, the Syrian Christians appear to have exerted a powerful predisposition among the Mussulmans to an accurate taste in letters.

Whether the repeal by Justinian, in the fifth century, of an ancient law granting public compensation to the philosophical and grammatical teachers of Athens and elsewhere, caused the dispersion of these literary scholiasts throughout the Orient, who in conjunction with Nestorian scholars,[12] moulded into practical shape Moslem enthusiasm for science and literature, cannot, perhaps, be established beyond a doubt. Other causes perhaps, co-operated with those stated, to propagate the embellishments of polite arts among the Arabs, since for centuries prior to the rise of Mahometanism, the Israelites throughout the east, which subsequently succumbed to the crescent and scimiter, on account of their academical institutes of learning, had obtained widely-extended celebrity. In the last year of the third century, this people maintained organized schools and colleges in the city of Bagdad, while in Sura a seminary of the highest culture was greatly renowned in the next age.[13]

Christian and Judaic civilization certainly assisted in developing the Arabic mind to that erudite culture afterwards so famous, and to which modern scholarship owes so much. To the Syrian followers of Christ, large numbers of Greek books were committed for translation into Arabic, and among these were the medical writings of distinguished scientists.[14] The

[11] "Todos sujetos á un moderado tributo gozarian el libre ejercicio de su religion, el uso y conservacion de sus iglesias: que se gobernariarn por sus leges y jueoces." Conde, Historia des Arabes en España, p. 20.

[12] Leo Africanus, De Virisque Illustratib., apud Arabos, cap. 1.

[13] Graetz, History of the Jews, pp. 237 and 266: and Leo African., De Medicis et Philosophis Hebraeis, p. 294.

[14] Abulfagus, Historia Moslem., p. 129. "Atque librorum, quæ scripta fuerunt

principal personage among these eminent scholars was a Chaldean Christian, John, son of Mesuach.[15] Syrian physicians, surrounding the sacred caliphs, were enabled to fan the intellectual fires which began to illumine these sovereigns, into a glowing, inextinguishable flame. Mahomet, himself, from whatever source originally drawn, perhaps from refugee scholiasts, was of high excellence in the art of medicine.[16]

His knowledge, similar to the elaborate system of Hippocrates, assumed the form of Aphorisms, but whether it originated in scientific examination and study, is unknown.[17] How swiftly the oriental caliphs advanced to an appreciation of the higher attractions of mental culture, appears from the fact that Ali Walid ordered Christian scholars, early in the eighth century, thenceforth to publish no books in Greek, but in the Arabic. This illustrious caliph, also distinguished for his fondness for architecture,[18] set an enlightened example, most assiduously followed by Almanazor, to whom astronomical science and due regard for men of letters, at that distant epoch, were under great obligations.[19]

Many mathematical works of the Alexandrian scholiasts or their predecessors, such as the writings of Menelaus and Euclid, were reproduced into the Arabic language from the original Greek, during his reign and that of Haroun al Raschid.[20] To the latter monarch, hero of the "Arabian Nights," lasting gratitude is due for his unremitting patronage of literature and

in artibus lingua Græca," etc. "Tunc segregati sunt boni, etc., sicut Medicina, Physica," etc. Leo Afric., De Virisque Illustr., apud Arabos, cap. 1.

15 "Posint supra traditionem linguæ Gracæ Ionnem filium." Mesuach, Natione Chaldaeus, et fide Christianus Nestorianorum secta, Ibid., cap. 1.

16 "Excelloit en particulier dans la Médécine." Gagnier, Vie de Mahomet, Tom. II., p. 405..

17 Gagnier, op. cit., Tom. II., pp. 405, 413.

18 Abulfagus, Histor. Moslem., pp. 123 seq; and 129.

19 Ibid., p. 160. Regular astronomical observations were established at Bagdad in the year 1129. Abulfagus, Annales Moslem., Tom. III., p. 441.

20 Leo Africanus, De Virisquibus Illustr., etc., cap. 1. Euclid was anonymously translated. Casiri, Biblioth. Hispan., Tom. I., pp. 339 and 345.

science, assisted by the ponderous favors of the caliphate. At a time when the Western Empire, under Charlemagne, was plunged into barbarism and groveling ignorance, when the mechanical skill of depraved Romans and uncultured Teutons utterly ignored rotary clock-work, a present from this illustrious eastern ruler of a horologe to the Frankish emperor, typifying the movements of time and seasons, combining intelligent action of horses and human figures, adjusted upon calculated pressure and counter-pressure, whose momentum was springs and weights, driven by wheels, so deeply stirred the imperial court and its chroniclers, that the annalists of this period fully describe the curious mechanism with the delight of youth and reverence of superstition.[21]

In addition to this, a gift by the same monarch to Charlemagne of an elephant, excited so great surprise and unparalleled interest at his court, that he dispatched a fleet to bring this absolutely novel specimen of natural history to the imperial residence,[22] and named it Abulabax, on account of its Oriental nativity.[23]

At the same period in the East, a young Nestorian, upon entering the famous city of Bagdad, was so profoundly impressed with the zealous devotion of both Mussulmans and Christians to the pursuit of liberal arts, that he, indeed, thought himself translated into a new world. This erudite scholar, the son of Mesuach, as stated, forthwith applied himself so assiduously to the acquisition of philosophy, astronomy, and medicine, that his profound learning quickly distinguished him as a suitable tutor for Almanazor, son of Haroun al Raschid.[24]

Upon the succession of this prince, in the year 813, the fervid desire for knowledge, characterizing the reign of his royal parent, developed in unrivalled splendor under the son.

---

21 Anony., Vita Carolimagni, sub an. 807.

22 Anonym., Vita Carolimagni, sub an. 807.

23 Eiginhardi, Vita Carolimagni, cap. XVI. This was the first animal of this colossal species ever seen in Germany. Ibid.

24 Leo African., De Virisquibus, etc., ap. Arab., c. 1, p. 259.

One of his first official acts was the formal invitation of the learned to the court; and from them he obtained the titles of such works in the Grecian, Syrian, and Persian languages, as had rendered their authors famous. For the purpose of advancing the intense ardor of the Saracen ruler for scholarly information, extensive explorations were directed to distant foreign countries, in order to procure written relics of the sagacious and wise of former ages.

When at length vast quantities had accumulated by the industrious zeal of his messengers, a convention under Almanazor himself decided upon those works worthy of translation. Among these the treatise of Galen[25] on Medicine and the writings of Aristotle were translated into Arabic. Similarly influenced as Cato, who feared the degrading tendencies of Hellenistic letters, the chief personages of this remarkable assemblage unanimously decided to commit to the flames whatever of this aggregation appeared antagonistic to Moslem faith. Many physicians employed at the Bagdad caliphate were Christians, and retained both at this period and in the twelfth century on account of their eminent surgical skill.[26]

Fired with zeal for knowledge, the Saracens pursued the sciences of mathematics, astronomy, and medicine, with an ardor which appropriated the treasures of foreign scholarship, and enlarged their own literary boundaries to include all. Euclid, Archimides, Apollonius, Diaphones, Hippocrates, Galen,[27] and Ptolemy,[28] were quickly reproduced into vernacular and made popular by astute and skilled commentaries, which opened the notable value of these exact sciences to the Arabic mind.[29] By the establishment of separate caliphates in

---

[25] "Traduxerunt Librum Galeni in medicina post quæ omnia Aristotleis Arabice," Ibid., cap. 1, p. 261.

[26] Abulfagus, Annales Moslem., Tom. III., p. 599.

[27] Voltaire, Essai sur les Moeurs et Usages, Tom. I., p. 333.

[28] Ibid., p. 334; and Heeren, Influence des Croisades, p. 51.

[29] Those by Alcindi were especially prized. Casiri, Biblioth. Hisp. De Medica, Tom. I., p. 355 seq.

Spain in the year 813, and in Africa, new seats of learning were created nearer the regions of Western Europe.

Under the prolonged though hotly contested reign of the Ommiades in Spain, the same line of literary and scientific research, provoking the admiration of strangers at Bagdad, was most zealously pursued. Here the revolted chieftains of Mahometanism obtained well-deserved celebrity for unfaltering culture of polite letters, and by a system of rewards and public commendation, allured the erudite to the rival courts of Moslem Spain. Although the royal library of the Fatimites at Bagdad is said to have contained at one time more than one hundred thousand volumes, including the entire range of ancient and modern scholarship, this collection was far transcended by those of Almeria, Malaga, Murcia,[30] and especially Cordova, selected by Abdelerham, and reached the enormous number of six hundred thousand manuscripts, whose catalogues swelled to eighty enormous tomes.[31]

From the year 711, when the Saracens first entered the regions of ancient Iberia and with uniform success to the portals of Tours established permanently their dominion, to the tenth century, a great and wonderful advance was made in those sciences which constituted the excellence of this strange people. In those countries adjacent to Europe, where such accomplishments were accessible to the north, the Arabians, through a stretch of two centuries, pursued with ardor that erudition which was to give new life and the mystic principles of unlimited learning to Western Europe.[32] In Cordova and elsewhere in Moslem Spain, Christians still adhering with an uncompromising tenacity to their ancient dogmas were permitted to reside with unmolested quietude, on paying tribute.[33] As a necessary medium of communica-

[30] "Complures per Universam Hispaniam Bibliothecas, constat." Casiri, Biblioth. Hisp., Tom. II., p. 38.

[31] "Bibliotheca Regia illo aevo ad sex centa volumina millia excrevit: quæ non nisi quadriginta ingenti mole catalogis recensebantur." Ibid.

[32] Voltaire, Essai sur les Moeurs, Tom. I., p. 325.

[33] Conde, Historia de los Arabes en España, p. 20.

tion these Mozarabes, as they were termed, acquired a fluent acquaintance with the Arabic tongue.[34]

In the year 756, the ruler of that portion of the Saracen government of which Cordova was the chief city, introduced the first palm-tree, which was planted in a botanical garden. In the same age academical institutes were established for instruction in various branches of human science, in this city. Sages attending the education of youthful Hixem, in striving for caliphate distinction, sought supremacy in these literary schools through erudite embellishments.[35] At this early period the Arabs in Spain appear to have devoted themselves largely to zoölogical studies, particularly at Cordova, where was an aviary fully stocked with rarest valuable specimens of falcons, which the Moslem princes enthusiastically used in unoccupied times for the delight and excitement of the chase.[36]

Abderaham, under whose reign the Spanish Arabs ascended the very apex of scholastic culture, signalized his occupancy of the throne by the establishment of numerous institutions of great sanitary value in the prolongation of life and the diminution of maladies, although at nearly the same epoch, 777, public hospitals were established under authority of the caliphs at Bagdad.[37]

Previous to his accession to the government of Spain, and prior to the transfer of its varied departments to Cordova, the citizens of this illustrious city, were provided with water according to the primitive methods of the Orient. In the year 826, Abderaham constructed several fountains in the open plazas, and supplied them with cold and refreshing water from the distant Sierras, conducted down the mountain slopes through leaden pipe.[38] At this epoch Saracen savans,

[34] Of these Eulogius, Memorialis Sanctorum, Lib. II., c. 1, mentions a Prefectus Presbyter at Cordova, distinguished for his Arabic learning, about the year 850; apud Bibl., Max. Patr., Tom. IX., p. 656.

[35] Conde, Historia de los Arabes en España, p. 100.

[36] Ibid., pp. 101 and 207.

[37] Abulfagus, Annales Moslem., Tom. II., p. 43.

[38] "Trajo á la ciudad aquas dulçes desde los montes con encañados de plomo." Conde, op. cit., pp. 132, 142.

before definitely selecting a permanent residence in Spain, pursued their academical education in celebrated schools of Africa, Egypt, Syria, and further into the Orient, where the advantages of literary and scientific accomplishments were added to those of foreign travel.

Towards the year 939, the savans of Cordova assembled regularly, under the presidency of a cadi, for the discussion of scientific questions propounded for elucidation, in which the highest nobility and princes of royal blood frequently participated. At the domiciles of Wazir Iza ben Ishor, and Caliph ben Abedel Zahrawi, both equally celebrated for their science and erudite treatise on medicine, stated conclaves were opened of such scholars as were famous for physical and astronomical learning.

The scientists designated were personal surgeons to the Saracen monarch.[39] In their leisure moments, where inclination and a cultivated taste directed, collections of rare and curious works on science and art were made, which sometimes became sufficiently illustrious to obtain specific mention by the Arabian annalists.[40] In the eleventh century, before the time Adam of Bremen, in amazed wonder, wrote that an ecclesiastic, thrice at Jerusalem and abducted to Babylon, after a heavy ransom returned to Europe,[41] an Arabic savan traveled from Spain to India, where he resided and accumulated there and in other Asiatic cities vast erudition.[42]

An adventurous Saracen vessel, in the first decade of this age, in exploring the hyperborean regions, was deterred in high altitudes by a viscid liquid, a fate which befel Northern explorers at a later period.[43] A century and a half prior to

[39] Conde, Historia des Arabes en España, pp. 212, 242.

[40] Ibid., p. 241.

[41] Adam Brem., Gesta Pontif., Hammaburg, Lib. IV., c. 68. Prior to 1068, occasional eleemosynary gifts were forwarded to pauper Christians in Syria and Egypt, at the close of the eight century, by Charlemagne—Eiginhard, Vita Carolimagni, cap. 27; and in the year 883 Alfred, Anglo-Saxon king, sent alms as far eastward as India. Flor., Wigior. Chronic., sub an. cit.

[42] Conde. op. cit., p. 293 seq.

[43] Ad. Brem., De Situ Danæ, cap. 39.

the composition by the nun Roswitha of Latin verses laudatory of Othonian battles,[44] many noble dames at the Ommiade court in Cordova had signalized themselves by the polished elegance of Arabic rhythm, as well as in the more laborious task of scientific investigation. Secluded life was prescribed by a law as rigid to Moslem women as the cloister regulations of Northern Europe; yet in defiance to such isolation, Saracen females obtained the honors of public recognition as a merited distinction for their poesies and the brilliant beauty of their written prose.

One of these performed the functions of confidential secretary to the king, while another attained celebrity for splendid transcription of books for royal use. Ayxsa, daughter of a famous savan of Cordova, excelled in literature; but her chief claim to renown arose from a marvellous collection of volumes treating of arts and sciences, which she had aggregated to the year 973.[45] At the houses of leading scientists in this vast metropolis, application for alms and medicaments could be made day and night. As a specific remedy in certain maladies thus presented, rose-water baths appear to have been frequently used, and with excellent results. In the tenth and eleventh centuries, the fame of Cordovan scholars had extended throughout the civilized globe, and attracted thither students of diversified sciences from Africa, Syria, Persia, and from France and the Roman provinces of the West of Europe.[46]

Before the close of the latter epoch, Soleiman ben Golghal had obtained universal repute on account of the profound erudition of his works on medical science. Equal scientific scholarship distinguished Ahmed ben Abdala, and so far East as Chorazan this superiority was admitted unreservedly.[47] How lasting was the interest of Moslem Spain in the unstinted culture of letters may be gathered from the fact that in the year

---

[44] De Gestis Odonum, p. 709 seq; Meibom., Tom. I.

[45] Conde, Historia de los Arabes en España, p. 211.

[46] Ibid., p. 263.

[47] Ibid., p. 277.

1051 the governor of Almeria convoked thither a congress of the most learned savans from the Orient, Spain and Europe, and submitted each week for discussion such propositions as came within the scope of their attainments.[48] Under the beneficent reign of Hixem, the hospitals and orphanages of Cordova were adjusted upon a superior arrangement, through personal supervision—a care extended to the public schools and colleges of his empire.

Oftentimes this wise and charitable ruler was seen in the infirmaries or hospitals of Cordova, inspecting the condition of diseased and infirm patients, to whom he directed the attentions of the royal physicians daily.[49] The accession of Gehwer to the throne of Mussulman Spain, early in the eleventh century, was marked by the promulgation of regulations so judiciously planned, touching medical science and its practice, that he deserves the highest commendation for the unwavering zeal with which he supervised this important branch of learning taught in the metropolis. Those evils which the provinces had suffered previous to his rule, through the practice of medicine by debased empirics, were quickly removed by this sagacious Caliph.

Upon the publication of his rescripts, such medical charlatans or ambulatory physicians as boldly announced themselves to be medici, without a knowledge of the science, were ignominiously expelled from the provincial towns. He decreed that a college of skilled surgeons should be forthwith organized, for the single specified function of rigidly examining into the assumed qualifications of applicants for licenses to exercise the curative art in municipal or rural departments, or sought professional employment as physicians in the numerous hospitals upon the Mahometan domains.[50] In the ensuing century

---

48 Ibid., p. 329.

49 "Sus mismos medicos debian visitar cada los almarestanes ú hospitales." Conde, Historia de los Arabes en España, p. 310.

50 "Echó de la provincia á los médicos charlatanes ó curanderos ignorantes, que se llamaban médicos sin experencia ni conocimentos, y ordinó un colegio de

the most celebrated medical scientists were selected by a Moorish king as his attending surgeons,[51] who, as hitherto stated, were not unfrequently Christians; and equal attention was given to the strict regulation of hospital service and colleges of students within the Spanish and African provinces.[52]

Before the thorough introduction of Arabic science into Northern Europe, the medical practitioners of Spain appear to have used certain medicaments, aqua vitæ or brandy, of which their European confreres were entirely ignorant. When the governor of Seville, in the year 1068, lost a daughter of great beauty and womanly excellence, so overpowering, indeed, was his grief as to provoke a grievous malady, which impaired the free action of the vital organs. To combat this, the physicians administered stimulants which restored their natural vigor, and for a brief period preserved his life; but suffering a relapse, in defiance of laxative remedies and cupping, death quickly ended his earthly existence.[53]

sabios que examinase á los pretendiensen ejercer la medicina y servir en los hospitales." Ibid., p. 316.

[51] Conde, Historia de los Arabes en España, p. 492 seq.

[52] Ibid., p. 487.

[53] Ibid., p. 337.

CHAPTER XVII.

Academies of Spain Offer Great Inducements to European Students—Christian Scholars Scoffed at in Cordova—Scientific Culture is Introduced to the North—Necromancy Taught at Seville, etc.—Abbots go to Spain to Learn Arabic Language and the Sciences—English Translator of the Alcoran in the Twelfth Century—Gerard of Cremorne Translates Arab Medical Books into Latin—Frederick II., of Germany, Patronizes Saracen Learning—Arab Savans in Sicily—Friar Bacon—Gerbert, Afterwards Pope, Studies in Spain—Constans Afer, the Illustrious Medical Writer and Translator—His Curious Adventures—Services to Erudition of Gerbert.

OFTENTIMES the Arabs formed alliances, both political and marital, with the Christians.[1] Touching the latter relation, the Moslem parent dying, the mother educated her son in the religion of Christ, and sent him to Arabic academies, as early as the ninth century, to be educated in Saracen literature and sciences; and indeed, at this period, Christian monks in Spain are alluded to in the chronicles, on account of skill in Arabic lore.[2]

One of the most brilliant rebels who invaded this territory in the eleventh century, was the son of a Christian mother; and another of this faith, wife of an illustrious Arab, became celebrated in Moslem annals, for her transcendent beauty.[3] Notwithstanding the regulations at Cordova admitted scholars of other creeds to the public academies, they were frequently maltreated and derided by Mussulmans whenever they appeared on the streets, while juvenile Arabs scoffed and amused themselves by throwing stones at them.[4]

[1] Conde, Historia de los Arabes en España, pp. 233, 278, 467 and 470.

[2] "Isaac Monachus litteris Arabacis imbutus." Eulogius, Memorialis Sanctorum, Lib. I., Prolog.; apud Bibl. Max. Patr., Tom. IX., p. 646.

[3] Conde, op. cit., p. 409.

[4] Eulogius, ap. Bibl. Max. Patr., Tom. IX., p. 218.

Uninterrupted amalgamation of Spanish Christians with Saracens from the ninth century, and unimpeded intercourse with the Saracen population during the Middle Ages, opened a way for the transition of Arabic literature, language and sciences, into different countries of Western Europe. To this, the most natural means, should be added the frequent assemblages in the princely courts of Spain of the most erudite philosophers, medical scientists and astronomers convoked from all nations,[5] which aided in transplanting these sciences to less favored people. It is, indeed, impossible to state with certainty, whether equal liberty of access to the schools and scientific colleges at Cordova was conceded foreign students, or whether the pursuit of such knowledge was restricted to private instruction, thus excluding them from public academies. The evident skilfulness of Arabic physicians in the preparation of medicaments, and dexterity of remedy, at the period under examination, may be inferred from the fact that the Catholic prelacy of this country entrusted their lives into the hands of Moslem scientists.[6]

In the eleventh century, when the Mussulmans, in their turn, redoubted the fanaticism of the crusaders, the relation of Europeans with the Spanish Moors had begun to reveal itself with increasing activity.[7] Scientific knowledge, thus imparted to the northern nations, was largely infected with magical superstitions—the application of which to medicine became an accessory to the curative art. The youth of Scandinavia, Bavaria, and other regions of Europe, flocked in great numbers to the schools of necromancy and the mystical sciences, opened in Toledo, Seville and Salamanca.[8]

In the thirteenth century, when Alfonso, surnamed the

[5] Conde, Historia de los Arabes, p. 278, gives an example of kindly treatment of Christian refugees among the Moslems at Cordova.

[6] Mariana, Historia de España, Lib. VIII., c. 7.

[7] Salverte, Sciences Occultes, p. 177.

[8] "Cum pluris ex diversis regionibus in eadem civitate suderent in arte necromantia, juvenes aliqui de Swedia et Bavaria." Heisterbach, Illustr. Miracul. et Hist. Memor., Tom. I., Lib. V., cap. 4.

Wise, established his university in the last-mentioned city, seeking to rival the Arab savans and their sciences,[9] he had recourse to Moorish learning in preparing the Alfonsine tables. The relations of this Christian prince with his Moslem competitors, and their erudite scholars, were uniformly of the most courteous character; so much so, indeed, that it was no unusual thing to meet Saracen scientists residing at the Castilian court under the public patronage of the king.[10] Gradually many persons of Europe, stirred by a sincere desire of thorough scientific culture solely possessed by the Spanish Arabs, sought their schools and colleges as early as the tenth century—an impulse continuing without interruption until towards the closing years of the Middle Ages.[11]

Of these, the first to avail himself of the intellectual treasures of the Moslems, were Gerbert, touching whose benefactions to this age we shall presently refer, and several residents of the British Isles; extending from the arrival of the latter in Cordova and other Spanish cities, early in the twelfth, through the ensuing century. Towards the end of the twelfth century, Peter, abbot of the celebrated Clugny monastery, journeyed to Spain, in order to acquire the Arabic language and make himself proficient in Moorish learning. At Toledo he procured an Englishman by the name of Robert, and a Dalmatian called Herman, studying astronomy or astrology, to translate the Alcoran into mediæval Latinity, which the abbot himself afterwards arranged according to its grammatical construction.[12] This was rendered necessary by the slight acquaintance of the translator with this dialect, and for this

---

[9] Voltaire, Essai sur les Moeurs, Tom. II., p. 270.

[10] Conde, Histor. de los Arabes en España, p. 557.

[11] Salverte, Sciences Occultes, p. 178.

[12] "Nihilominus ex Arabice ad Latinitatem perduxi interpretantibus scilicet, etc. Roberto Retenensis de Anglia, etc.; Hermano quoque Dalmeta," etc. "Quos in Hispaniam astrologicæ arti studentes inveni," whom he prevailed upon by urgent solicitation—"multo precio"—to undertake their erudite task. Machumetis Saracenorum, etc., Bibliandri, p. 4 seq.

cause a notatorial writer, also denominated Peter, was detailed as coadjutor in these labors.[13]

Gerard of Cremorne, observing the extreme penury of the Latins in Arabic literature, especially such as related to medicine, expatriated himself to Toledo, where he acquired profound knowledge of the language, and made several versions of medical text-books, and others on astronomical subjects.[14] The Englishman employed by the Clugniac prior was liberally rewarded by his patron, and as an additional claim upon Western scholars, translated a collection of Saracen laws and letters.[15] Athelard of Bath, whose works are still extant in the public libraries of England, was in Spain about the year 1135 pursuing Arabic studies, some of which were cognate with medicine,[16] upon returning to England, through the medium of a correspondence with his nephew, he was induced to publish to the British people certain details touching the successful acquisition of Saracen learning.[17]

Other valuable contributions to the study of natural sciences in England were made by this laborious student while studying among the Spanish Arabs. Under the patronage of Frederick II., Emperor of Germany, Michael Scott, celebrated in the annals of England as the Wizard of the North, wrote a treatise upon his imperial patron's prayer,[18] and was sufficiently learned in the Arabian language to translate for the Hohen-

---

13 "Sed quia lingua Latina none ei adeo familiaris vel noto erat, ut Arabica, didi ei coadjutorem, bene cognitum, doctum virum dilectum Petrum notarium nostrum." Ibid.

14 "Tunc medicinæ opera ex Arabica in Latinum conversa." Murator., Antiq. Ital., Tom. III., p. 936.

15 These appear to have been translated, or at least some of them, by a Toledo professor. "Feci autem eam transferri à perito utriusque linguæ viro magistro Petro Toletanto." Machumet. Saracen., Bibliandri, p. 4 seq.

16 In the Tractabus ejusdem ad Nepotem, cap. 41, Athelard sagaciously argues why married women cannot be infected with leprosy.

17 Athelardi, Questiones Naturales Perdifficiles, Prologus, Ed. 1489.†

18 "Quem secundo loco breviter compilavit a ejus precio." Muratori, Antiquitat. Ital., Tom. III., p. 945; and Sarti, De Professorib., Bonon., Tom. I., p. 511.

stauffen monarch Avicenna's commentary on Aristotle's De Animalibus—a work used by the celebrated lexicographer, Du Cange, to great advantage.[19]

How rapidly and with what eagerness the European mind seized upon Arabic science thus imported from the Spanish provinces, may be gathered from the fact that before the close of this age the commentaries of Averroes[20] on Aristotle were actually made the subject of public scholastic lectures near Cambridge.[21] The writings of Almanazor on the medicinal virtues of plants and the Herbarium of Dioskorides were possessed in the same era, 1194, by a Peterborough abbot, or transcribed, together with a treatise on medicine, by Panteginus,[22] while in the ensuing age an archbishop formally donated to this church the treatises of Avicenna.[23] In the year 1094, an Arabic manuscript volume was presented to the Corvey abbey in Germany; but the annalist in recording this noteworthy event does not state the name of it, of which doubtless he was ignorant.[24]

In the twelfth century, Roger of Sicily, at whose court many famous Arabic savans and scientists were constantly entertained in royal pomp, caused the writings of Essouph to be translated from the Arabic into Latin,[25] for use of his scholarly subjects. In the year 1219, while the Crusaders were before the city of Damietta, a work written in the Arabic language appears to have circulated among these hardy war-

19 Muratori, op. cit., III., p. 945.

20 Freind, Historia Medicinæ, p. 544; and Leo African., De Virisquib. Illus. Arab., cap. 20, p. 282.

21 Ingulph., Croyl. Hist. Continuat., p. 114.

22 "Ars physica Pantegini, et practica ipsius in uno volumine, Almasor et Dioscorides, de Virtutibus Herbarum," Rob. Swaph. De Libris ejus, circ. 1194; ap. Sparke, Histor. Anglic. Script., etc., p. 99.

23 "Dedit etiam ecclesiæ suæ duas libelles quorum una gallice scripta Avicenna," Walt. de Whytles, Cœnobii Burg. Histor., p. 170; Sparke, Ed.

24 Annales Corbeiensis, sub an. 1094.

25 Leo Africanus, op. cit., cap. 14, p. 278.

riors, some of whom were sufficiently conversant with this language to interpret its contents.[26]

About this period Friar Bacon and his ecclesiastical friend, whose contribution to magic remedies will be adverted to hereafter, bishop Grossteste displayed amazing familiarity with the entire range of Arabic authors, including Averroes, Avicenna the great scientist, the equally celebrated Alharen and Alcindi.[27] The scholastic monk wrote an elaborate treatise on the mistakes of physicians—De Erroribus Medicorum,[28] and exhibited remarkable knowledge of Saracen pharmacy.[29]

Although it has been doubted whether Europe really owes to the Arabs that practical acquaintance with chemistry, which under the searching investigations of modern scientists, has become the foundation of medical economy[30]—a doubt shared by the illustrious Petrarch himself—as early as the ninth century Alcindi, alone, had composed twenty-two seperate works on medicine, about twenty-nine on chemical and physical sciences,[31] while Rhazes of Chorazan, in the ensuing age, swept the entire circle of medical science and its kindred filiations, in his treatises on medicine, botany, oculism, surgery and chemistry, and commented the anatomical and medicinal writings of Hippocrates, Galen, Oribasius, Aetius, Pauli, etc.[32] To the Arabs high commendation is due for many valuable discoveries, such, for example, as numerical

---

[26] Oliveri, Historia Damiantia, cap. 20.

[27] Bacon., De Arte Chymica, cap. VI. of Excerpta, p. 56. The Tractatus de Speculis Illustratis, seems to be almost an entire reproduction of Alharen's principles of refraction of light. On Bacon's knowledge of Arabic authors, vide De Retardandis Senectutis Accidentibus, cc. 1, 2, 4, 5 and 6.

[28] Apud Bale, Scriptores Brittannicæ, Pars I., p. 343.

[29] De Compositione Elixir, p. 70. The writings of Avecenna are largely used in his Specula Mathematica, Dist. I., cap. 3; and Dist. II., c. 2.

[30] Whewell, History of Inductive Sciences, Vol. I., p. 256 seq; and Voltaire, Essai sur les Moeurs, Tom. I., p. 334.

[31] Casiri, Biblioth. Hispan., Tom. I., p. 353.

[32] Freind, Historia Medicinæ, p. 484 seq.

figures, and the art of dyeing.[33] Among the first to make known to Europe the vast resources of Saracen learning in the science of medicine and philosophy, was Gerbert, although his efforts may not have had the general influence, at so early a period, which characterized the contributions of Constans Afer, in the next century, to the medical and surgical knowledge of southern Italy.

Inspired with an inextinguishable ardor for a solid learning, this Carthagenian scholar proceeded, in the first years of the eleventh century, from his natal city to the great literary metropolis of the eastern Moorish empire—Babylon, in order to acquire a profound insight into that erudition for which, in its multifarious nature, an equal has been seldom produced. During a prolonged residence in this illustrious city, he applied himself with diligent assiduity to the careful acquisition of grammar, dialectics, physics, and necromancy, which constituted at this epoch in Spain an important branch of liberal education,[34] geometry, arithmetic and medicine, to which he added a thorough theory of the musical art of the Chaldæans, Arabians, Persians, and Egyptians.[35]

Having exhausted Babylonish science, he went to India, urged by the same spirit of inquiry prevailing among the western Moors, in order to master the learning of the Indians; and after an absence of thirty-nine years, returned to Africa, where he practiced, or rather taught, his vast scientific and literary culture to disciples eager to learn it.[36] As usual, in those distant ages, when Gerbert and Roger Bacon were no exception to popular superstitious hatred, Constans was immediately exposed, upon domiciling himself in the city of his

[33] Heeren., Sur l'Influence des Croisades, p. 53.

[34] Heisterbach, Illust. Miracul. et Hist. Mem., Lib. II., c. 4.

[35] Petrus Diaconus, Chronicon Casinense, Lib. III., c. 35.

[36] "Nec non physica Chaldæorum, Arabum, Saracenorum, Egyptorum ac Indiorum plenissime eruditus est: completis in ediscendis istiusmodi studiis trigenta et novem annorum curriculus ad Africam reversus est." Ibid., Petr. Diac., Liber. de Viribus Illustratibus Casinensis, cap. 23.

birth, to a literary martyrdom by the citizens of Carthage, who, startled by the immense learning which he possessed, fearing that he might possess the power of a magician, determined to assassinate him.[37]

On learning the sinister preparations against his life, he secretly fled to Salerno, where for a considerable period he sought safety in the privacy of a mendicant costume, evidently as a strolling physician. The arrival there of a brother to the Babylonish monarch, disclosed the secret presence of Constans, and was the means of his becoming attached to Robert Guiscard, king of Sicily, in the official position of confidential secretary.[38] Wearying at length of this subaltern function, he abandoned the Sicilian court, and withdrew to Monte Cassino, in refuge with the prior Desiderus, from whom he received monastic vestments in the year 1086. In this monastery he passed the remainder of his days, employed in translating medical works from Greek and Arabic into the Latin language, and in composing books and treatises on this science.[39] He finally attained so great distinction as to receive the cognomen of Master of the East and West.[40]

Among other translations, one on fevers, rendered from Saracen into the vulgate, was particularly commended.[41] Notwithstanding the highly eulogistic encomium without stint accorded this celebrated scientist, there are excellent reasons for assuming that outside of his own treatise on surgery his medical influence on the age was either dwarfted to the contiguous territory of Salerno, or expanded within narrow circles beyond.

---

37 "Quem cum vidissent Afri, ita ad plenum omnium gentium studii eruditum, cogitaverent occidere eum." Paulus Diacon., Liber. de Viribus Illustr. Casinens., cap. 23.

38 Petr. Diac., Chronic. Casinens., Lib. III., c. 35.

39 "De diversarium gentium linguis," Ibid. Among other writings thus translated were the works of Plato, and Hippocrates, and the Simplic. Medicam., of Galen. Ibid.

40 Ibid.

41 "Librum febrium quem de Arabica lingua." Ibid.

The remarkable impluse given by Gerbert, a century previous, to nations of the North, had perhaps laid the groundwork upon which future development of accurate taste in science might be expected, while, indeed, the energizing forces of Constans Afer were impotent to accelerate zealous assiduity in sound erudition, outside the limits of his Italian domicile. Nearly contemporary annalists, as cited, have established the fact that the Carthagenian refugee translated Arabic and Grecian medical books into mediæval Latinity;[42] but it is equally historical and curious, that these reproductions in the Middle Ages were held in trifling esteem.

In the thirteenth century, the famous Florentine physician and professor, Thaddeus, wrote an expository work on the Aphorisms of Hippocrates, and in the preface dwells upon the translation of this treatise in terms of profound contempt, asserting a preference for the version made by a native Italian.[43] Thaddeus excuses himself for using the African's translation, as necessitated by familiar references and common usage: "Et translationem Constantini persequar, non quia melior est, quia communior: nam ipsa pessima est, et superflua, et defectiva." He then charges the "insane monk with violating the original in quantity and quality"—"nam ille insanus monachus in transferendo peccavit quantitate et qualitate."[44]

Considerable activity seems to have manifested itself in vulgate versions of Hippocrates at this period, when a Genoese by the name of Simon, in cautioning students against the slothful and suspicious interpretation of Constantine, alludes in the most contemptuous manner to a version of the Aphorisms by

---

[42] Vide Fabricius, Bibliotheca Græca, Tom. X., cap. 205.

[43] "Tum translatio Burgundinis pisani melior est." Thaddei, Epositiones Oper., Hippocrat., Præfatio, p. 1.

[44] Thaddei, op. cit., p. 1. This distinguished professor himself slumbered in mental inactivity until his thirtieth year, when he awoke from the sale of trifling souvenirs, to become the chief of a great science. Sarti, De Profess. Bonon., Tom. I., p. 467.

a certain Isaac, perhaps an Israelite: Et si aliqua ex libris Isaac, etc., nam ejus translatio satis est nihi suspecta.[45]

It may be added here, that the Spanish Jews were far in advance of Western Christians at the era before us in their knowledge of useful sciences, and largely aided in publishing to the nations of Europe many valuable discoveries of medicine and surgery, by transporting Arabic manuscripts with them to the principal trading towns of the North and West, particularly Montpelier,[46] long before this municipality was known for its schools of law and medicine.

One of the earliest Europeans to explore the intellectual treasures of Spain, and to introduce these to contemporary notice was Gerbert, afterwards Pope under the name of Sylvester II. His adolescent education was superintended at the convent of St. Gerard Aurillac, in which he had assumed monastic vows of abnegation and celibacy. Here for several years, by close assiduity to grammatical and other liberal arts, he obtained the unrestricted commendation of his superiors.[47] At length Borrelus, duke of a Spanish province, arriving at this monastery to offer humble prayers, was accosted by the youthful scholar, as to whether the culture of science and art among the Arabs was of higher grade than prevailed in schools of the Latin Church; and upon an affirmative answer, through the abbot, he besought the ducal visitor to assist him in procuring from the Moors that erudition to which he fervently aspired. This urgent request was granted, and finally, committed to the care of Hatto, bishop of Ausonia, he quickly illustrated his studies in geometry, music, magic, and astronomy—classified by the chronicler as Mathesi.[48]

Pending his residence near the Saracen savans, a frequent epistolary correspondence attests the rapid progress of this

---

45 Tiraboschi, Storia della Litteratura Italiana, Tom. III., p. 398.

46 Cuvier, Histoire des Sciences Naturalles, Tom. I., p. 387.

47 Richerius, Historiarum, Lib. III., cap 43.

48 "Apud quem etiam in Mathesi plurimum et efficaciter studuit." Richerius, Historiarum, Lib. III., cap. 43; Du Cange, Glossar., sub v. Mathesis.

scholar in these sciences, then the exclusive possession of Oriental sages. In writing to a Barcelona ecclesiastic, he begs of him the perusal of a work on astrology, then, and at a later period of the Middle Ages, regarded as a branch of the curative art, and which it seems, had been translated by the Spanish scholastic from Arabic sources, and at the same time alludes to the arithmetical treatise of a certain Joseph the Spaniard.[49] On another occasion, he distinctly avows the great obligation he was under to Moslem philosophy, and affirms an intention to seek the superior culture of Saracen courts, in order to obtain the finest scholarly facilities. In this letter, Gerbert adverts to the commencement, by him, of a celestial sphere upon which were delineated the heavenly bodies,[50] which, astrological orreries frequently performed important functions in medical prognostics.

On returning to his native land, the contemporary annalist becomes the panegyrist of Gerbert, and declares this movement was by divine command, to dissipate the profound darkness of ignorance, beneath whose sombre gloom lay the whole of France.[51] Five years subsequent to his return—in the yea 970, imperial patronage preferred him to the priory of the Bobbio monastery.[52] An early attestation of rising fame in Western Europe was the remarkable affluence of foreign students, attracted thither by this prelate's scholastic accomplishments.[53] The fame of this great scholar spread to the Germans, throughout Italy, and extended indeed, to the Tyrrenean and Adriatic seas.[54] Among the contributions of Arabic science, which Europe owes directly to Gerbert, are numerica

[49] "De multiplicatione et divisione numerorum, editum à Josepho Hispano Gerberti, Epistolæ, Ep. 17 and 25.

[50] Ibid., Ep. 148. Gerbert's treatise on astrology was eagerly sought. Ibid Ep. 24.

[51] Richerius, op. cit., Lib. III., cap. 43.

[52] Tiraboschi, Storia della Litteratura Italiana, Tom. III., p. 258.

[53] Gerberti, Epistolæ, Ep. 13.

[54] Richerius, Historiar., Lib. III., cap. 55.

figures,[55] whose application, even in this pontiff's age, to higher mathematics, quickly revealed their value in the construction of more elegant and graceful edifices. Richerius, a resident of Rheims, the archiepiscopal see, coeval with its occupancy by this scholastic,[56] distinctly asserts that to Gerbert "was due the introduction of the abacus,"[57] the description of which is fully given by the mediæval chroniclers as an object of striking wonderment.[58] After his vexatious expulsion, towards the close of the tenth century, from his pontificate, he sought the protection of Otho, emperor of Germany, and while there constructed a sidereal clock.[59]

In regulating the exact chronometer movements of this horologe, which was placed in the city of Magdeburg, in the year 999, the learned scientist found the precise time by observing the polar star through a telescope—per fistulam.[60] Notwithstanding mathematical science and its cognate branches of astrology and geometry were the predilection of Gerbert, he had obtained profound insight into the theory and practice of medicine, as understood and professed among the Saracens of Spain. On this subject his epistles contain numerous and important references.[61] Similar to the scholars of that period, Gerbert, under the nomenclature of Mathêsi,[62] directed an inquiring mind into the possibilities of magical science,[63] for

---

[55] Gerberti, op. cit., Ep. 17 and 25; and Richerius, op. cit., Lib. III., cc. 57, 58. Vide on this interesting subject, Matter, École d'Alexandrie, Tom. II., pp. 52, 126; and Gouget, Origin des Artes et Sciences, Tom. III., p. 110.

[56] Voltaire, Essai sur les Moeurs et Usages, Tom. II., p. 22; and Tiraboschi, op. cit., Tom. III., p. 258.

[57] Richerius, op. cit., Lib. III., cap. 54.

[58] Wm. Malmsb., Gesta Pontif. Angliæ, Lib. II., p. 65.

[59] Dithmar, Chronicon, Lib. VI., sub an. 999, p. 196; and Richerius, op. cit., Lib. III., c. 55.

[60] "Illud recte constituens considerata per fistulam quadam Stella Nautarum duce." Dithmar, op. cit., Lib. VI., supra.

[61] Gerberti, Epistolæ, Epp. 17, 92, 124 and 151.

[62] Du Cange, Glossar., sub v. Mathesi.

[63] Tiraboschi, Storia della Litteratura, Tom. III., p. 259.

which the Arabians preserved their renown until the fifteenth century.

The inculpation of these dark arts against this prelate was first urged by the enmity of Cardinal Birno, under the papacy of Gregory VII. After struggling to discredit the papal dignity of Sylvester II., the official title of Gerbert, and failing, he was entirely successful in this bold accusation of magical practices,[64] which in the Middle Ages was universally accepted as a demoniacal power. Mediæval chronists elaborated with much prolixity these diversified charges.[65] As early as the time of Adam of Bremen, the haruspici or soothsayers of Curland, in Scandinavia, were visited by persons from Spain and Greece, seeking prognostications or health,[66] while at the same period identical enchanters among the Spanish Arabs, whose puissance was able to resurrect even the dead by certain characters placed under their arm-pits, were sought by Europeans.[67] A definite allegation against the erudite pontiff was his fabrication of human effigies, which, it was asserted, he had endowed with the virtues of gesticulation and speech.[68]

This extraordinary mechanism was, however, confined to an affirmative or negative response to specific questions;[69] but, according to the credulous narrator cited, the figure used by Gerbert was composed by him in perfect adjustment by astronomical calculations, and possessed the power of predicting its maker's death, which, if the chronicler be accredited, actually happened.[70]

Such effigies, actually fabricated with a self-moving energy,

---

64 Ibid.

65 Herman, Corneri Chronicon, sub an. 998.

66 De Situ Danae, cap. 16.

67 Gervais. Tilburn., Otia Imperialia, Lib. I., c. 20.

68 "Christiani Tholetum, et Saraceni Hispalim urbem, quam Sibiliam vulgariter nominant, caput regni habentes, divinationibus et incantationibus student." Herman., Corner., op. cit., an. 998.

69 Wm. Malmsb., De Gestis Pontif. Angliæ, Lib. II., c. 40.

70 Wm. Malmsb., De Gestis, Pontif. Angliæ, Lib. II., c. 50.

according to a writer of the thirteenth century, by Dædalus,[71] recede in their preternatural virtue before the power of Gerbert to walk with ease upon the surface of deep water.[72] The construction of these puissant images, perhaps a development of the idolatrous mandragora figures of the early Carlovingian period, was a standing incrimination against ecclesiastic scholars hated and feared for eminent erudition, down to the time of Albert Magnus, who, it is asserted, successfully compounded one of clay.[73]

During the Middle Ages it was devoutly believed, and as scrupulously written by pious chronists, that Gerbert had sold himself to the devil. As late, indeed, as the year 1418, an annalist, whose register of events is of the most commendatory character, hesitated not to reaffirm this demoniacal transaction, and to detail the articles of the compact, which aid in elucidating Malmsbury's intimations.[74]

---

71 Gervasii Tilburnen, Otia Imperialia, Lib. I., cap. 19.

72 Chronicon Halberstadense, sub an. 998; and Herman Corner., Chronicon, sub an. 999.

73 Panciroli, De Rer. Rec. Invent., Tom. II., Tit. X., p, 230.

74 Gobelin. Personæ, Cosmodrom., Aet, VI., cap. 51.

CHAPTER XVIII.

Maladies Traced to Demoniac Sources—Holy Curatives Sanctioned by the Church—Social Troubles and Bodily Ailments Caused by Demons—Flowers Grown on Martyred Tombs of Great Sanitative Power—Healing Force of Prayers—Imbeciles as Tenements of Foul Spirits—Curative Virtue of a Saint's Hair—Monastic Treatment of Sick—Separate Division for the Infirm—Eagerness of Monks to go on the Sick List—The Mediæval Lancet—Sorts of Medicaments in Vogue.

THE case of Gerbert is particularly elaborated, in order to attest the ineradicable faith of those ages in the doctrine of diabolical potency, which, it was accorded, included the causation of maladies; and as a corollary to this proposition required saintly or magic interference to vanquish these manifestations of the arch-enemy or his demons. At a time when popular credence asserted that sudden death was purely a direct revelation of a decedent's evil nature, and that such events were a divine testimonial of judgment inflicted upon a vicious man,[1] it may be assumed that the dogma of demoniacal origin of diseases flourished into luxurious expansion among the ecclesiastics above, and rooted itself profoundly in the vulgar mind beneath. An unequivocal doctrine was finally reached and enunciated—inasmuch as Satan caused not only sickness and death, under the restrictive stipulations hitherto designated as dictated by Deity, as a logical sequence saints and martyrs, or their material representatives, could heal the diseased and revive the dead.

Legends of these sainted beings announced the resistless potency of their cure of maladies, together with the spiritual remedies of sinful and irreligious actions. Such virtues emanated, in the traditions, to cure hemorrhages, aches and pains

[1] Anglia Sacra, Tom. I., p. 12 seq.

of the head, caused by demons,[2] or of the body; readjusted luxations, united fractures, removed calculus, moderated the agonizing pangs of parturition, restored vision to sightless eyes, and renewed the sense of hearing to the deaf. Such remedies were both mediatory and immediate, or represented by tangible objects.

Thus, for instance, Franciscus de Paula succored an anchylosed joint, which the malevolence of the person afflicted had alone provoked, by the energetic surgery of three dried figs, which he gave the suffering patient to eat.[3] Like potency was displayed through the powerful properties of certain herbs, restoring to robust vigor a maiden grieving under a cancerous disease, when surgical skill had frankly admitted the impossibility of medicinal cure.[4] Hugo the Holy abstracted from the infirm body of a female a serpent by consecrated water, and Saint Melanus revived a child suffocated by the Devil. Coleta, the saintess, awakened from the dreamless slumber of death more than a hundred slain infants by the efficacy of a cross.[5] We have previously stated the strange forces attributed to the sepulchres of the sainted dead, whose curative prowess was universally accorded to survive their earthly dissolution; consequently, when the humble hunchback bowed the knee in adoration at the tomb of Saint Andreas, this irresistible faith instantly released him from his unnatural rotundity.[6]

The frequent cure of calculus seems to have been a favorite subject for the exercise of this holy expulsive power, summarily removing the painful disease. The same curative energy which immediately checked the aching throbs of a disordered head, reappeared in the vastness of magic power.[7]

---

[2] Annalista Saxo, Chronicon, sub an. 891.

[3] Acta Sanctorum, Bolland., Apr. 2, Tom. I., p. 98.

[4] Ibid.

[5] Acta Sanctor., Bolland., Apr. 29, Tom. III., p. 331; and Mar. 6, Tom. I., p. 626.

[6] Ibid., Mar. 19 and 6, Tom. I., pp. 14 and 19.

[7] Vita S. Præjecti, Januar. 25, Tom. II., p. 636.

Thus when the quenched light, which added to the sombre pomp with flaming rays before the sarcophagus of Saint Severin, had revived in the splendors of renewed fire, it was understood the vivifying sparks flashed forth directly from that occult source which fired the extinguished tapers in the crypt of Saint Gall.[8]

The lapsing of a tower in the Winchester cathedral attributed to divine vengeance for the contiguous interment of the unshrived William Rufus,[9] and the falling walls of Leicester to a nearly similar reason,[10] together with the horrors of famine and pestilence to an amazing defiance of the Holy Mother,[11] equally belong to that identical faith according the immensity of curative powers to entombed relics. Cognate with this principle of celestial visitation, through diabolical agencies, was the decree that the same William should immediately descend to hell, in case he retained the great see of Canterbury in his own hands.[12]

With the water in which Saint Sulpicius washed her hands, and with the flowers blooming in aromic beauty at the tomb of Bernard, aggravated infirmities were instantly cured.[13] The devout application to Saint Martin's pall, by Gregory of Tours, as an energetic medicine, has its singular counterpart in the puissant touch of the funebral bier of the above saintess, or by actual contact with the mortuary cloth enclosing her mortal remains.[14] Hairs of saints in the thirteenth century, especially of Boniface, the famous Teutonic evangelist, were endowed with the virtue of a medicinal purge;[15] and therefore

[8] Walafr. Strabo, De Miraculis S. Galli, Lib. II., c. 46.

[9] "Peccatis illius contigisse." Anglia Sacra, Tom. I., p. 270.

[10] Wm. Neubrig., Histor., sub an. 1196, Tom. I., p. 192.

[11] Scriptores post Bedam, p. 382.

[12] Eadmer Monachi, Histor. sui Saeculi, Lib. VI., p. 17.

[13] Acta SS., Jan. 23, Tom. II., cap. 8, p. 178 seq. Healing potency of Bernard, Helmoldi Chronicon, sub an. 1146, Lib. I., cap. 49.

[14] Acta SS., Jan. 24, Tom. II.; and Jan. 23, Tom. II., cap. 2, p. 454.

[15] "Pilos barbæ: pilli illi in aqua benedicta sibi darentur ad libidinum."

when a deeply grieved parent hung this sainted relic in the face of her moribund daughter, the divinized force was instantly exerted to cure the suffering infant.[16] This capillary remedy was of extraordinary potency when compounded with the hairs of saintess Coleta, not only to quickly eject heart disorders, but the possession of such objects enabled an innocent person accused of crime, subjected to torture, to pass with a peaceful smile through his agonizing proofs, as though reposing upon a downy bed. Fragments of her veil and the use of a well-worn cloak immediately cured a terrible luxation, and a cataleptic patient was restored to sanity by drinking from her cup.[17]

As a practical part of this mediæval medicine, the sick were taught the curative powers of liberal gifts to such ecclesiastical objects as the priestly physician indicated. Eadmer distinctly affirms the gigantic influence of the devil and his evil spirits, for ill, when he states that Anselm's return to England was delayed by advice of the demoniacal hosts, in order to crush out the vestiges of British Christianity.[18]

In all epidemics during the Middle Ages, such persons as were afflicted with pestilential diseases were declared contaminated by the Devil,[19] and carried to churches and chapels, a dozen at a time, securely bound together and thrown upon the floor, where they lay, according to the attestation of a pitying chronicler, until dead or restored to health.[20] Astrological prognostications for future health, and as a formal guide in the affairs of diurnal existence, were at an early period adopted by both Saracens[21] and Christians indifferently.

Matth. Paris, Annales, sub an. 1244. Essayed with effect by a Canterbury barber who had cut them from the saint's face.

[16] Acta SS., Febr. 19, cap. 3, Tom. III., p. 146.

[17] Ibid., Mar. 6, Tom. I., p. 626.

[18] Eadmer Mon., Histor. sui Saec., Lib. IV., p. 80.

[19] "In æstate grassavit quadam enormis infirmitatis acsi esset de temptatione malorum spiritum." Knyghton, De Eventibus Angliæ, Lib. IV., sub an. 1355; apud Dec., Script. I., p. 2609.

[20] "Ubi vincti jacebant donec à Deo relevationem acciperent." Ibid.

[21] Conde, Historia de la Dominacion des Arabes en España, pp. 378, 381.

The chamber described in the acts of Saint Sebastian was composed exclusively of glass, through which was visible a celestial sphere upon whose convexity was delineated the starry universe, with lines and admeasurements, designed to indicate the heavenly bodies.[22] Such orbs appear to have been used to fix certain days during mediæval times for taking physic, a custom carried down to the sixteenth century, when persons as a medicinal act throughly inebriated themselves, in order to secure the purification of the resultant emetic.[23] Oftentimes saintly remedies were applied to curing suffering animals, and frequently this exercise of preternatural power displayed itself in freeing captive birds and animals.[24]

To the Devil were attributed powers of evil, which popular belief admitted to be within the possibilities of magic; while on the contrary miraculous exhibitions of saintly and canonized martyrs were devoutly thought to possess advantages of unbounded good to mankind.

Holy Agnes, upon the pitiful prayer of a friar, saved him from suffocating by a fishbone, and a like invocation to Saint Peter prevented a woman from drowning.[25] Magical puissance of saints was, as we have seen, not restricted to the living body, but the inanimate type of the dead was endowed with forcible energy by contact or petition. Thus at a banquet presided over by emperor Henry of Germany, a costly vitreous urn was exhibited as a notable specimen of Alexandrine fabric, and during its passage around the table, by careless handling of the ecclesiastics, it was broken. Odilo, in attendance at the feast, fearing imperial anger against the clergy, proceeded to a conventual chapel, where by certain prayers and psalms he obtained the divine force which restored the fractured vase to its original integrity.[26]

---

[22] Du Cange, Glossar., sub v. Holivitreus.

[23] D'Aussy, Histoire de la Vie Privée des Français, Tom. I., p. 332.

[24] Acta SS., Bol., Mar. 5, Tom. I., pp. 318–31, 333. Dead raised by prayers. Ibid., Apr. 2, Tom. I., p. 94.

[25] Acta SS., Boll., Jan.21, Tom. II., p. 362.

[26] Ibid., Jan. 21, Tom. II., p. —.

In the year 1243, a Ferrara writer was at Padua for solemn vespers, and while attending these at the tomb where reposed the sainted body of the Minorite Anthony, he affirms that he saw a person, mute from birth, recover his voice and speak audibly. This man, according to the attestation of trustworthy Paduans, had been absolutely voiceless, and they expressed their amazement at this miraculous cure, which was performed by the defunct saint in the presence of the chronicler cited.[27]

Through the vicious agency of an enchantress in Regensburg, Satan professed to obtain unquestioned control over persons of evil character. Unsound mind was universally accepted as the specific distinction of diabolical power, and caused by the corporeal presence of an impure spirit. In this instance, Godehard, connected with the above mentioned city and its monastery,[28] one day journeyed along the municipal streets on cloister business, and met a personage so afflicted. Close scrutiny and peremptory interrogatories revealed to the saint the foul presence of a demon, whom, by the resistless power of divinity, he ejected from the enchantress' body, which restored her health to its former sanity.[29]

Imbeciles and the insane were, throughout the Middle Ages, especially conceded to be the abode of an avenging or frenzied demon. In aggravated cases actual presence of the medicinal saint was necessary; in less vexatious maladies the bare imposition of hands, accompanied by plaintive prayer, quickly healed the diseased.[30] Inasmuch as diseases during this period were attributed to Satanic origin, according to the direct transmission from the early Church, the principal, and in many

---

27 "Vir natus mutus, ut omnium civium erat assertio, dum orasset, vesperis sub illius sepulchro, loquelam et auditum recipit, quem vidi et audivi loquentem." Ricobaldi, Historia Imperatorum, sub an. cit.; ap. Eccard. I., p. 1170. In the year 1283, a chronist asserted he saw blind restored to sight by saintly surgery—"oculisque nostris vidimus." Lerbeccii, Chronic., Epp. Mind., cap. 35.

28 Anon. Chronic., Stedensberg, sub an. 1010.

29 Acta SS., Boll., May 4, Tom. I.

30 Ibid., Mar. 22, Tom. II.; Ibid.,—, Jan. Tom. II., § 5, p. 259 seq.; and Ibid., Vita S. Marci, Ap. 28, cap. 2, Tom. III., p. 584.

cases the only remedies applied, were drawn from the reliquiaries, or procured from materials assumed to contain a divine puissance—objects which the departed saints had used in daily occupation, incidentally touched, or, more powerful still, well-preserved bones, finger-nails, hair, and other fragments of the human frame.

When certain fevers were apparently too obstinate for treatment with medicaments, the immersion in water of a ring worn by Saint Remiginus, conveyed to it such magic force that it instantly became an infallible potion for such troublesome disorders.[31] It was doubtless a logical sequence from the premises stating the diabolical origin of maladies, that suitable cures must be sought in those types whose energy transcended the disabling force of Satan, because it was inspired by Deity; therefore, relics performed the most important functions in exorcising these impure germs. Thus, for instance, the wine washing such sacred objects, given to an imbecile, forcibly ejected an evil spirit from his mouth; while another tainted with idiocy was restored to instant health by simply transporting the fragments of Saint Anastasius.[32]

A single hair from the beard of Saint Vincent, placed about the neck of an idiot, drove away a vicious spirit which had withheld the sanitary operation of the imbecile's brain.[33] In the year 1244, Louis IX. of France, almost in the agonies of earthly dissolution, with rigid body, rigorous limbs, and fluctuating spirit, was brought to full health by the application to his moribund body of a piece of the true cross.[34]

How profoundly a belief in the actual presence of evil angels, as causes of bodily sickness, was current in mediæval society of lay and cleric, appears in the curative operations of Saint

---

31 "Annulus autem à digito ipsius extractus ab aquis intinctus potum febricitantibus varisque languoribus ægrotantibus salubrem dedit." Girald. Cambrenes, De Vita Episcop., Lincol., cap. 10; apud Angl. Sacr., Tom. II., p. 416.

32 Acta SS., Bolland, Jan. 17–22, p. 437 seqq.

33 Acta SS., Apr. 5, Tom. I.

34 "Aptavit corpori rigido et frigido, et redeunte spiritu, revivit." Matthew Paris, Annales, sub an. 1244.

Catharine. A woman possessed of the devil was presented to the immaculate saintess for prompt remedy: by the virtue of divine magic a demon was forced from each part of her body where he had taken refuge, but resisting absolute ejectment from this carnal abode, made a desperate conflict in the throat, when by uninterrupted scratches he reproduced himself in the form of an abscess.[35] Mediæval monasteries and cloisters, in possession of sanitary relics, were custodians of an inexhaustible source of riches and adoration.

We have hitherto stated the greed with which these sacred objects were struggled for by force and fraud in sacking the Byzantine city, and how swiftly the renown of their invincible virtues expanded throughout the West, which rapidly returned in a swelling tide of affluence to conventual treasuries. Thriving incomes were readily derived from them when carried about cities or provincial towns, and urged upon the grievously sick and infirm as containing transcendent curative power. In such proffers, enormous sums of money were demanded by the bearers of these sainted fragments, to furnish access to such as aspired to test their lauded remedial properties.[36]

For such purposes defunct saints inspired the same puissance into a limb or other fragmentary member, attributed to their whole bodies.[37] Slothful indifference of pontifical authorities, urged on by the rising necessities of denuded cloisters or impoverished nunneries, easily provided suitable methods of acquiring ecclesiastical fortunes, or remedying prelatial indigence by facile canonization. In such cases an official promulgation of miraculous properties in new saints was procured from the Archbishops,[38] and when this notice had issued to the public, the way was opened for traffic. Under specific circumstances conjuration formulas were used as a saintly

[35] Acta SS., Boll., Apr. 30, Tom. III.

[36] Decem Scriptores post Bedam, p. 25.

[37] Eadmer, Monach., Histor. sui Saeculi, Lib. IV., p. 78.

[38] Du Cange, Glossar., sub v. Preconizare.

medical cure for such diseases as impure spirits caused. Frightened priests resorted to these soothing curatives when afflicted women besought them to exorcise[39] a demon provoking maladies.

Oftentimes the formulary book contained no sufficient potency to expel the diabolical disease, although in unnumbered instances solemnly adjudged synodal exorcisms, by Church or Carlovingian authority, readily furnished desired remedies.[40] Laurentia, a maiden of youthful years, placed by her father within the sheltering walls of a cloister, to assume ultimately monastic vows, was quickly captured by an errant demon. As an irrefutable demonstration of the impure origin of her infirmity, an annalist asserts, this spirit promptly answered in elegant Latinity all questions propounded; but the strongest confirmation of this belief was the miraculous ability which enabled her to disclose the most secret thoughts of others, and divulge the mysterious affairs of her associates.

In this evident superiority of the afflicted girl may be traced a sly satire against erudite clerics, who ordinarily were inculpated with Satanic assistance in the ranking distinction of learning. Saint Catherine at length liberated the suffering female from her diabolical tenant.[41] Frequently the presence of a saint averted a catastrophe; or in their hands, by the magical stroke of a cross, an efficacious remedy was administered to diseases causing sudden death.[42]

Flowers reposing upon the tomb of a saint, when steeped in water, were regarded as endowed with mirific sanitary power.[43] Impostors were everywhere met, according to the annalists of

---

[39] "Qui cum per Bened. Petrum Martyr. dæmones adjuratus est, duo protinus exierunt." Acta SS., Boll., Apr. 29, cap. 14, Tom. III., p. 718. For similar cures, Ibid., p. 716.

[40] Baluzius, Formulæ Exorcisor., Tom. II., col. —, p. 639 seq.

[41] Acta SS., Boll., Apr. 30, Tom. III.

[42] Ibid., Apr. 30 and 22.

[43] "Quasdam de herbulis, quas devotis populi sacrum jecit in tumulum," etc. "Nam discerptis de his particulis, et frigoriticis cum aquæ potu porrectus, protinus cum haustu salutem invixit." Ib., Apr. 2, cap. 3, Tom. I., p. 98.

the Middle Ages, perambulating the different holy places in Germany, asserting most impudently that they were formerly deprived of sight, speech, hearing, and possessed of devils; but, in the presence of an excited multitude, swiftly flitting to and fro, as idiots, and with clenched fists pounding their hardy chests, proclaimed themselves the objects of saintly cures.[44]

Nuns and consecrated women residing in convents, whose time was employed in embroidering fine textures and attiring themselves in bridal vestments to attract the attention of strange men,[45] after having glided down the fascinating slope of human impulses, instead of relying upon the presumed puissance of religion, had recourse to the more practicable method of restoring their virginity by medicinal potions—a practice placed under the ban as early as the year 798, by a Carlovingian rescript.[46] In some instances erring sisters bore amulets or applied the preventative talismanic influence of a sacred shirt or girdle, to suppress the manifestation of conventual irregularities. The bold recommendation of mediæval medical professors against the legitimate results of these frailties, attests the extent of an evil justly regarded by the Church as a most heinous crime.[47]

At an early period, as we have seen, in the construction of monasteries, a regular appartment was set apart for a hospital or infirmary surgeon. Of these chambers devoted exclusively

---

44 "Personas, quæ in nostra patria, usitato more per sacra loca discurrentes, se aut cæcos, aut debiles, vel elingues, vel certe obsessos temere simulant, et ante altaria vel sepulchra sanctorum, se coram populo volutantes, pugnisque tundentes, sanatos illico proclamant," etc. Vita Godehardi, Ep. Hildist., cap. 7.

45 An inculpation by Beda, Histor. Eccles., Lib. IV., cap. 25, against Anglo-Saxon nuns as early as the year 679. Simeon, Dunhelm., Histor. Eclles., Lib. II., cap. 7. The cartulary of 789, by Charlemagne, evidently contemplated the secret principle involved in the text. Cap. 3, Baluz., Tom. I., col. 243.

46 Lex Salica, Tit. XXI., lex. 4.

47 "Si mulier bibat quodlibet mane per tres dies duas minas aquæ, in qua ferrarii extingunt forcipes suas steriles sit in perpetuum." Arnold Villannov., Breviarii Additiones, Lib. III., c. 5, col. 1338. To obtain this result Constans Afer advises "stercus elephantinum cum melle mixtum et in vulva mulieris positum." De Chirurgia, p. 320.

to cloister maladies or stranger infirm, usually designated by the name of Infirmary, there were several kinds. In the hospitals which, in the year 845, in Scotland, were placed under ecclesiastical protection by synodal canons,[48] specific divisions were made according to the nature of the diseases to be treated—one of which was solely directed to the care of bed-ridden patients—another received and attended those whose maladies, elsewhere subject to successful manipulation, rapidly approached convalescence, while the last gradation included aged, infirm, blind, and otherwise physically incurable, whose time was passed in carefully nursing monastic sick.[49]

An official specially deputed by the abbot, entitled Infirmerius,[50] was charged with the supervision of patients in this department. These rooms were provided with a chapel annexed to the infirmary itself, where the disabled brethren were obliged to appear for religious services so far as their disordered condition permitted.[51] Here divine celebration was performed from a breviary placed permanently in this structure.[52] Added to the sacerdotal functions of this charitable establishment, other practical adjustments contributed to the ease and comfort of cloister sick.

Private chambers, distinguished as antexenodochium, were often used as duplicate hospitals for the reception of aggravated diseases, requiring removal from the regular infirmary.[53] Notwithstanding the abbey Regulæ were so dexterously drawn as to repress, in great measure, fraudulent accessions to the monastic Infirmary, frequently young and robust, but indolent

---

48 Mabillon, Annales Ord. S. Bened., Tom. II., p. 660.

49 Du Cange, Glossar., sub v. Infirmarius.

50 Ibid.

51 Ibid., sub v. Lobium.

52 Anglia Sacra, Pars I., pp. 393, 399. In the year 680, it appears that moribund sick were carried into a special chamber to die—"autem in proximo casa, in qua infirmiores et qui prope morituri esse videantur, induci solebant." Beda, Histor. Eccles., Gent. Angl., Lib. IV., c. 24.

53 Du Cange, sub v. Antixenodochium.

monks, gained a relaxation of severe discipline by blinding the prior, thus obtaining entrance to the hospital. This eagerness of recluses to procure access to the domum infirmorum, is made the subject of biting sarcasm by the illustrious prior of Clairvaux abbey, in the year 1120.[54] When, however, the malady was slight, it received medical treatment in the Oriel.[55] The principal motive in procuring admission on frivolous pretences to this apartment, appears to have been a meat diet or other delicacies,[56] which were given when the disease threatened rapid progress.[57]

Among other necessary appurtenances to the infirmary was a stone slab on which the dead were washed for funeral rites.[58] Medical assistance was provided the brethren and visiting monks, by the communal organization of the convent, whenever such medicines were essential.[59] If it happened, which was indeed rare, that suitable medicaments could not be furnished by an abbey, leave was granted to obtain them from other sources. According to the architectural plan of Saint Gall, in the eighth century, which may be accepted as uniform with subsequent edifices till the close of the Middle Ages, the Benedictines kept a botanical garden, not alone for growing medicines and remedial herbs, but a regular pharmaceutical depôt, or, as in the case of San Vitalis, a Ravennate cloister, maintained a complete assortment of surgical instruments, adapted to great diversity of operations.[60]

Minute regulations by ecclesiastical authority, in conformity to earlier Carlovingian and synodal canons,[61] prescribed phle-

---

54 "In domo se infirmorum, qui non sunt infirmi, collocare." Apologia ad Guillelmum, cap. 9, § 22.

55 Du Cange, Gloss., sub v. Oriel.

56 Chronicon Novalense, Lib. II., cap. 1.

57 Matthew Paris, Annales, sub an. 1009.

58 Matth. Par., cit. 1045.

59 Vadiani, De Collegiis Monasteriis, Lib. I., p. 23.

60 Observations sur l'Italie, Tom. I., p. 323 seq.

61 Baluz., Cartular, cap. 11, Tom. I., p 581.

botomy as a sanitary precaution or certain curative, and aided in developing a filiation of medical economy, which survived most obstinately to modern practice. The lanceola or knife which performed this important function was thus denominated on account of its resemblance in miniature to the military lance of the age; and the operation was designated commonly minution, originally incised by a monastic servant or barber.[62] Dugdale reproduced a curious contract with the founder of Piperville abbey, by which he should receive four blood-lettings a year.[63]

Constans Afer not only gives precise directions touching the construction, shape, and length of this lancet, but advises the utmost precaution in such operations,[64] and urges the surgeon to cultivate such skill as to be able to distinguish by the touch what portion of the person holds the veins, nerves, etc., necessary to be known in these operations, which should besides be treated in connection with golden pellets once a week.[65] Monasteries of enormous numbers, including regular monks and conversi, appear to have had a small edifice exclusively devoted to this principal surgic operation of the Middle Ages,[66] and dangerous oftentimes by a dexterous hand,[67] especially if performed, according to the sagacious Bede, in the moon's first quarter.[68]

The act of minutio, or cupping, is oftentimes referred to by mediæval chroniclers, under the general classification of phlebotomy, as performed by the most exalted personages in soci-

---

62 Du Cange, Glossar., sub v. Lanceolus.

63 "Item vendicat quator minutiones per annum infra abbatiam." Monastic Anglic, Tom. I., p. 818.

64 "Neque in tenebrose id faciendum est loco." De Chirurgia, p. 324.

65 "Item Chirurgici utantur," etc.; "et semel in hebdomada pillulis aureis. Phlebotamor discat tactu digitorum venas, carnem, nervum agnoscere." Ibid., p. 325.

66 Du Cange, sub v. Phlebotamus.

67 Walafr. Strabo, De Miraculis S. Galli, Lib. II., c. 37.

68 Histor. Eccles., Lib. V., c. 3.

ety,[69] both sacerdotal[70] and lay, for purely medicinal purposes.[71] When it became evident that a monk in the Infirmary was approaching earthly dissolution, notice was sent to the prior and convent by the official in charge.[72] Thereupon a monastic servant placed beneath the agonizing friar a hair cloth, enclosing consecrated ashes,[73] and in the last utterances of death two anchorites on watch by the dying brother's side hastened to the cloister portals, and struck a table with a hammer, which was a signal of death agony.[74]

Instead of frequent medication, physical exercise on foot with staff in hand,[75] or sawing wood, were recommended in the abbeys as of the highest sanitative efficacy—closely resembling the advice of Galen in the second century.[76] The gradual increase of secular patients in monastic hospitals, attending for medical treatment, bathing and healthy diet, rendered the influx at times so great that the troops of restless valetudinarians and impostors became troublesome, and intensified this grievance by liberal interchange of public scandal. This tumultous crowding finally reached to such objectionable features, that strict ordinances were promulgated restricting actual presence in Infirmaries to the sick, physicians, and lay servants attending by medical direction upon helpless inmates.[77]

If the vehement satires of Burton be accepted as indicating the usage of medicaments during the Middle Ages, it would seem that the physic most gladly followed was found in a liberal diet for the robust people of country towns, while sur-

[69] Conrad Ursperb., Chronicon, sub an. —.

[70] Paul. Diacon., Chronic. Casin., Lib. IV., c. 100.

[71] Du Cange, sub v. Minuere.

[72] Ibid., sub v. Infirmarius.

[73] Du Cange, Glossar., sub v. Cinis.

[74] Ibid., sub v. Ferula.

[75] "Baculos in manibus sortare jubentur aegrotantes." Bernard, Apologia ad Guillelmum, cap. 9, § 23.

[76] Galen, De Sanitat. Tuenda, cap. 8.

[77] MS. Cotton, Claud. E., fol. 245.

feited courtiers and idle gentry resorted to frequent medications.[78] Whether mediæval dentists reached the skill of their more ancient precursors, in the dexterous use of the dentiducium, there can be no doubt touching the inferiority in the preparation of powders and gold filling of the seventh century, when indeed artificial teeth appear to have been used.[79] In the eleventh century Constans Afer advised the preference to file down rather than extract teeth as a cure for the dolorous pangs of tooth-ache,[80] with which, in an epidemic form, the doughty crusaders were frequently afflicted, so severely indeed, as to become mortal.[81]

Vagrant monks, in Wickliffe's age, habitually studied the physiological constitution of women from the works of Hippocrates and Galen, and when possessed of sufficient knowledge to give apparent reason to their medical argumentations, persuaded wives, in the absence of their husbands, that certain bodily ailments could be alone corrected by permitting them the right of administering the remedy as they pleased.[82]

In a manuscript diary of Gerald Cambrenesis,[83] two wily cenobites are described as deserting conventual rules and abandoning themselves wholly to a vagrant life, who, after struggling for an indefinite period to maintain an existence honestly or otherwise, finding the effort too severe and unprofitable, turned their attention to the art of medicine, apos-

---

[78] Burton, Anatomy of Melancholy, fol. 36.

[79] Lessing, Geschichte der Medezin, Th. I., p. 175 seq.

[80] "Deinde vero super dentem nisi dolor accedat, melius est limare, quam ex trahere." Liber de Chirurgia, cap. 35, p. 339.

[81] Amelrici, Historia Pontific. Roman., sub an. 1243, Ecc. 11, p. 1775.

[82] "Docentes, cum illis concubere in absentiis maritorum, maxime esse contra varias ægritudines salubre." Wickliff, De Hypococrasi, Pars I., p. 475, Ed. Bale.

[83] MS. Cotton, Tib. B. 13. This MS., published by Brewer, at p. 19, Vol. I., Rer. Brit. Med. Ævii Scriptores, entitled De Rebus à se Gestis, according to the terminal note on the parchment, lacks nearly a hundred chapters. Fosbroke, British Monachism, p. 236, evidently reproduced the citation in the next note from an unverified source, at second hand, because this portion of the text was destroyed in the last century.

trophized as a most lucrative profession in the twelfth century—pecuniosam artis medicinalis peritam—and began with impudent boldness to practice medicine, without, as the writer indignantly declares, having ever heard or read of Galen or Hippocrates, or other books of this avocation, in schools or elsewhere.[84]

[84] "Et pecuniosam artis medicinalis peritam profitere non minus imprudenter præsumpserunt, cum tum Hippocratem aut Galeni cæterumque librorum facultatis illius, nunquam in scolis aut alibi lectionem unnam audissent aut legissent." Gerald, Cambr., De Rebus à se Gestis, cit.

CHAPTER XIX.

Medical Astrology—Its Adaptation to Ordinary Social Events—Charms for Expelling Disease—Astrological Treatises of Friar Bacon—Virtue of Magic Words—Alchemy—Extraction of "Spirits"—Medicinal Energy of such Extracts—Curative and Preventative Puissance of Stones or Gems—Necromancy—Mediæval Scientists Admit the Power of Charms and Letter Characters—Potency of Angelic Names for Cures—Enchanters' Spell—Amulets in the Middle Ages—Prayers or Invocations Inscribed on Leaves, etc.—Sanitary Angels—Stellar Influence Applied to the Curative Art—Effigy of Diseased Part Fabricated to Obtain Remedy.

IN close and intimate connection with the curative art, throughout the entire period of the Middle Ages, was the science of astrology. During the earliest eras of civilization, astronomical influences over the destinies of mankind appear to have been universally accepted, and its details, according to more elevated refinement of the people, reduced to rigid rules. As remote, indeed, as the Babylonians, certain calculations were made to determine the movements of celestial orbs, the subtle essence of which was presumed to be an integral force in the operations of the human body.[1]

Notwithstanding the fact that the Fathers of the Church, soon after its development and organization under imperial recognition, altered the plan somewhat of medicine[2] and astronomy, in order to reduce them to a Christian basis,[3] the vital power supposed to inhere within these heavenly bodies was perpetuated under the form of magic and its diversified operations. In the second century Gamaliel astonished the crew of a forlorn vessel, on which he was a passenger, by an

---

[1] Matter, École d'Alexandrie, Tom. II. p. 80.

[2] Cuvier, Histoire des Sciences Naturelles, Tom. I., p. 366 seq.

[3] Bossuet, Histoire des Mathematiques, Tom. I., p. 160 seq.

abstruse calculation of exact location from the sight of a comet revolving in an orbit of seventy years.[4]

Judicial astrology maintained a tenacious vitality in the popular mind in Europe to the very close of the Middle Ages —a function to which the terrible Tamerlane himself seems to have abandoned his reason and discretion, although requiring his sons to be instructed in the science of astronomy in the academy of Samarcand, where this abstruse art was taught.[5] Beyond the limits of magical circles, the human mind eagerly sought, by means of subjective powers, unlimited pleasure, constant health, and uninterrupted affluence. Although astrological science in its medicinal application was currently practiced from an early period of the ages under examination, in the fifteenth century, after the fall of the Byzantine empire before Ottoman forces, it was vigorously developed through duplicate Greek manuscripts, explanatory of this curious subject, mainly derived from corrupt Arabic sources, where such calculations were made at birth and carefully recorded.[6]

In the year 968, when the envoy of Otho I., Emperor of Germany, was in Constantinople, he found the Greeks using Saracen astrological books, in which prognostications touching future events of that empire were written and awaiting verification.[7] Through these various avenues, the potency of astrology was encouraged and essayed, as appears, successfully in the cure of diseases. Robert Grosteste, bishop of Lincoln, hitherto alluded to as the scientific friend of Friar Bacon, in the first part of the thirteenth century, while at Oxford, certainly utilized his Arabic knowledge to construct charms for expelling maladies.[8]

[4] Graetz, Hist. of the Jews, p. 33 seq.

[5] Voltaire, Essai sur les Moeurs et Usages, Tom. II., p. 477.

[6] Conde, Historia de la Dominacion de los Arabes en España, p. 326.

[7] "Habent Græci et Saraceni libros quos vocant, ego autem sibyllanos; in quibus scriptum repositur, quotannis imperator quisque vivat, quæ sunt futura, eo imperante, tempora," etc. Liudprandi, Legatio, cap. 39.

[8] "Invenit voces, quibus allevare solebat
Ægrorum morbos, subsidiumque dabat."

De Vita Grostest., cap. 19.

Bacon himself, notwithstanding his studies and researches in Arabic medicine and pharmacy,[9] was not exempt from professing a firm belief in the omnipotence of astrology to cure maladies, while Gerbert most unequivocally reduced the operations of nature to hazard.[10] The progress made in mathematical science from the time of Hermanus Contractus, a monk of Saint Gall, in the year 1050, to the Hohenstauffen Emperor Frederick II., advanced in an exact proportion to the movement of astrology. Independent of the private historical writings[11] of this illustrious author, and his services to geometry at the period designated, he was equally famous for an astrological treatise known as Tractatum Astrolobii.[12] Frederick II., one of the most munificent patrons of solid learning and science in the thirteenth century, in the translation of the Ptolemaic Almagest, permitted the version to be drawn up on an astrological basis, similar to the errors contained in the Alfonsine tablets, the conjoined labor and erudition of Jewish, Moslem, and Christian scholars.[13]

At a time when the best minds of Europe were engrossed with Arabic sciences, whose application aided in the delineation of the metallic plate with the system of Ptolemy's universe, in the possession of Croyland abbey,[14] Grosteste, pontiff of Lincoln, essayed the practical adaptation of his Oriental learning to inventing words for exorcising fiends, and other equally mystical characters of medicinal puissance, which, as manifestations of this exalted power, were engraven on valuable gems.[15]

---

9 Bacon. De Compositione Elixiris, c. 6. p. 70.

10 "Sors omnia versat." Gerberti, Epistolar., Ep. 15. On his astrology, Ibid., Ep. 8 and 24.

11 According to Otto Frisingen, Chronicon, Lib. VI., c. 33, this was an account of the acts and virtues of Henry, Emperor of Germany, for private circulation—"quem ipsi destinavit."

12 Andræ Ratisbon, Chronicon, c. 157.

13 Bailly, Histoire de l'Astronomie Moderne, Tom. I., p. 299.

14 Henry, History of England, Vol. VI., p. 109.

15 "Deque characteribus fuit auctor quos pretiosos.
Inscripsit geminos, mira potentur agens,"

De Vita Grosteste, cap. 19.

The use of names for speedy curatives was charged upon the Christian evangelist, Saint Swibert, in the seventh century, by the Frisian sacerdoty, who alleged the restoration to sanity of a stricken paralytic was accomplished "not by medicaments and iron," but by the magic word.[16]

Gervaise, of Tilbury, affirmed the Tetragrammaton of the Jews was sufficiently potent to revive a cadaver after long burial,[17] and that the exorcising prowess of Solomon's ring was omnipotent.[18] Of the species of minerals most industriously sought for remedial or other properties was the philosopher's stone, to which transcendent wisdom, unremitting health, and the certainty of wealth were ascribed.[19] From the ancient doctrine, that beneficient or malevolent angels peopled the universe, was gradually developed an unquestioned belief that in all things, animate and inanimate, were contained these demons, who, by the superior energy of magic or formal incantations, could be subjected to human control; and that within the hidden recesses of metals or minerals resided the subtle essence or spirit, whose divine powers were manipulated by cabalistic combinations for the benefit of the possessor.

This system of extracting the energetic beings domiciled in these mystic abodes, was apparently introduced as early as the time of Gerbert in the tenth century, and pursued in the retired pharmacies of convents, upon formulated prescriptions procured from Spain[20]—an operation partaking a union of ecclesiastic or theological process, sanctioned by authority, and performed with pious but ardent prayers during the tests. The holiness with which this was originally invested, either through neglect or despair, vanished when the invocations of divinity during the alchemical labors had been forgotten and

---

16 Vita S. Swiberti, cap. 18; ap. Leibnitz, II., p. 234.

17 Otia Imperialia, Dist. III., cap. 112.

18 Ibid., Dist. I., cap. 20.

19 Liebig, Chemische Briefe, Th. I., p. 51; and further, 3d Briefe, Tom. I., p. 46 seqq.

20 Delrio, Disquisit. Magicar., Lib. I., cap. 5, § 1, p. 29.

fallen into desuetude towards the thirteenth century, a period wholly engrossed with the superiority of Satan over deified angels—consequently the enthusiastic alchemist or astrologist sought refuge in adjuration of evil demons to consecrate the secrets of this mighty art and render his essays satisfactory.[21]

Medical and alchemical writers of the Middle Ages, in recommending the use of minerals, minutely described their sanitary properties, which made them objects of zealous research. The diamond rendered a man wholly invisible; the Indian agate provided him with eloquence, prudence, and an agreeable amiability. For its preventative virtues against inebriety, the amethyst was greatly cherished; and the hyacinth was an infallible cure for sleeplessness. The amber was a a sovereign panacea against cerebral troubles and fevers, the jasper cured epilepsy and for such purposes was unrivalled, while the pulverized magnet taken as a potion with milk, prevented melancholy. The bezoar was an instant antidote for poisons.[22]

Coral hung about the neck as a talisman, strengthened the body, and peculiarly so if held in the mouth—the efficacy of which was attested by experience.[23] Constans Afer advised dog-teeth as a specific remedy for rabies.[24] Solomon's ring controlled demons.[25] Noblemen wore the smargdum attached to a chain, in the belief of its potential virtues against epilepsy.[26] The sard prevented terrible dreams, and the cornelian worn on the finger or suspended from the neck pacified anger and provoked contentment. Onyx superinduced troubled sleep, but fastened to the throat, stimulated the salivary glands.[27]

---

[21] Roskoff, Geschichte des Teufels, Th. II. p. 107.

[22] Panciroli, Rer. Memorabil., Tom. II., Tit. 3, p. 117.

[23] Arnold Villannova, De Distillatione Medicinorum, cap. 11, çol. 591. On this subject Galen, De Composit. Medicam., Lib. IX., cap. 5, §§ 19 and 29.

[24] Constans Africani, De Incantat. et Adjurat., Epistol., p. 318.

[25] Gervas. Tilburn., Otia Imperialia, Dist. III., c. 28.

[26] Const. Afric., op. cit., p. 319.

[27] Ibid.

Saphirs cured internal ulcers and excessive perspiration, when taken as a potion dissolved in lacteal fluids.[28] The gaygetes and ætite stones were urged as a certain remedy for difficult parturtion,[29] while others prescribed the smaragd mixed with honey, in cases of strabismus.[30]

Spider webs constituted an important article of medication to cure superficial ulcers.[31] It was urged that the green jasper, to possess the proper endowments of sanitary amulets, must be engraved with a dragon figure and radiated mane, according to the counsels of an ancient Egyptian king, Nicephorus.[32] When these gems changed color, it was considered a sure and reliable test of the presence of poison.[33] One of the most curious features of this systematic extraction of spirits or divine essences enclosed within these stones or metals, was the perfect good faith with which famous alchemists and astrologers persisted in their declarations of possessing such diabolical beings thus obtained, and carried them around in glass bottles.[34]

Chemical extracts, or essences procured by mysterious processes and designated spirits, when liberated and free to exert their natural energies, might, indeed, deceive venerable scientists in those obscure ages, and pass for bottled demons. Mediæval soothsayers fabricated images in which captive spirits were placed, to suitably instruct their possessors touching doubtful affairs in an uncertain future.[35] Divination, or augury, as a well-defined branch of astrology, was much used as a means of predicting events and prognosticating maladies.

[28] Aëtii, Tetrabili, Lib. I., Sermo 2, cap. 38.

[29] Ibid., Lib. I., Ser. 2, c. 24.

[30] Ibid., cap. 39.

[31] Ibid., cap. 165.

[32] Ibid., Lib. I., Ser. 2, cap. 33.

[33] Dec. Scriptor., p. 2435.

[34] Kopp, Geschichte der Chemie, Th. II., p. 161 seq. Alchemy zealously patronized by Spanish Sultans in 1190, Ib., p. 193.

[35] Du Cange, Glossar., sub v. Imaginarii.

For such purposes, cups, basins, swords, mirrors, glass, or other smooth surfaces, were largely used for the prophetic voice.[36]

Early synods of the Church specifically defined this sortilege by a Christian as incantation, and consequently forbidden as a nefarious usage, especially to Irish converts.[37] Enchanters were sufficiently adepts in occult sciences in the thirteenth century to compel demons to appear by the puissant energy of certain rites, and reveal at the intersection of public highways on sacrificing a pair of pigeons at midnight,[38] urns, ships, towers, immense treasures, and other paraphernalia, usually conceded to Arabic jugglers.[39] As early as the latter part of the sixth century, medical soothsayers were called upon to cure vexatious and obstinate diseases. Their system appears to have included murmured incantations, throwing of dice or hazards, perhaps prophecy, and the suspension of ligatures to the neck.[40] As a direct emanation of alchemical processes, which extracted essential elements from metals or minerals, subsequently imprisoned in crystal flasks under the generic term of imps or evil spirits, was the accusation charged upon certain scholastics of maintaining familiar demons under the common-place form of cats.[41]

A profound impress was given at a remote epoch to the specific remedies designated for the cure of disorders, and they were constantly used throughout the Middle Ages. Hu-

---

36 Ibid., sub v. Specularii.

37 Synodus Patricii, Canon. XVI.; and Gratian, Concilia, Decr. II., Causa XXVI., Qu. 5, c. 12.

38 Notices et Extraites des MSS. du Biblio. Roi, Tom. V., p. 506.

39 "Quendam incantor et urnes et navem et domum cum immenso ostendit." Annales Eccles. Wigiorn., an. 1287; ap. Anglia Sacr., Pars II.; p. 509.

40 "Ariolum quendam invocant, ille verò venire non differens accussit ad ægrotum et artem suam exercere conatur. Incantationes immurmurat, sortes jactat, ligaturas collo suspendit." Gregor. Turones, De Miraculis S. Juliani, Lib. II., cap. 45. Also, Vita S. Præjecti; ap. Acta SS. Bolland., Januar. 25, Tom. II., p. 636.

41 "Quidam scriptor Jonnes habens murelegum sibi familiorem." Knyghton, Dec. Script., p. 2535.

man figures, military tessera—evidently the dice employed by medical enchanters—sortes jactat, and certain words, were of universal application instead of medicaments, so much so, indeed, that Maimonides, of Cordova, the illustrious Jewish physician and scholar, in the twelfth century, in the most denunciatory epithets, while admitting the curative properties of certain mineral or metallic essences, asserted the absolute folly and mendacity of predicting restoration to health upon the use of images, written letters, or magic vocables, with which the very air was startled as by the repercussion of thunder.[42]

The mediæval scientists of Western Europe, however, were not so free from superstitions as the Israelitish savan of Spain. Villannova abundantly recognizes the power of lettered characters when sprinkled with blood in the hands of an unforgiving rival, to totally transform the enticements of the nuptial chamber.[43] Equally famous surgeons of the eleventh century admitted their adhesion to the salutary benefactions, to suffering patients, of incantations.[44]

Magicians professed to have at their command a triple kind of effigy, whose potency through the incantation or adjuration of fifty-four angelic names was irresistible.[45] Manuscript books on such subjects, explicitly stated, that when Deity granted proper nomenclature to persons or material objects, he simultaneously inspired certain offices and forces to the names and things, correlatively, which being aggregated evolved an energetic puissance, not by reason of the image or pronunciation, but by virtue of that inherent force with which God had endowed both upon calling them into existence.[46]

Therefore magic rings and sanitative seals or gems, on which were skillfully dilineated the potential names of Raphæl, Macchabees, Solomon, Eleazer, Zacharias, and Constantine the

[42] Ductor Dubitant, Lib. I., cap. 60, fol. 24.

[43] "Ne coeant in lecto jacintes; quædam de characteribus scriptis cum sanguine vespertilionis." De Maleficiis, col. 1529.

[44] Constant. African., Liber de Chirurgia, p. 318.

[45] Delrio, Disquisit. Magicar., Lib. I., cap. 4.

[46] Ibid., p. 18.

Great itself, to which—especially the last, on account of the cruciform figure and symbol of Deity, extraordinary powers were attributed.[47] To this class of enchanters is to be ascribed an Israelitish physician or medicus, in the year 876, who exhibited in the presence of Ludwig, emperor of Germany, the vast resources of the art. He could call forth the sounds of an army moving with heavy tread and hastening march through the invisible regions of space, and evoke the rarest flowers, magnificent gardens and choicest fruits.

When, indeed, under his enchanting spells, a person advanced one foot, the other must follow.[48] Notwithstanding, controversial writers of the Romish Church with explicit denial repudiated the curative forces of words or letters of the alphabet, which by the system of Joseph of Castile, as explained in his Isogoge, combined with the fifty executory spirits, aggregated seventy-two essences, or the Shemhamphorash, it was expressly avowed that the consecrated exorcisms, formulas of saints, ecclesiastical prayers, were charged by Divinity himself with a vital energy for transcending magic or demoniacal rites.[49]

Upon the accepted principle that those portions of the human body devoted to tender sentiments were in close astrological connection with celestial orbs whose invisible essence or spirit controlled corresponding elements of the terrestial sphere, therefore a skilled magician, physician, as we shall presently see, or alchemist, in its relation to medical economy, was enabled to provoke, through his superior science, those subtle and resistless forces which blindly performed their functions with the certainty of a mathematical problem.[50] The use of amulets for the prevention of disease and other pur-

---

[47] "Par ratio est de annulis et sigillis magicis quantumvis præferant speciosissima nomina Raphaëliis, Machæborum, Salominis, Elizei, Zachariæ, Constantini, et quorundamundam sanctorum." Ib., Lib. I., cap. 4, Qu. 1, p. 18.

[48] Ibid., p. 17.

[49] Delrio, Disquisit. Magicar., Lib. I., cap. 4, Qu. 3.

[50] Ibid., cap. 4, Qu. 4, p. 27. "Quidam voces ex verborum conjunctione vires adipisci existimant." Vairius, De Fascinatione, Lib. I., cap. 5.

poses, is of high antiquity. Greek athletes before hazarding their physical forces in the struggles of the arena wore amulets or phylacteries, as charms against the magic devices of an antagonist.[51]

Cognate with access to reliquaries as curatives for maladies, was the custom sanctioned by the mediæval church, of carrying consecrated objects as talismans suspended from the neck. Certain formulas of prayer inscribed on vellum, leaves or tessera, were regularly borne about as amulets against sickness, wounds, dangers by fire and water, at a period as late as the sixteenth century.[52] Of this nature was the agnus dei, for which especial potency was claimed.[53] Church synods distinctly inculpated this medicinal adoption of Paganistic customs, and classified the ursarii, addicted to suspending tinctures to the head or body of bears, and having clipped the hair from the animal's hide a potion was made of it, which it was alleged had the mighty property of expelling disease or arresting evil influences of "fascinating eyes."[54]

The name of Raphael for such purposes was presumed to be omnipotent, and largely used by Gallic peasants during the Middle Ages.[55] The principle by which these celestial beings were set in motion was perpetuated from distant periods, consisting of that mutual correlation existing between the names, when rightly understood, and the essential power of heavenly personages, whose puissance extended to presaging fatalities and predicting the future.[56]

During the pontificate of Zacharias, a council at Rome, presided over by the pope, after publicly reading a treatise of Adalbert, proceeded by solemn vote to condemn the sanitary

---

[51] Juvenal, Satyra, Lib. III., v. 1.

[52] "Alia quoque amuleta succini ant alterius materiæ contra morbos gestitabant." Delrio, op. cit., Lib. I., cap. 4, p. 27.

[53] Vairius, op. cit., Lib. III., cap. 10.

[54] Delrio, Disquisit. Magicar., Lib. I., cap. 4, p. 28.

[55] Legrand D'Aussy, Histoire de la Vie Privée des Français, Tom. II., p. 195.

[56] Cornel. Agrippa, De Occult Philosoph., Lib. II., cap. 26.

use of the words Uriel, Raguel, Tubuel, Michael, Adimis, Tubuas, Simihel, and Sabaoth.[57] Of these, the last appears to have represented typically the superior and exalted power of the Hebrew tetragrammaton.[58] Like magical and sanitative force was presumed to dwell within images fabricated to resemble celestial beings, whose gracious care was thus conciliated.

If it were desired to provoke a favorable event, either of health or fortune, the right side of a statuette was specifically operated; while, on the contrary, malevolence of body, mind, or wealth, was irresistibly evoked upon an enemy by the reverse of the effigy.[59] The preparation of such figures for good or ill, is certainly traceable to the universal medical endowment accorded mandragora images by pagan Norsemen, for the expulsion of diseases,[60] and at a later epoch of the Middle Ages—A. D. 1190—such sanitary effigies appear to have constituted an important element in the curative power attributed to Sicilian baths.[61] The vitality of this singular credence, when practiced to cure disorders, was sanctioned by secular authority through an interdict against the use of charms and herbs in judicial duels.[62]

Touching the details of the pathology or curative system for aggravated diseases, the mediæval astrologers, into whose hands the care of infirm and suffering patients was committed, asserting astral influences, divided this art in mathematical departments, where chronology united its force to restore health jointly with medical astrology.[63] For instance, in this

---

[57] Delrio, op. cit., p. 28 seq.

[58] Cornelia Agrippa, op. cit., Lib. II., cc. 7 and 8.

[59] Delrio, op. cit., Lib. I., p. 6.

[60] Rothii, De Imagin. German., p. 52.

[61] Arnoldi, Chronica Slavorum, Lib. V., c. 19.

[62] "Si quis culpabilis ingravante Diabolo, corde indurato, per aliqua malificia aut per herbas contegere peccata sua voluerit." Goldast, Alaman. Antiquitat, Tom. II., p. 139.

[63] Cornelia Agrippa, De Occult. Philosoph., Lib. II., cc. 36 and 37.

solemn function, when the operations were rendered infallible by mystic rites and potent words to conjure the most obstinate malady, a planet, in accord with the invalid's age, was selected as directly in conjunction with the sickness sought to be cured.

The great mediæval physicians urged with much vehemence and amazing elaboration the necessity of practitioners familiarizing themselves thoroughly with the profound and obscure principles of medical astrology, and for such, prepared erudite treatises governing the practical application of this curative art.[64] Thus the puissance of Saturn was manipulated for dotards, Mercury for adolescents, and Jupiter for manhood. To these planets, when properly subjugated by mysterious ceremonies, other virtues were accorded, by which qualities or affections might be superinduced.[65]

In such emergencies, Mars inspired hatred, and the tender Venus the sentiments of love. From Aries, at the head, to Pisces, or fishes, upon the feet, corresponding virtues were under the control of the dexterous astrological physician. In their atmospheric influences—an important element of medical economy, and fully appreciated by mediæval practitioners—these orbs were exactly graded: Saturn was asserted to be a planet of dry and frigid action, and contrary to vitality; Jupiter, in his warmth and humidity, was favorable to life; Mars, though tepid and dry, contained the elements of destructive energies, and the Sun, combining heat and dryness, possessed benevolent forces.[66]

Erudite and learned medicists of the Middle Ages, in defiance to ecclesiastical authority, devoutly adhered to this system of remedies.[67] Oftentimes physicians, in strict harmony with the method of astral treatment indicated, performed the

---

[64] Arnold Villannova, De Judiciis Astronomicæ, cc. 5 and 9.

[65] Cornelia Agrippa, op. cit., Lib. II., cap. 26.

[66] Arnold Villannova, De Judiciis Astronomiciæ, cap. 10.

[67] Delrio, Disquisitio Magicar., Lib. I., cap. 1, p. 7; and Condromachi, De Morb. Venefic., Lib. II., cap. 6.

surgical operation of phlebotomy or blood-letting on certain critical days—dubius criticus, as they were denominated—and administered potions or philters prepared upon similar notions, equally drawn from the postulated assumption that the time fixed for these important events was rendered propitious by the planets controlling the particular disease, and that medicaments thus compounded were of especial power in expelling sickness.

So great, indeed, became the abuse of medical astrology, whether by the direct juxtaposition of stellar influence, or through apposite images,[68] that a celebrated Church Council at Paris declared that images of metal, wax, or other materials fabricated under certain constellations or according to fixed characters—figures of peculiar form, either baptized, consecrated or exorcised, or rather desecrated by the performance of formal rites at stated periods which it was asserted, thus composed, possessed miraculous virtues set forth in superstitious writings—were placed under the ban and interdicted as errors of faith.[69] In the ninth century (A. D. 875), it was yet a usage in provoking a remedy for otherwise incurable ailments, to fabricate an effigy of the diseased member and consecrate it for supernatural cure somewhat after the earlier Teutonic pathology. Thus, for instance, if it were a sightless orb to be restored, the similitude of an eye was formally presented.[70] When, therefore, Theetmar's son, a sufferer with a disordered head, for many years after the eleventh century surgeons confessed, after numerous operations, their utter impotency, an image of the stricken member brought a permanent cure.[71] In the Sicilian baths mentioned, the figures of bodily parts, for

---

[68] " Efficaciores tamen largiuntur imaginibus virtutes, si non ex qualibet, sed certa materia fabricientur." Cornelia Agrippa, De Occult. Philosoph., Lib. II., cap. 35.

[69] Delrio, Disquisit. Magicar., Lib. I., cap. 1, p. 7.

[70] "Quædam matrona dolore occulorum gravabatur, occulos argenteos sanctis transmisit et salvata est." Lerbeccii, Chronic. Epp. Mindensis, cap. 3.

[71] Vita Bernwardi, Ep. Hildish., cap. 58.

the diseases of which the waters were a remedy,[72] evidently assist in elucidating this curious inquiry. Benno's parent, for many years afflicted by the sterility of his dame, secured the joyous consummation of long-deferred hopes by fabricating a silver effigy of a boy at an early period of the eleventh century.[73]

More enlightened scientists during the Middle Ages, distinctly denied the medical energy of these material representatives, evoking planetary spirits,[74] although Maimonides otherwise avows the talismanic quality of stones.[75] To this class of mineral pussiance, so ardently sought by erudite alchemists, may be ascribed the Lapis Mizoris or Mozor stone, which had the amazing energy of evoking the most majestic demon of the celestial sphere, and by it the mirific name of this being was procurable, which, conjoined with the stone, was of transcendant efficacy in conjurations. Strange methods were pursued by the diseased Alsatians, in order to ascertain to what saint a malady should be assigned. When the discovery was perfected a suitable specific quickly dispelled the disorder.. The punishing saint was found by lighting as many tapers as saintly emissaries, to each of which a proper name was given. The blazing candle, the first consumed, was an unanswerable accusation and conviction of the injurious personage.[76] Pregnant women in the Middle Ages usually consulted female obstetricians in advance of accouchement, in order to ascertain whether labor would be prolonged. These feminine haruspices, by a dexterous inspection of nodules and particles adhering to the umbilicus of slaughtered animals, provided ready responses.

---

72 Arnold, Chronic. Slavor., Lib. V., c. 19.

73 "Fieri jubent unius simililitudinem pueruli ex argento purissimo." Vita Bennonis, cap. 1. But the most singular part of this affair is, the figure was ordered to be made as near like the father as possible. Ibid.

74 Maimonides, Ductor Dubitant, Lib. I., cc. 60 and 72; and Ibid., De Idolatria, cc. 11 and 12.

75 Ibid., More Nevochim, Pars I., cap. 61, p. 108.

76 Delrio, Disquisit. Magicar., Tom. II., Lib. IV., cap. 2, § 1, p. 287.

CHAPTER XX.

Chemistry and Mediæval Pharmacy—Medicaments—Alchemists Prepare Salutary Remedies for Maladies—Notable Discoveries of these Enthusiasts—Subtle Powders—Distillation and Research for Essences—Aqua Vitæ, or Eau de Vie—Discovered by Villannova—Thaddeus, the Great Florentine Chemist of the Twelfth Century—Pharmacists in this Age—Venetian Glassware—Their Chemical Acquisitions—Extracts of Gold Water, of Sovereign Potency—Albert Magnus and his Nickname—Lully, the Renowned Alchemist—Agrippa's Familiar Demon.

OF all appliances closely identified with medicinal art, the one rendering the most signal returns for efforts strenuously devoted to penetrating and exploring the secrets of nature, and boldly appropriating the principles thus obtained to scientific curatives, alchemy is certainly entitled to unstinted laudation. Out of that burning frenzy of mediæval alchemists and astrologers to fabricate the "philosopher's stone,"[1] arose, towards the fifteenth century, the exact science of chemistry, and from absurd notions of astrology originated a more perfect astronomy.[2]

Alchemy, vigorously pursued with unremitting energy by illustrious scholiasts, and after the accumulated learning of years pronounced by a famous scientist to be a mendacious fraud,[3] in its medical association, may justly claim the high commendation of establishing that system of extracting essential principles from metals or minerals, whose energetic forces abundantly assisted the cure of maladies. Whether derived

[1] Cornelia Agrippa, De Vanitate Scientiarum, cap. 90, p. 206 seq.

[2] Liebig, Chemische Briefe, Th. I., p. 46 seq.

[3] "Ars suspecta probis, ars ipsa invisaque, multis
Invisis etiam cultores efficit artis.
Mendaces adeo multi manifeste videntur,
Qui seipsos, aliosque simul frustantur inertes."

Cornelia Agrippa, De Vanitate Scientiar, cap. 90, p. 206.

directly from Arabic sources,[4] or traceable to Egytian hierarchy, as a portion of those hidden sciences exclusively possessed by the ancient sacerdoty, doubtless its medicinal adaptation should be awarded the Saracens.[5]

It would seem that the Christian clergy of an early age understood sufficiently the operations of chemistry to be able to control the results of the judicial hot iron and water adopted as tests of enormous crimes.[6] The general principles of this science were certainly known in Diocletian's time, by the order of whom Egytian books on this subject, as previously stated, were given to the flames.[7] Alchemical art was from the first directed to extracting spiritual beings or essences supposed to reside within metals, or minerals and plants; in the prosecution of this process "drinkable gold"—aureum potabile—was obtained.[8] In Villannova's day, it was usual for the prelacy and nobility to boil golden petals with their food;[9] others sweetened it with syrups—electuariis, or converted it into a drinkable form, and imbibed it as a potion.

Taken in this dissolution, it was asserted to prolong life and act as a preservative of health, although our authority frankly admitted it was difficult to accredit such belief.[10] A mediæval alchemist of somewhat earlier period, equally skilled as a physician, cautions practitioners of medicine against the use of gold fabricated by alchemy or artificially.[11]

Among the earliest discoveries developed from the ardent

[4] Pancirolus, Rerum Memorabil. Rec., Tom. II., p. 134.

[5] Goujet, Origin des Arts et Sciences, Tom. I., p. 228; and Voltaire, Essai sur les Moeurs et Usages, Tom. I., p. 334.

[6] Voltaire, op. cit., Tom. I., p. 507.

[7] Suidas, Lexicon, sub v. Χημια.

[8] "Spiritus enim subtilissimus ex metallis, geminis plantisque educens; quo subtiliora," etc., "hoc efficaciora remedia præbat." Delrio, Disquisitio Magicar., Tom. I., Lib. I., c. 5, p. 20.

[9] "Bullire petias auri cum cibis." Villannova, De Vino, col. 591.

[10] "Ut difficile sit credere." Ibid.

[11] "Quod ipsi caveant ab auro facto per artem alchemiæ sine præparando naturam." Raymund Lulli, Testamentum Novissimum, Lib. II., cap. 21.

zeal of these dreamy enthusiasts, in their untiring efforts to compound an elixir which should prolong human life,[12] and, in conjunction with the philosopher's stone, provide a certainty of undiminishing happiness,[13] may be designated a subtle powder, which combined with brass produced most brilliant flames in consumption, causing the original metal to re-appear intact.[14] By mystic prescriptions mediæval alchemists coated the saphir with a suffusion of alien matter, which so closely assimilated it to adamant that connoisseur Venitians were unable to detect the deception. This invention, so valuable to the mediæval mind in its eagerness for medicinal gems, was supplemented by another process imitating metallic silver so dexterously that in spite of tests and heavy percussion the impurity was beyond disclosure.[15]

Perhaps the highest practical discovery of these pharmacists, was that of the essential force of aquafortis, by whose solvent virtues brass or copper was readily separated from gold or silver. This system of purging valuable metals from useless dross was utterly unknown to the ancients, according to the utterances of an illustrious jurisconsult, who declared when brass became amalgamated with gold it was impossible to separate them.[16] Chemists, in the Middle Ages, were so profoundly skilled in these operations, disuniting the elements indicated, that oftentimes silver in alloy, when disintegrated, under the soluble virtue of aquafortis, ascended in columnar shape, emitting variegated colors, and when thoroughly laved, and nothing of this substance was visible, in a vase of water the pure gold was found resting at the bottom.[17] An additional purifying element largely used in those ages was the cupella, fabricated by a chemical process from bones, which enabled

---

[12] Delrio, Disq. Magicar., Lib. I., cap. 5, p. 31.

[13] Cornelia Agrippa, De Vanitate Scientiar., cap. 90.

[14] Pancirolus, Rer. Memorabil., Tom. II., Tit. III., De Alchymià, p. 136.

[15] Ibid., p. 136 seq.

[16] Ulpian, De Rei Venedicat., Lib. V., § 3.

[17] Pancirolus, op. cit., p. 135.

gold and silversmiths to purge their wares of every particle of impurity or alloy. It appears to have been operated by covering the finer metals with laminated sheets of lead, beaten very thin, and placing them in a crucible exposed to intense heat. When liquefaction had melted these substance, the above preparation was mingled with the molten mass, which caused a precipitate of pure gold, and denominated aurum de cupella by Italian alchemists.[18]

The great and specific property for which the philosopher's stone was estimated at such transcendent worth, was its power to transmute base metal into gold and silver. On this subject Agrippa confessed absolute confidence. Especially when these efforts where subordinated to spiritual essence of astral bodies and the demon or spirit had been properly extracted, transmutation would be instant[19]—for which Pancirolus records a receipt.[20]

Medicine, at the earliest introduction of the results developed from the enthusiastic researches of these pharmaceutical scholastics, appropriated the discoveries—not indeed, as grounded upon systematic science, so much as sharing a moiety of its visionary zeal—but adopted the medicaments thus compounded, under the propulsion of exalted laudation.[21] Notwithstanding the more erudite of mediæval scholars ascribed unbounded virtues to remedies they prepared and used in extraordinary maladies, towards the close of this period, Petrarch, who, as we shall presently discover, coöperated by the pressure of personal influence and the prestige of an illustrious name, to advance medicine towards the plane of an exact science, most unequivocally affirms that alchemy, in the fourteenth century, according to the methods pursued and its

---

[18] Pancirolus, Rer. Memorabil., Rec. Inven., Tom. II., pp. 136, 139.

[19] De Occult. Philosoph., Lib. I., cap. 14.

[20] "Frugiferum *auri semen*, cujus drachma si in ducentas quinquagenta liquati plumbi aut stanni drachmas infundatur, id universum in aureum purissimum converteret." Op. cit., Tom. II., p. 147.

[21] Pancirolus, op. cit., Tom. II., p. 150.

slender results contrasted with the panegyrics of devotees, was an impudent scheme of deception and falsehood.[22]

He further incriminated the physicians of his day, for their mendacious ignorance in locating fevers in the body when their proper location was in the soul.[23] It was doubtless fortunate for chemical science that the enlarging necessity for solid and rational culture, conjoined with the extraordinary intellectual activity following the great Reformation, enabled critical minds to ridicule the fallacious and impudent assumptions of these zealots, while exercising judicious discretion in discriminating the meretricious elements among priceless utilities.[24]

Processes of distillation were used at remote periods of the Middle Ages, in order to procure medicaments in such suitable and attractive forms as to admit of readier acceptance by the sick. Among these may be designated the aqua vitæ, or eau-de-vie—as its name implies, life-potion—oil of cinnamon and herbal extracts, such as chickory, etc., with precipitates in the nature of medicinal salts—all were applied to the cure of diseases.[25] The preparation of these oils and waters is certainly traceable to the year 1080, and perhaps to the second decade of the eleventh century.[26] In the year 1160, Mesue had already made distillations of absinthe and rose-water.[27] Touching the period of the discovery of spirit of wine, or, perhaps, its importation to Europe from Saracen sources, it has been

---

[22] Petrarca, De Remed. Utriusque Fortunæ, Dialog., Lib. I., Dial. III.

[23] Ibid., Lib. I., Dial. IV. On his notion of herbal remedies, vide Ibid., Dial. III.

[24] Pancirolus, Rer. Memor., Tom. II., p. 150 seq, quotes a stinging diatribe on alchemical zealots, of which we reproduce the opening lines:

> "Ars fallax invisa bonis, dulcedine captos
> Jucundè ut perimis! dementibus improba Siren.
> Naturam superare putas te posse per ignem?
> Stulta, quid insanias."

[25] Pancirolus, op. cit., Tit. VIII., p. 152.

[26] Ibid., p. 154.

[27] Rubens, De Antiquitate Distillationis, Lib. I., cap. 4.

claimed to be due to Arnold Villannova, whose medical writings we have freqnently referred to, the date of whose death is fixed in the year 1313; but sufficient proofs attest that anterior to this famous professor of Montpelier, the Florentine Thaddeus, tutor of Villannova,[28] actually used this distillation as a remedy for certain bodily infirmities.[29]

To Villannova should be accorded the praiseworthy adaptation and first precise description of eau-de-vie, or brandy, prior to the end of the thirteenth century. In his treatise on the preservation of youth, he explicitly states that the virtues of this potion were already fully known to many by actual experience.[30] Then describing its amazing properties, Arnold exclaims: "Who would believe that from wine can be extracted a fluid which requires different processes, having neither the color, nature, or effect of wine! This eau-de-vie, or life-potion," which he alleges, "is called by some eau-de-vie, abundantly justifies its name, since it prolongs human life."

He proceeded to add, that "its tested qualities preserved health, dissipated superfluous humors, revived the heart, prevented decay of youthful vigor."[31] Conjoined with other remedies, or alone, it was an infallible curative against hydropsy, paralysis, quartain fevers, calculus, operating certain restoration of sanity to the insane, and healing lepers.[32] Rival physicians of the fourteenth century exhausted the entire range of panegyric, in order to enlarge the use of eau-de-vie as a medicament. So great, indeed, was its celebrity, that before the conclusion of the era mentioned it came to be regarded as

[28] Villannova, Breviarium, Lib. I., cap. 14, col. 1086.

[29] Sarti, De Professor. Bononiensis, Tom. I., Pars 1, p. 467; and Ibid., Pars 2, p. 227.

[30] Villannova, De Conservanda Juventate, cap. 3, col. 833.

[31] Ibid., col. 833.

[32] "Habet enim virtutatem confortandi cor, desiccat superfluitates," etc., "ut juventutem nutrit, proprie illis, qui sunt in ingressu senectutis vel in ea positi prolongat vitam," etc. Ibid. Nearly equal properties were claimed for the tinctures of gold. Villannova, De Vino, p. 590 seq; and De Distillatione Medicinarum, col. 398.

a universal remedy, and applied indifferently, either externally or inwardly. This liquor was prescribed for a malady of Charles the Bad, king of Navarre, and, by a singular casualty, provoked his death in the year 1387. In order to rejuvenate this exhausted royal libertine, physicians ordered him enwrapped in linen bandages saturated with brandy, sewed closely to his body. A servant charged with this duty, lacking scissors to cut the thread, sought to sever it with a lighted taper; instantly the inflammable texture was fired, and quickly terminated in inexpressible agony the life of this prince, stained with infamous debauches.[33]

In the Italian monasteries, and doubtless elsewhere, until after the Middle Ages, the conventual pharmacies were well supplied with this active stimulant, used almost exclusively in grievous maladies, and prepared by the monastic distillery. As usual in the administration of remedies to the poor,[34] this medicine was freely given to the impotent and impoverished, consequently large quantities were ever ready for emergencies.[35] The personages entrusted with the custody of curatives or medicaments in the cloister pharmacy, were distinctively named from an early period as apothecarii—a perfunctionary service of so great importance as to receive, from time to time, specific regulations by the principal church synods.

The storage of medical supplies seems to have approximated the pharmacy in the twelfth century, although even earlier the word apothecary appears to have been interchangeable with the booth where assorted wares were offered at public sale.[36] Henry, king of England, anterior to the year 1198, maintained a functionary apparently the exact type of the modern pharmacist, upon whom the name of apothecarus

---

[33] Le Grand D'Aussy, Histoire de la Vie Privée des Français, Tom. III., p. 77.

[34] Montalembert, Les Moines d'Occident, Tom. III., p. 170.

[35] Le Grand D'Aussy, op. cit., Tom. III., p. 77, Not. 1.

[36] Du Cange, Glossarium, sub v. Apotheca.

was bestowed, an officer evidently of high repute in those days, as in this instance he was bishop of London.[37]

The apothecarii or pharmacopilæ, were exposed to the just resentment of patrons, on account of offering for sale diversified drugs, whose energetic virtues were so earnestly eulogized that a single medicament possessed the power of curing the most infinite range of diseases, and by such indiscretion, in their eagerness to vend noxious wares as simple medications, excited defiance and an unprofitable suspicion.[38] The Venetian Republic, in order to encourage the development of alchemy to a practical use, was influenced by identical reasons of monopoly which forced the government into a bitter contest with Roger king of Sicily, in the twelfth century, to ruin the factories of silk,[39] established by that sagacious monarch at Palermo in defiant rivalry to the weaving of these goods by the people of Venice.[40]

Doubtless immense advantages were obtained by this maritime nation, whose knowledge of dyeing rapidly extended the fame of their fabrics, through valuable immunities granted them in the capital of ancient Egypt,[41] where thorough insight into alchemy was procured from the Saracens, earlier than the people of Western Europe. Venetian traders in the century above noted were also attracted to the Tyrian coast for its admirable glassware, eagerly sought by the Latins.[42] Unrivaled indeed, for many ages, were the productions of their laboratories in the preparation of alum, borax and cinnabar, largely utilized in finishing dye stuffs, and ultimately an important part

---

37 "Richardus, Regis Henrici Apothecarus," Notices et Extraites du Bibl. Roi, Tom. V., p. 507.

38 Cornelia Agrippa, De Vanitate Scientiar., cap. 83.

39 Otto Frising., Gesta Imper. Frederici, Lib. I., c. 33.

40 Daru, Histoire de Venise, Tom. I., p. 298.

41 Daru, op. cit., Tom. I., p. 31.

42 "Sunt illac vitrarii artifices qui vitrum conficunt Tyrium dictum præstantissimum, et maximi in omnibus regionibus æstimationis." Benj. Tudelensis, Itinerarium, p. 36.

of medical compounds imported by them from the Levant or the remote East, and again exported to Occidental nations.[43] Before the conclusion of the Middle Ages the corporation of dyers published a complete treatise under the name of Mariagola dell' arte dei Tĕntori.

An active and scrutinizing mind, Giovanni Ventura Rossetti, discovered a chemical method of fixing superior colors in textures. One of the first results of Venetian alchemy was a dexterous fabrication of ornate leather in such perfection that for ages it constituted a most profitable monopoly, of which the yearly sales reached a net profit of a hundred thousand ducats.[44] From remote periods, long anterior to the beneficial impulse of the Crusades upon this traffic,[45] the citizens of the great Italian Republic had directed their attention to the practical compounding of medicaments for consumption in Western Europe.

These pharmaceutical commodities developed into a vast commercial export, and for centuries they possessed almost exclusive control of the sale of theriacs, not alone to the larger cities of the Levant, but everywhere throughout the West—to the Netherlands tartar, and to France terebinths. A leading article of exportation, whose uses became famous, was that saline matter known by the name of borax, so largely applied to chemical or medicinal purposes, and especially to metallurgy, where its specific virtue promoted the liquefaction of metals.[46] This substance, obtained by the Venetians from Egypt, where, from the eleventh century, they had acquired a monopoly of trading privileges, and in China, required a preparation to render it of practical use, of which the secret was

---

[43] Daru, Histoire de Venise, Tom. I., p. 299.

[44] Ibid., p. 299 seq.

[45] Heeren, Sur l'Influence des Croisades, p. 421.

[46] Ibid., and Pancirolus, Rer. Memorabil., Tom. II., p. 135 seq. The artificial silvering of counterfeit coin in Edward First's reign indicates skillful use of chemical properties of silver, copper and sulphur—"erant artificialiter compositæ de argento, cupro et sulphure." Hemingburg, Chronicon, sub an. 1299.

preserved by these enterprising artisans.[47] While the occidental nations were still slumbering in slothful indifference, or with amazement began to perceive the faint rays of ascending light, the Venetian artificers turned to commercial account that knowledge of chemistry already known to a few enlightened Europeans, characterized as useless magicians or dreamy enthusiasts, and had advanced far along the plane of successful manufacture of glassware and optical instruments, the fabrication of which alone occupied over two thousand five hundred workmen.

In the skillful compounding, however, of chemical wares for medicinal or textile purposes, nearly the entire metropolis was employed; and in all commercial relations with Oriental ports drugs of the most diversified assortment were made a specific object of merchandise for sale in Western Europe,[48] for which, during the Crusades and subsequently, the people of the West exhibited the greatest eagerness.[49] To the zealous and investigating anxiety of alchemists for subjugating the spirit or essence hidden within the inmost recesses of metals and minerals, must be ascribed numerous discoveries advantageous to medicine.

In Villannova's time certain professors of this art pretended to have extracted a liquid styled aqua auri or water of gold, whose curative elements were claimed to be infallible.[50] This tincture uninterruptedly for six centuries maintained a vigorous vitality as a popular medicinal drink or tonic, and such devotion may be attributed to that excessive zeal among erudite scientists to compound a sovereign elixir, elevating its possessor above the necessity of resorting to other remedies.[51]

---

[47] Daru, Histoire dé Venise, Tom. I., p. 300.

[48] Ibid., Tom. I., p. 302 seq.

[49] Heeren, Sur l'Influence des Croisades, p. 421.

[50] "Et est sciendum quod innovatio et confortatio cutis fit cum potatione aquæ auri purissimi propriæ." Arnold Villannova, De Juventate Conservanda, cap. 2, col. 818. Here its use is signified as intended to heal epidermic, perhaps leprous troubles.

[51] Le Grand d'Aussy, Histoire de la Vie Privée des Français, Tom. III., p. 87.

In its general color this liquor closely resembled the famed aurum potabile or drinkable gold, and was subrogated as a potion to produce infinite wealth and undying youth. This metal thus transmuted, according to the flaming philippics of Agrippa, was endowed with irresistible energy; but he plainly states his incredulity in its magic virtues or unfailing energies.[52] Fascinated and provoked by the enchanting power ascribed to this liquid, ardent and frenzied alchemists sought to dissolve gold or transmute it into drinkable fluids, in order to obtain the amazing medical puissance evolved by the metamorphosis. Towards the thirteenth century, alchemy was pursued exclusively within cloistered solitudes, and its professors were for the most part ecclesiastics, of whom many attained illustration for their solidity of intellectual culture and undisputed distinction as chemists.

Of these may be designated Albert of Bollstadt, usually cited as Albertus Magnus, who died about the year 1282, whose Historia Animalium, professedly an imitation of Aristotle,[53] is a work of admirable utility; his disciple, Thomas Aquinas, who is said to have translated the Greek Diaclectian,[54] and celebrated for a treatise on meteors; Michael Scot, Roger Bacon and Raymundus Lully—the most famous of the mediæval alchemists. Albert Magnus was universally accorded this appellation by the learned of his day, but the rabble of Ratisbonn do not appear to have shared such veneration for the great scholastic—on the contrary, they followed him about the streets whenever he was visible in the city, hooting and yelling after him the nickname of "Lace-shoe," on account of his wearing closed or laced shoes, customary with preacher monks. The chronicle of this episcopate unequivocally alleges that the distinguished scientist resigned the mitre through the willful perversity and malevolence of the people.[55] An annalist,

[52] Cornelia Agrip., De Vanitat. Scientiar, cap. 69.

[53] Heeren, Sur l'Influence des Croisades, p. 421, No. 1.

[54] Fabric., Biblioth. Græca, Tom. III.; De Barbar., Aristotl. Versio, p. 305.

[55] "Resignavit episcopatum propter gentis proterviam et populi vanitatem." Chronicon Episcop., Ratisbonensium, cap. 30.

who provides an excellent and sagacious resumé of Albert's writings, urges that he was doubtless justly charged with necromancy.[56] The alchemists of the Middle Ages, as a necessary adjunct to monastic education, cultivated medicine.

Lully was particularly famous for an alphabetical method of inculcating the entire range of philosophy,[57] a system adopted by the equally scholastic Agrippa.[58] Lully expresses himself repeatedly against the possible procuration of immortality by medical compounds, one of the principal factors in the great alchemical problem, and mournfully agrees "they have occasion to grieve over it."[59] In his medical treatise he advises physicians, or rather earnestly adjures them, to practice their profession upon the basis of a science.[60] As late as the closing years of the sixteenth century, a professor of medicine, commenting on the alchemical writings of this scholastic, wrote: "On inquiring, he had found among the English that Lully, as asserted, by chemical processes had obtained a pure and unalloyed gold, which by order of the king was produced at the Tower of London."[61]

This, in form of an effigy, was exhibited to the medical writer, who "alleges it was genuine metal, and named after its fabricator, Nobile Raymunde."[62] By a papal bull, in the commencement of the fourteenth century, the pursuit of alchemy was placed among forbidden practices, as detrimental to the church and provocative of heresy. Notwithstanding this sweeping interdict, the works of Lully were distinctly exempted from the list of heretical books.[63]

---

[56] Hermani Corneri, Chronicon, sub an. 1265.

[57] Fr. von Raumer, Geschichte der Hohenstauffen, Th. VI., p. 423 seq.

[58] Occult, Philosoph., Lib. I., cap. 74.

[59] "Et in isto posso Alchemistæ dolent et habent occasionem." Lullius, Ars Magna, De Novem Subjectis, cap. 52.

[60] Ibid., Testamentum Novissimum, cap. 10.

[61] Delrio, Disquisit. Magicar., Lib. I., cap. 5, p. 37.

[62] Delrio, Disquisit. Magicar., Lib. III., c. 5; and Mariana, Historia de España, Lib. XIV., c. 9; and Lib. XV., c. 4.

[63] Delrio, Disquisit. Mag., Lib. I., c. 5, p. 37.

During Henry IV's reign in England, in the year 1404, a law was enacted forbidding the further pursuit of this science. Towards the close of this era, the council of Venice, likewise, subjected the art to legislative forbiddance.[64] At this late period of the Middle Ages, the power of necromancy was firmly believed to be attainable; and, notwithstanding the gradual extension of knowledge, the art of transmuting metals into gold or silver, and preparing elixirs of immortality, was pursued with unextinguishable ardor, and under the patronage of enlightened princes at various European courts. In the year 1416, John III., bishop of Verdun, was distinguished for alchemical skill.[65] Although the English king's rescript alluded to may have tended to retard or repress unlimited practice of this visionary avocation, the attempt at necromancy was permitted by Henry VI., in the middle of the fifteenth century, under the protecting sanction of royal patents.[66]

Thus, indeed, in the years 1449 and 1452, a license was signed by the king's own hand—per ipsum regem—to transmute metals and make that priceless medicine, denominated by some the mother of philosphers and imperial medicament, otherwise the inestimable glory, while some alchemists named it quintessence, "philosopher's stone and elixir of life." [67] A few years later, a patent was granted for similar purposes, and sealed with the royal warrant of England, valid for a limited period.[68] The futility of scientific inquiry into the possibility of composing such omnipotent mineral is pithily portrayed by Agrippa, after his abandonment of the art.[69] The mystical principle which oftentimes coöperated to render necromantic efforts of this and earlier ages an apparent success, was the direct devel-

---

64 Kopp, Geschichte der Chemie, Th. II., p. 192 seq.

65 Chronicon, Epp. Verdeniens, cap. 46.

66 Rymer., Foedera, Tom. XI., pp. 240, 379.

67 Entitled, "Licentia ad Conficiendum Elixir Vitæ et Lapidem Philosophorum." Rymer., op. cit., p. 379.

68 "Per biennium duraturas." Rymer, Foedera, Tom. XI., p. 379.

69 De Vanitate Scientiarum, cap. 90.

opment of a faith in the actual existence and irresistible puissance of unseen spirits.

Although invisible, these mighty beings could be subjected by secret ceremonies, and imprisoned within the bodies of animals or men, the master of whom, consequently, possessed the appliances of vast and energetic forces. The speaking heads of Albert Magnus[70] and Gerbert appear to have been assigned to the custodian of familiar spirits. It was the corporeal envelope in which the mighty demon of Agrippa was enclosed, by which the transcendent potency of this skeptical scholastic was revealed;[71] while the famous alchemist, in practically conceding the attendance upon Socrates of a familiar spirit, most unequivocally asserts an assumption of such personal imp to be fraudulent, and practiced for imposition to captivate the ignorant rabble.[72] In direct opposition to what appears to be a clear and unmistakable opinion of this famous scientist, at the close of his age it was currently believed the many mysterious events savoring of supernatural power attributed to Agrippa were alone traceable to demoniacal assistance.

Delrio himself, in the sixteenth century, seriously discussing the lawful possibility of evoking demons subject to human will, narrates the following curious history as a vindication of an allegation that magicians by compact were enabled to control such diabolical beings:

"Cornelius Agrippa, similar to an earlier ecclesiastic,[73] had a commensal or servant of great curiosity, to whose wife he usually entrusted the keys of his laboratory or museum while absent, expressly interdicting the entrance to any one. The husband, of youthful age, having at length found an opportunity, importuned the woman to assist him in entering the mystic chamber. In this apartment he found a book entitled 'Libellum Conjurationum,' which he began to read. Engrossed in

---

70 Delrio, Disquisit. Magicar., Lib. I., c. 1, p. 2.

71 Ibid., Lib. II., p. 164.

72 Agrippa, op. cit., cap. 45.

73 Knyghton, Decem Scriptores, p. 2535.

the perusal of this curious manuscript, he was aroused by a slight blow on the door, to which no attention was given, when another knock startled the reader, likewise ignored. The familiar demon of Agrippa entered, and demanded why he was invoked, and what he should perform. The adolescent intruder, in timorous consternation, opened not his mouth, and frigid with fear, spake not a word. He thereupon suffered the dolorous consequence of an indiscreet curiosity. Upon the return of the Archimagus Agrippa, he beheld demons exulting around his domicil; quickly learning the cause, he ordered the cadaver of the young man, possessed by these impure spirits, to arise and pass into the forum or court-yard. This was instantly accomplished, and after perambulating the enclosure a few times, the actuating demon fled the body, which immediately assumed the rigidity of death. At first the inculpation of suicide was propounded as a solution of this mysterious event; but indications of suffocation being discovered, the sombre affair was finally divulged, and acknowledged by the alchemist's flight."[74]

Nearly at the same epoch, in the year 1483, the royal alchemist of Louis XI. of France, pursued with devoted avidity the composition of aurum potabile or potable gold, and received from the king ninety-six ecus to reimburse him for an outlay of precious metal absorbed in making this famous beverage, which had been prescribed by court physicians as an infallible medicament.[75]

Mediæval pharmacists assumed to instruct in the proper preparation of this priceless medicine. Certain alchemists, actively influenced by their visionary notions, sought to impregnate table potions with an aureated solution. An ancient medicinal treatise, of the year 1372, prescribed the following method to obtain the proper compound of this beverage:

---

[74] Delrio, Disquisitio Magicar., Lib. II., Qu. 29, p. 157.

[75] "En remboursement de quatre-vingt seize écus d'or vielz, quil a mis pour ledit seigneur Roy à faire certain breuvage appellé aurum potabile à lui ordonné pour medicine." Le Grand d'Aussy, Histoire de la Vie Privée des Français, Tom. III., p. 87.

Heat strips or lamina of pure gold almost to liquefaction, and immerse them in this state forty times in spring or filtered water. The liquid should then be carefully sealed in a glass bottle and drank without diluting or with excellent wine.[76] Physicians of those distant ages professed an unshaken faith in the unfailing power of crude golden pellets to remedy with instant results the most obstinate diseases, if swallowed or eaten with food in a pulverized form.

Others, indeed, not less credulous, were so profoundly impressed with the curative properties of this royal substance that they fabricated gold pills and gave them to capons, on the implied principle that the digestion of these fowls would absorb into their edible flesh sufficient of the divine metal, which skilled cookery caused to reappear in tempting, savory soups.[77]

Prejudices provoked in favor of the chemical power of this material, dissolved for medicinal purposes, by the pretended miracles of Paracelsus, were strictly maintained throughout the sixteenth century. This charlatan, vaunting his puissance of prolonging human life, and dying at the age of forty-eight, asserted as an incontrovertible fact that he had repeatedly cured lepers by a dexterous use of gold. As a consequence, golden elixirs and drops of gold were everywhere sought with frenzied research, on their assumed remedial sovereignty over most vexatious and unsightly disorders. Among scientists of the age who combated the potential efficacy of such tinctures should be especially distinguished the illustrious Palissy, whose exquisite good sense and thorough familiarity with natural sciences elevated him far above fanatical enthusiasts of his day.[78]

---

[76] Ibid., p. 88.

[77] Ibid., p. 88 seq; Delrio, Disquisit. Magicar., Lib. I., p. 33 seqq., may be consulted for elaboration of this subject, and to great advantage.

[78] Le Grand d'Aussy, Histoire de la Vie Privée des Français, Tom. III., p. 89.

CHAPTER XXI.

Hospitals in the Middle Ages Developed from the Conventual Infirmary —Hospitia of Cloisters first used for Sick Strangers—Public Institutions of this Character in the Tenth, Eleventh and Twelfth Centuries—Corps of Trained Nurses—Regular Organization of Hospital Assistants—Use of Sugar in Syrups at an Early Period in the Orient—Thorough Equipment of Hospitals at Bagdad in A. D. 1173—Salaried Physicians and Complete Stores of Pharmacy—Insane Asylum for the Cure of Patients There—Mediæval Digest of Regulations for Church Hospitals—Charity Institutions and Rules for Admissions—Leprosy—Seclusion of Lepers—Reverence for this Disease—Cures of Varied Assortment—Lazarettos for Lepers near City Entrances—Revolt of the Lepers—Jews Classed with these Infects.

FROM the monastic Infirmary and Hospitium was developed a system for the regular aggregation and treatment of sickness and diseases, under rules and ordinances whose careful execution contributed to practical mediæval philanthropy. Touching the nature of Infirmaries, sufficient has been written in this treatise, but of the Hospitium or Hospitale, which has furnished a fitting nomenclature for the edifice where indigent or stranger infirm were gratuitously attended, exclusive of the monastery, it may be stated the idea involved in its original conception was fraternal welcome to pilgrims or homeless travelers seeking accommodation in cloisters at a time when inns and hosteries were too remote, or offered less security to life and property than the inviting threshold of a structure generally constructed by the side of public thoroughfares,[1] and from the special purpose of its establishment, designated as above written.[2]

In that signification, this department of conventual organization is of high antiquity,[3] and as early indeed as the age of

[1] Fosbroke, British Monachism, p. 297.

[2] Wm. Neubrig., Historia Anglicana, Lib. IV., cap. 14.

[3] Du Cange, Glossar., sub v. Hospitium.

Charlemagne, such separate apartments were used exclusively for sick persons.[4] They afforded a practicable means of exhibiting in practice the fundamental principles of conventual charity in providing food for the impoverished, lodging for the houseless, and medical treatment for diseased strangers. Different countries altered or modified the uniformity of the meaning of these hospitia by diverse interpretations.

While the original sense of lodging-house for travelers still attached, it was used by English jurists of the Middle Ages to signify students' chambers near the great Universities, where, indeed, as we shall presently discover, they were regularly domiciled in large numbers.[5] By whatever series of eventualities this monastic institution passed from the strictest interpretation, and survived as a hospital, or edifice entirely set apart for reception and cure of maladies, may perhaps be gleaned from notions touching its more ancient purposes, which, under ecclesiastic manipulation, necessarily were remodelled toward the end of the twelfth century.[6] In the year 1059, a hospital exclusively for sick girls had long been extant at Durham, and was highly eulogized by the conventual historian.[7]

At a much earlier period, however, there were organizations of this character among the Spanish Arabs,[8] together with poorhouses solely occupied by the indigent and pauper people entirely supported by public funds in the year 976.[9] Before the year 1006, the Venetian Republic possessed a hospital erected at the private expense of the ducal Urseolo.[10]

---

[4] Vita Idæ Ducissæ, cap. 1.

[5] "Sunt namque in eo decem hospitia minora, et quandoque vero pluraque nominantur hospitia cancellariæ." Fortescutus, De Laudib. Angliæ, cap. 49, p. 113 seq.

[6] Wendover, Flor. Historiar., Tom. III., p. 227.

[7] Sym. Dunelhm., Historia Ecclesiæ, Lib. III., c. 46. Touching this form of charity, vide Giselberti, Chronicon Hanoniense, sub an. 1194.

[8] Conde, Historia de la Dominacion de los Arabes en España, p. 310.

[9] Conde, Historia de la Dominacion de los Arabes en España, p. 261.

[10] Daru, Histoire de Venise, Tom. I., p. 27.

When Benjamin Tudelensis was at Jerusalem in 1173, the Christian people maintained an institution of this character exclusively for their own sick.[11] Eight years later, Roger de Moulin promulgated a series of regulations for these eleemosynary organizations in this city, which may have been suggested by earlier rules, and perhaps constituted a safe norm to guide similar philanthropic bodies elsewhere. By these ordinances each hospital should have four physicians skilled in diagnostics, pharmacy, etc., and a like number of surgeons. To these were added nine *sergens*, or assistants as menials, to provide ready service for the feeble and wounded.

Knights of the Hospital Order, whom these regulations principally controlled, were detailed to a day and night watch over the sick, and, indeed, for this attendance the Hospitallers of either sex were liable.[12] For ready use syrups or electuaries were applied as potential curatives.[13] These compounds, it has been stated, were unknown to the Western monasteries at this period, and their existence in this venerable ordinance attests the rapid appropriation of Arabic drugs by crusading adventurers. It is, doubtless, correct to assume the limited usage of such excellent specifics directly derived from the Saracens, although a more ancient code, the Jerusalem assises, drawn up about the year 1090, distinctly mentions this medicament,[14] while certain grades of Oriental spices—classified as aromati—were freely used in Europe after the year 1138,[15] perhaps exported by Venetian merchants during uninterrupted voyages to the Levant.[16] A substantial diet of pork and mutton was provided for the sick and suffering males and females

[11] Benj. Tud., Itinerarium, p. 40 seq.

[12] "Hospitalarii utriusque sexus, qui in hospitalibus ægrorum ac pauperum obsequiis addicti Regulam S. Augustini profitentur." Du Cange, Gloss., sub v. Hospitalarii.

[13] Lessing's Ed., p. 550.

[14] "La medicato con tal medecine, e siropi, per li quali," etc. Le Assisse et Bone Usanze del Reaume de Hyerusol., cap. 218.

[15] Annales Bosovienses, sub an. 1138.

[16] Daru, Histoire de Venise, Tom. I., p. 16.

of the hospital in Jerusalem, at least thrice each week. Another clause directed that two patients should have one pair of shoes to the twain.[17]

Notwithstanding the ordinance alluded to exacts that all foundling children—quetez—shall be received and nourished by this Hospital, there were institutions in Western Europe of a more remote period where abandoned infants were taken and sustained. Some of these are mentioned by Italian writers,[18] while others were already, thus early, in vigorous operation in Switzerland, Germany, France and elsewhere.[19] In the form of gratuitous attendance upon the sick and diseased, the Eastern Arabs in the eighth century possessed a regularly organized system of public Infirmaries in the great metropolis of Bagdad.[20]

In the time of Benjamin, the Hebrew traveler, A. D. 1173, a most efficient and practicable scheme had long existed in this city, for the reception of the disabled and infirm poor into hospitals, thoroughly equipped with sixty salaried physicians and completely furnished with pharmaceutical supplies.[21] But transcendent and above this form of philanthropic benefaction, called into existence by enlightened Moslem economy, was a most thorough organization of a public establishment at Bagdad for the custody and cure of the insane, brought thither from all parts of the Persian empire.

This asylum and curative institution in the Saracen tongue was denominated Dak Almaraphthan. Here the inmates were subjected to scientific medical treatment until sanity was restored, when the patient returned to his domicile, where he received professional attendance for several months to prevent a relapse into the malady of which he was cured.[22] That the

---

17 Lessing's Ed., p. 550.

18 Muratori, Antiquitat. Ital., Tom. III., p. 591.

19 Von Raumer, Geschichte der Hohenstauffen, Th. VI., p. 533, N. 4.

20 Abulfagus, Annales Moslem., Tom. II., p. 43.

21 "Construxit Xenodochia, ægrotatibus pauperibus curandis idonea." Benj. Tudel., Itinerarium, p. 62.

22 "Palatium quod Dak Almaraphthan vocatur, hoc est domus misericor-

crusades indirectly opened to the Western nations a practical acquaintanceship with natural science, cannot be successfully controverted; although wherever the details of this useful erudition were known they appear to have been accepted for qualities of utility in fabricating real necessities, or as indulgences for the refinements of luxury.[23] Little indeed, if anything, was gained for general science.

Touching increased knowledge of medicine as practiced in eleemosynary establishments of this era, doubtless an identical conclusion should be deduced. The crusades provided ample opportunities to apply a knowledge of this art, although the movement towards a theory based upon rational principles made trifling progress. For ages anterior to that ardent zeal which precipitated the whole of Europe upon the Orient like the fall of an irresistible avalanche, pilgrimages to the countries of Syria provoked the construction of Hospitia or lodging houses, heretofore described, where sick and infirm pilgrims received treatment for their bodily ills.[24]

In an era when long voyages on foot constituted a chief claim to divine pardon to old and young,[25] of both sexes,[26] the affluent and indigent, and when as stated hostelries and inns were either objects of defiance to peaceful travelers, or at so remote intervals along the public highways, the establishment of these hospitals at the side of the great routes of travel became indispensable, which the religious authorities quickly recognized and promptly supplied.[27]

---

diæ, furiosis omnibus in regionibus inventis includandis, vinciendis et curandis destinatum: donec ad mentem redeant: tunc enim singuli in domum suam reverti permittuntur, curantibus id examinantibus per singulos menses viris." Benj. Tudelensis, Itinerarium, p. 62 seq.

[23] Heeren, Sur l'Influence des Croisades, p. 421.

[24] Ibid., p. 422.

[25] Albert. Stadens. Chronicon, sub an. 1212.

[26] Nude women in great numbers, professing to be pious pilgrims, boldly perambulated mediæval cities. Ibid.

[27] Heeren, Sur l'Influence des Croisades, p. 423.

At the commencement of this swelling tide of pilgrims to Palestine, such charitable structures were erected as a compulsory adjunct to accommodate voyagers from the north of Europe[28] to the city of Jerusalem.[29] In their primitive arrangement these hospitals, whose subsequent development in the west reflected lustre and aided in the progress of medicine and surgery, were regularly attended by conventual brethren, who furnished medicines and nursing to disabled pilgrims and suffering wanderers.

Simple piety and unskilled attendance by monastic friars were the first offerings instead of educated practice, conjoined usually with the potency of sainted reliques or experimental alchemical essences. The Hospitallers[30] were consequently scattered along the highways of travel, to the very gates of Jerusalem, and wherever these philanthropic abodes opened to welcome the weary and diseased, the limited resources of a prostrate science were humbly applied to the cure of maladies.[31] They were indeed ecclesiastics and zealous soldiers of God's militant forces, priests and cavaliers—at once physicians, nurses, defenders and consolers of the sick and lowly.

Hospital regulations, digested by ecclesiastical authority, doubtless contemplated the presence of professional practitioners during the Middle Ages, although at their earliest inception the only skill produced was furnished by the monks, whose knowledge of medicine consisted usually in the use of traditional recipes, which they applied with excellent intentions, and independent of simple maladies were inefficient.[32] The Clugniacs appear to have pushed their saintly cures quite to the exclusion of terrestrial medicaments.

Odo, abbot of this illustrious monastery, in response to the demand of a pair of sick friars for medicine, quaintly informed

---

28 Ad. Brem., De Situ Daniæ, cap. 35; and Annalista Saxo, sub an. 952.

29 Heeren, op. cit., p. 423.

30 Du Cange, Glossar., sub v. Hospitalarii.

31 Heeren, op. cit., p. 423.

32 Heeren, Sur l'Influence des Croisades, p. 423 seq.

them in conceding their request, "the same remedy had been tried for a similar disorder and found useless!"[33] It was fortunate for medical science that such opinions were not accepted in the establisment of hospitals in the west of Europe, where this charitable system was introduced in advance of the ordinances of Roger de Moulin.

Hospitals for the sick, orphanages for foundlings, and great institutions for the proper care of paupers, developed with immense strides, under the thoughtful and judicious zeal of their founders, and during the twelfth century expanded into gigantic proportions.[34] Usually the endowments of these eleemosynary organizations emanated from the accepted dogma of the atoning virtues of voluntary contributions to the poor, or from the equally energetic propulsion of a belief in possible catastrophes resulting from a haughty indifference to the wants of this afflicted class.[35]

In the ensuing age, the mediæval mind was fired with a faith in the efficacy of unstinted charity; members of society, from holy pontiff himself to the humblest cloistered recluse by the way-side, rivalled each other in gratuities of clothing and food, founding of hospitals, and endowment of beneficent public institutions.[36]

Saint Louis' highest claim to pious glory arose from his restless and unstinted charities to the indigent and sick. The intercourse of this king with the diseased in hospitals, where he entered to administer personal consolation, utterly oblivious or indifferent to the dangers of such nursing, may be taken as an important attestation of the extension of this virtue toward benevolent enterprises during the Middle Ages.[37] The internal arrangements, and thoroughly practical nature of the

---

[33] "Ac medicamenta eis dari præcipit, præfatus, ea simul morbo tentatus antea nihil profuisse." Mabillon, Annales Ord. Bened., Tom. III., sub an. 937, p. 437.

[34] Du Cange, Glossar., sub v. Eleemosynarii.

[35] Fr. von Raumer, Geschichte der Hohenstauffen, Th. VI., p. 533.

[36] Vita S. Ludovici, apud Duchesne, Tom. V., p. 452.

[37] Ibid.

ordinances to which the mediæval hospitals owed their existence, excite surprise and demand unreserved admiration. Ordinarily, attendants and nurses, after a probation of definite time to test their abilities for this function, were required to obligate themselves with spiritual vows, similar perhaps to the oblati and conversi,[38] in order to exalt the dignity of the avocation, although hospital goods were administered by the more practical laity.[39] To this rule there were exceptions, when both civil and canonical authority managed certain kinds of personal property, as early as the year 1038.[40]

A rigid ordinance of the Brussels hospital interdicted access to its benefactions to any diseased person able to procure a livelihood by personal effort, or through the aid of others.[41] The original and thoroughly religious character of these charitable asylums may be gathered from a requirement that each applicant should, similar to postulants of monastic chapters, solemnly confess and abandon, or quit claim to the hospital, his entire possessions. If the invalid was restored to health, he could withdraw and receive everything back again, and as a salutary concession it was ordained whatever remained over the costs and charges incident to medical care of such inmate, by testamentary disposition might be willed at pleasure after death; but in case the decedent died intestate, the institution inherited his property to the exclusion of all heirs.

Identical with the Jerusalem Hospital regulations of 1181, patients were to receive three times each week fresh meat, and if sanitary economy demanded, other food was freely provided. Women in pregnancy and foundlings were susceptible of admission, although under such scrutinizing restrictions as tended to prevent the entrance of disreputable persons. In

---

[38] Du Cange, Glossar., sub vv. Oblatus and Conversus.

[39] "Persona idonea ac sacerdotalis eligetur, quæ et debitum," etc., "pauperum quoque et infirmarum qui in hospitali curam genere possit, anno 1126." Miraeus, Opera Diplomatica, cap. 47, Tom. II., p. 964; Ibid., Tom. I., p. 210.

[40] "De laicis vir boni testimonii socius eligetur, ad dispositionem temporalium." Ibid., cap. 51, Tom. II., p. 966; and Ibid., Tom. III., p. 104.

[41] Ibid., Tom. III., p. 609.

the Brussels Hospital, entrants upon their reception formally donated earthly goods to the eleemosynary corporation in perpetuity, together with the legal rights which they possessed, and professing an entire abjuration of civil society, assumed the clerical costume of brown or gray.

No married person was admissible, and all trades or secular occupations were formally interdicted, and no one without imperative reasons was allowed to descend into the city.[42] In the year 1341, an asylum, partaking of the nature of a hospital, was erected in London, for impoverished and aged goldsmiths, out of the public moneys and by charity.[43] In the treatment or succoring indigent sick, benevolence was in some instances carried to excess; and oftentimes in administering funds appropriated or donated for such purposes, the monks, as almoners of these gifts, were influenced in their disbursements by a partisan impulse, or diverted them to different uses.[44] Romish pontiffs by personal example, and the vast machinery of the Episcopacy with its priestly subordinates, largely aided in a proper distribution of church alms.[45] which gave especial vitality to proper medical attendance upon the distressed and suffering sick.

Of all afflictions entailing the severest misery during the Middle Ages, and necessitating a sagacious economy, both of medicine and legislation, leprosy was preëminently the most baleful. This dread disease, in its worst form, was fully known to professors of the curative art in the last days of declining Rome, and recognized as difficult of treatment. From the application of simple cosmetics to heal cutaneous discoloration

---

[42] Miraeus, Opera Diplomatica, A. D. 1235, cap. 137, Tom. III., p. 116.

[43] "Pro aurifabris Londonis fumo argenti viri coecati." Rymer, Foedera, Tom. V., p. 246. Access to this asylum appears to have been restricted to such as were blinded by the fumes of metal.

[44] Von Raumer, Geschichte der Hohenstauffen, Th. VI., p. 535. Ambulances and refrigerators were used by Frederick II., in 1256, in his army, for sanitary purposes, and to add comfort to wounded soldiers. Gesta Frederici Imper., sub an. 1256.

[45] Otto Frising., Chronicon, Lib. VII., c. 35.

preceding graver types of this disintegrating infirmity, to severer methods of emasculation, the entire range of medicaments and surgery was unsuccessfully essayed. The foundation of this abhorrent treatment appears to have originated in a professional asseveration that eunuchs and women were exempt from the disease—a notion maintained by the Arabic scholar, Athelard, in the twelfth century.[46]

Although leprosy seemingly assumed not the importance of an infectious disorder, nor became sufficiently extended among the nations of Western Europe to merit serious attempts at repression prior to the vast movement eastward and the reflex action of the Crusades, there can be no doubt of its existence in an aggravated form, dormant or confined to isolated invalids in the Occident, long before the middle of the eleventh century. Legislative enactments in the year 757, by Pepin, Frankish ruler, forbidding by rescript conjugal relations between a leper and a healthy woman,[47] and the enforcement by Charlemagne thirty years later of sequestration against this terrible malady, interdicting contact with robust people,[48] attest the full knowledge and dread of this disease among the early Teutonic races.

A century or more anterior to Pepin, hospitals, under monastic management, exclusively set apart for the care and quarantining of lepers, were erected at important points on the colossal extension of Carlovingian territory. In the year 720, Othmar, abbot of the cloister of Saint Gall,[49] directed the construction of a small edifice—hospitiolum—not far distant from those buildings abandoned entirely to indigent and weary travelers, and isolated or quarantined it so completely that none but the leprous were admitted,[50] who, it was distinctly decreed,

---

[46] Athelardi, Questiones Perdifficiles, cap. 41.

[47] Baluzius, Cartularia, cap. 16, Tom. I., p. 184.

[48] Ibid., Capitulare Tertium, A. D., 789, cap. 20, Tom. I., p. 244.

[49] Vadiani, Chronologia, Abb. Monaster. S. Galli, sub an. 720.

[50] Walafrid Strabo, De Vita S. Othmari, Lib. I., cap. 2. Voltaire, Essai sur les Moeurs, Tom. I., p. 429, argues the lack of linen vestments as a possible cause

were compelled to live disjoined from the society of other men.[51] It may be added, the pious prior hesitated not to lave the feet of these infects, and to purge their eruptions of prurient matter, at the same time serving them with delicate food.

Under religious influences, this dreaded disorder was the object of especial reverence from the time of Saint Martin, who cured a leper by kissing him,[52] to Eberhard, under the Hohenstauffen rulers, whose humility found pious expression in personal attendance upon these unsightly beings,[53] shunned, indeed, by all excepting saints and saintesses. Towards the middle of the sixth century, Saint Radegonde displayed her faith in first washing these repulsive sores, and afterwards applying her sainted lips to them. An insolent leper, indeed, asserted unless his putrefying limbs were kissed by this candidate for canonical honor, he could not be cured.[54]

In the time of Charlemagne, Saint Boniface, the evangelist, in a letter to a German bishop, requested him to forward heavy stuffs with which to wipe his feet, and to this evident lack of linen the spread of this malady has been attributed.[55] To accept this suggestion, based upon the implied absence of such vestments, would be gratuitous and groundless. It is doubtless true, the use of linen wear in the Middle Ages did not approximate its adaptation in modern times, neither was the paucity of it so general as stated in those periods.

We have seen the constant usage of the camisa or underwear by Charlemagne himself. At later epochs this article was oftentimes donated to indigent paupers as a gift of high charity with other clothing.[56] Frequently the camisa consti-

---

of leprosy, which he says was general throughout Europe four centuries after Charlemagne.

[51] "Nam ad suscipiendos leprosos, qui cæteris hominibus sejunctim manere semotim consuerunt, constituit." Walafrid Strabo, op. cit., Lib. I., c. 2.

[52] Sulp. Sev., Vita S. Martini, cap. 18.

[53] Otto Frising., Gesta Frederic I. Imp., Lib. IV., c. 73.

[54] Montalembert, Les Moines d'Occident, Tom. II., p. 353.

[55] Voltaire, Essai sur les Moeurs et Usages, Tom. I., p. 429.

[56] Vita Meinwercki, Ep. Paderb., cap. 32, § 8.

tuted a portion of a tax or rent in kind, in payment of the leasehold by tenants,[57] a fact which confirms the more universal wear of this linen garment late in the eleventh or beginning of the twelfth century. In the next era, Italian wives wore linen outer vestments, which custom is, indeed, mentioned by Ricobaldi as of long continuance.[58]

Crusaders, unquestionably, provoked contagious diseases, on account of which the Levant for ages had been celebrated. Some of these were mainly generated in the West by infected vessels, dissolute armies, filthy bands of pilgrims, returning from the Orient. Leprosy, with other malignant disorders, engendered by unchecked license, excessive indifference to sanitary rules, and almost total indifference to civil precautions, was spread throughout Europe as a vast epidemic anterior to the year 1179,[59] to the rapid extension of which the criminal use by several of the same baths, when publicly established in the West, largely contributed.[60]

In the year 958, the mortality by this disease was so great as to attract the attention of annalists,[61] and in the year 1019, the biographer of a famous ecclesiastic recounts the bitter quarrels of the insane, the blind, the lame and lepers, who crowded the chapel dedicated to this Saint, for precedence to saintly cure.[62] The horrors entailed by these infectious disorders rendered it absolutely indispensable that extraordinary safeguards against the spread of this particular infirmity should be taken. In addition to causes assigned for the rapid expansion of leprosy about the time of the Crusades, it was apparently well understood in the Gallic provinces, that the flesh

---

57 Ibid., cap. 32, § 52.

58 Ricobaldi, Historia Pontific. Roman., sub an. 1234. Du Cange, Glossar., sub v. Camisia, has valuable facts touching the general use of linen vestments at the era designated.

59 Labbe, Concilia Lateran III., sub an. 1179, cap. 23, Tom. XXII.

60 Heeren, Sur l'Influence des Croisades, p. 424.

61 Annalista Saxo, sub an. 958.

62 Vita Heimeradi Presbyteri, cap. 34; apud Leibnitz, Tom. I., p. 575.

of swine promoted cutaneous maladies resembling this great affection, early in the history of the Frankish kings, who appointed inspectors of this food whose duty it was to examine and declare the sanitative condition of slaughtered swine.

Those exercising this function were designated languyanos, or tongue-inspectors, because this member was scrutinized to detect the impurities of the meat. As late as the year 1375 an ordinance required these officials to perform the duty only, after a master of the guild of butchers had made such examination. If any signs indicated the presence of disease, the suspected beasts were marked on the ears in order to apprise purchasers.[63] In some portions of Europe, however, medical practitioners freely advised bacon as a sovereign remedy against the disease of leprosy, when, indeed, paupers were exposed to infection from tainted bathing water used by lepers, and at a time when bleeding and use of the bath, as anciently prescribed,[64] were rendered doubly dangerous by common diet of pork and wine, urged as infallible cures.[65] In general this excellent sanitary system of bodily lotion was regarded graciously by mediæval chronists.[66] The waters near Naples,[67] mineral springs at Bath,[68] England, and at Arles, which cured gout,[69] were especially famous. Frederick I. of Germany, freely adopted this remedy by advice of his surgeons.[70] It was apparently inevitable, to prevent serious results from repeated use of identical water by filthy vagrants and leprous bathers, which, combined with greed for pork as a standard diet,

---

[63] Le Grand d'Aussy, Histoire de la Vie Privée des Français, Tom. I., p. 316.

[64] Baluz., Cartular., A. D. 817, cap. 7, Tom. I., p. 581.

[65] Lessing, Geschichte der Medezin, Th. I., p. 270, No. *

[66] Beda, Histor. Eccles., Lib. I., cap. 1.

[67] Arnold, Chronic. Slavor., Lib. V., c. 19; and Gervais Tilbur., Otia Imperialia, Dec. III., c. 15.

[68] Anon., Gesta Stephani, p. 38.

[69] Gervais Tilb., op. cit., Dec. II., c. 126.

[70] Gothofred, Gesta Fred. I., cap. 29, v. 760 seq. Bruno contemned the bath. Rusoger, Vita Brunonis, cap. 30.

aggravated the types of epidermic eruptions. This meat was regarded by pilgrims as a great delicacy in their distressed famishing peregrinations to Palestine,[71] and a mediæval romancer recites, with gleeful melody, how Richard the Lion-hearted demanded bacon when prostrated with fever in the East, and in the absence of the real was given a generous cut of a boiled Saracen. Upon discovering the substitution, he admitted that Turk flesh was of finer flavor than swine.[72]

Villannova treats leprosy purely from a professional view, and asserted it was propagated by generation or transmission, and provoked by unnatural food, infected pork, etc. He urges against the use of pure, undiluted wine, the certainty of causing this disease, and makes the following singular reproof: "The French and Burgundians, on account of their immoderate potions, are more numerously leprous."[73]

He however recommends the free application of Gallic soap, already celebrated as a curative.[74] According to this medical professor, a sure test of a leprous condition was cupping the arm for a slight quantity of blood, into which should be cast a trifling amount of pulverized lead. If this floated on the surface, the absence of a taint of this disease was verified; but in case it sought the bottom, the proof of leprosy was incontestable.[75] Mediæval annalists show the presence of this infirmity among the higher clergy and prelates, long anterior to its alleged introduction from the Orient. Thus in the year 1029, Thurgot, the laborious bishop of the Bremen Episcopacy, one day, while assisting the archbishop, was stricken with this loathsome disease, which finally ended his life.[76]

About the year 937, in Germany portents of unusual significance were visible on the garments of many persons, in the shape

---

[71] Wipon, Vita Cuonradi, an. 1027, cap. 23.

[72] Romance Richard Cœur de Lion, vv. 3190–3200.

[73] Villannova, Breviarii, Lib. II., cap. 52, col. 1313.

[74] Ibid., col. 1316.

[75] Ibid., Additiones, col. 1317.

[76] Adam Bremen, Gesta Hammaburg. Pontific., Lib. II., c. 62.

of a crucifix, which appears to have been in some way at that remote period associated with the dress of lepers. For this reason prognostications predicted great mortality among the diseased, which actually happened.[77] In the year 882, the disorder with which the impious Anglo-Saxon king, Halfden, was punished, has a close resemblance to leprosy.[78] The extent to which this calamitous affliction followed European pilgrims and Crusaders returning from the Orient,[79] necessitated compulsory medical attendance and a more general adoption of the sagacious hospital regulations of Saint Othmar, in the erection of hospitals for such invalids, in order to prevent serious catastrophe to the human race.

Isolated houses, distant from the abodes and settlements of men, remote from highways of travel, were constructed to receive pestifers and inoculates, obliged to repair thither voluntarily or by force.[80] In the year 1179, the third Lateran Council decreed lepers should have private chapels and cemeteries,[81] although the city of London, as early as the year 1118, established a Leprosarium for absolute sequestration of such patients.[82] Knights of the Order of Saint John, in the different countries of Europe, had consigned to their care and especial attention eighteen thousand lepers.[83] The same necessity which erected these pestiferous huts and cabins, as an active agent in mediæval medical economy, forced the practical appliance of such methods as were efficient obstacles to the inroads of pestilence in sea-port towns. The first, indeed, to essay sys-

[77] Witchindi, Annales, Lib. III., c. 61.

[78] Symeon Dunelhm., Historia Ecclesiæ, Lib. II., cap. 28.

[79] Sismondi, Histoire des Français, Tom. I., p. 429.

[80] Heeren, Sur l'Influence des Croisades, p. 424.

[81] Labbe, Concilia, cap. 23, Tom. XXII; and Neubrigeus, Historia Anglicana, Lib. III., c. 3.

[82] Rog. Wendov., Flor. Historiar, sub an. 1118.

[83] Matthew Paris, Annales, sub an. 1244. In the Auctiarium Additimentum, p. 161, of the same author, copious extracts are reproduced from the ordinances Hospitalis de Sancto Juliano, touching dress, reception, etc., by which this organization was incorporated.

tematic prevention was the Venetian Republic in the year 1423, at which time a fully equipped and furnished Lazaretto or Quarantine was constructed by the government.[84]

Lazarettos, also denominated ladreries, for the seclusion of lepers, were, in the Middle Ages, sometimes located near the entrance of municipal towns, where such as were infected by this awful disorder were detained in custody and maintained by funds charitably contributed.[85] From the order to whom the care of pestifers was assigned, nurses and attendants in these sequestered hospitals were named lazzaretists.[86]

In some cases this sorrowful service was faithfully performed by Augustine monks, whose regulations present a striking identity with those of Saint Julian.[87] Oftentimes cities by communal ordinance interdicted Lazzaretto establishments in order to avoid possible contamination, while Zurich with extraordinary integrity declared this disease should not render lepers uninheritable,[88] although usually the Ladrerie regulations admitted testamentary disposition by a leper of his property.[89] These infects were forbidden entrance to towns and villages, and required to avoid possible contact with the healthy, for fear of propagating the hideous malady; and to make such rule efficient they were obliged to carry a bell to sound an alarm upon the approach of travelers.[90] When marching to church, their dress prescribed consisted of a close fitting mantle with cape attached, drawn tightly about the head, of a somber, perhaps wholly black, color.[91]

---

[84] Daru, Histoire de Venise, Tom. I., p. 202; Heeren, op. cit., p. 425, for quarantine of later date.

[85] Sismondi, Histoire des Français, Tom. I., p. 429.

[86] Cibario, Studi Istorici, p. 382 seq. Nobility often attended lepers as nurses. Ibid., p. 180.

[87] Designated "Pauperes Christi videlicet Lazaris." Dugdale, Monasticon Anglicon, Tom. II., p. 376 seq.

[88] Von Raumer, Geschichte der Hohenst., Th. VI., p. 534.

[89] M. Paris, Auctor. Addit., p. 163.

[90] Möhsens, Geschichte der Wissenschaft, in Mark. Brandenberg, Th. II., § 22.

[91] "Cum ad ecclesiam exierint ab hospitali, copa clausa ad modum mantelli de nigro panno; cum capucis ejusdem coloris." M. Paris, op. cit., p. 162.

Whole villages were composed of these outcasts, and a person suspected of touching a pestifer was immediately secluded.[92] Quarantine, in modern times, doubtless is executed upon more exact principles of science; but it has never been as inflexibly maintained, both by civil and canonical law, as during the Middle Ages. Churches and cemeteries were formally set aside for exclusive use of these afflicted beings,[93] and to the world of life and happiness around them they were as thoroughly dead as though sheltered beneath an eternal tomb. In the time of Louis VIII. of France, this disease had made such rapid progress in its sinister movements that at his death, in the year 1225, he bequeathed a sum of money to each of the two thousand lazzarettos in actual existence in his kingdom at this period[94]—a figure still undiminished at the middle of the fifteenth century.[95]

Doubtful manifestations of excessive charity aided in rapidly extending leprosy, and contributed to preserve its virulence unimpaired. Thus the priest Thermes actually stole garnered grain for indigent sufferers, and in the strange revelation of divine presence received the undisputed attestation of the purity of his motives,[96] while the daughter of Fulk, king of Jerusalem, purged suppurating leprous sores, and when her spirit was daunted by the horrible putrefaction, to vanquish this repugnance she calmly filled her mouth with water from the bath-tub.[97]

---

[92] "Ut ubicunque tot simul sub communi vita fuerint congregati, quod ecclesiam cum cœmetaris sibi constituere." Labbe, Concilia, A. D. 1179, cap. 23, Tom. XXII. From some of these communities married lepers were excluded. M. Paris, op. cit., p. 161 seq.

[93] Neubrigeus, Historia Anglicana, Lib. III., cap. 3; Giselberti, Chronic. Hanoniense, sub an. 1195; and Baluz., Concilia Narbon., Tom. I., p. 168.

[94] "Item donamus et legamus duobus millibus domorum leprosorum decem millia librorum videlicet cuilibet earum centum solidos." Testamentum Ludovici VIII., Reg. Francor.; ap. Duchesne, Tom. V., p. 325.

[95] Heeren, Sur les Croisades, p. 424.

[96] Helmoldi, Chronic. Slavor., Lib. I., c. 66.

[97] Iperius, Chronic., p. 643; ap. Martene Thesaur., p. 441.

The necessities of their seclusion apparently provoked a desire of vengeance on the part of the abhorred recluses. In the month of June, 1321, the awful announcement was made to Philip V., king of France, that deputies from all the Ladreries in Christendom had convened at four general councils,[98] and in accordance with a treaty solemnly compacted with the Saracens, they had agreed to poison all Christians everywhere dispersed, the method of which plan was to place poisons in springs and fountains.[99] In its original scope, this sinister conspiracy seems to have been restricted to the robust and healthy of the race, as an impressive vindication of the frightful sufferings of these outcasts.[100]

Superior toxicological knowledge of the Israelites, it seems, caused them to be suspected of complicity in this systematic assassination; at all events, Jews were arrested and incarcerated, charged with furnishing aid and counsel to the vengeful infects.[101]

Although not a single well or fountain was proven to be poisoned, nor one human being to have perished, by means of two or three sachets of alleged venomous contents, including an adder's head and the feet of spiders, all lepers however, and those tainted with the disease, were seized throughout the French kingdom and in the Provençal provinces.[102]

Thereupon the entire force of the Gallic judiciary was set in relentless motion—prelates, barons, municipalities and royal arbiters, authorized by an ordinance of August 18, in that year, "to cleanse the earth of the criminal and superstitious leprous fester." By this most inhuman and calamitous edict all perished in the flames[103]—a result impossible to record without a shudder.

---

98 Sismondi, Histoire des Français, Tom. I., p. 429.

99 Ad. Murimuth, Chronicon, sub an. 1320.

100 Sismondi, op. cit., p. 429.

101 "Et Judæi detenti et incarcerati, propter auxilium et consensum eis præstitum ut publice dicebatur." Murimuth, Chronicon, sub an. 1320.

102 Ad. Murimuth, op. cit., p. 32 seq.

103 Sismondi, Histoire des Français, Tom. I., p. 430.

The utter impotency of such diabolical measures to eradicate a disease which for centuries was indigenous to France, may be gathered from the fact previously stated, that a century later an equal number of Ladreries was to be found in this kingdom.[104] In the year 1368, a Narbonnese synod ordained that lepers should be forcibly prevented from entering public markets, communal churches, walled enclosures, hostelries, or other places frequented by healthy persons.

They were further directed to discontinue the use of variegated colored clothes, nor should they wear their hair or dress it so as to resemble the untainted,[105] as an unmistakable stigma. These unhappy people were ordered to fasten a mark on their garments by which the uninfected might the more certainly shun them.[106]

---

[104] Heeren, Sur l'Influence des Croisades, p. 424.

[105] "Nec pannos portent varigatos seu coloris, nec pilos nec comas." Concil. Vaurens, cap. 21; ap. Baluz. I., p. 167 seq.

[106] "Signoque in vestibus diferant per quæ à sanis patenti differentia cognosceret per diocesanos ordinanda." Concil. Vaurens, cap. 21.

CHAPTER XXII.

Abandoned Women: their Relation to Medical Economy in the Middle Ages—Legislation against Them—Resort to Barber Shops—"Ambulatory Maidens"—Low Grading of Actresses and Laundresses—Mayor Owns a House of Prostitution—Attire of Degraded Females—English Cardinal Landlord of a Bordello, or Bawdy House—Great Number of these Women among the Crusaders—Forbidden to Enter Wine Houses—Prescribed Dress—Scholars Especially Liable to their Fascinations—Municipal Ordinances—Attempts to Reform—Husbands Sought and Obtained by Money.

PERHAPS the most important matter of medical economy which next to the isolation and quarantining of lepers, during the entire stretch of the Middle Ages arrested the attention of both secular and sacerdotal authorities at a comparatively early era, was the subjection of unfortunate prostitutes to such discipline as would best repress the propagating of disorders of aggravated types, of which some, even in the time of Villannova, seem an exact counterpart of syphilitic maladies.[1]

Doubtless the inspiriting anxiety for their improved condition, attested by pontifical regulations and ecclesiastical canons, strongly coöperated to a higher elevation of the disreputable class than the lot assigned them in Imperial Rome. A favorite illustration of the unmeasured rapacity and sordid greed of these women, under the declining Roman government, was aptly drawn from the Egyptian sphynx, whose facial effigy delineated a human head, while the balance of the body hieroglyphically represented powerful claws, typical of the avarice and tyranny exercised upon admirers.[2] In the

[1] Villannova, Breviarii, Lib. II., cap. 43.

[2] Panciroli, Rer. Memorabil. Deperdit, Tom. I., p. 106.

imperial city the licentia stupri operated a loss of heirship,[3] a law re-established with all its inflexible rigor, in the establishments of Saint Louis.[4]

Church legislators in mediæval times assumed control of abandoned women, and encouraged such organizations among them as promoted a healthier internal polity, designed to check the spread of disease. Consequently from the bordello,[5] or houses solely frequented by these females and their paramours, to Magdalen orders, pontifical vigilance traversed the entire distance for medical or sanitary purposes.

Parisian barbers appear to have provided apartments convenient to their shops where the dissolute of both sexes regularly met—a nefarious connivance, threatened with severest punishment, but without correcting the mischief.[6] At an early period of municipal governments in Europe, women of fair repute organized themselves into a secular corporation, under the designation of "ambulatory girls," whose ostensible object was performing domestic and other services at annual fairs, imperial diets, church synods, and as Focariæ,[7] or fireside menials, sought attendance upon spiritual magnates.

These feminine guilds of the thirteenth and fourteenth centuries were constructed in all points similar to those of other trades, and had their ordinances, judges, and their jurisdiction.[8] At the great mediæval fairs in Europe, where the women of doubtful virtue abounded, bargains were struck on the basis of a package of bodkins or lace-needles,[9] or aiguil-

[3] Ibid.

[4] "Quand se fait depuceler, elle perd son heritage par droit." Establiss. de S. Louis, Titr. I., c. 12, an. 1254.

[5] In 1168, the eighth of Henry II., Stow, Survey of London and Westminster, Vol. I., p. 7.

[6] Ordonnance de Troisiéme Race, Tom. V., p. 441.

[7] Du Cange, Gloss., sub. v. Focaræ, furnishes full explanation of this word.

[8] "Les femmes amoureuses formaient alors, une corporation comme les gens des autres métiérs, quelles avaient leurs statuts, leurs judges et leur jurisdiction." Lacroix, Prostitut. au Moyen Age, fol. 9.

[9] "Le prix était un paquet d'aiguiellettes." Ibid., fol. 31.

lettes, which they usually carried as a distinctive badge upon the shoulder, a custom surviving to Rabelais' day.[10] Annalists of the Middle Ages classified actresses,[11] female joculatores[12] or minstrels, laundresses or lotrices,[13] as meretrices or prostitutes.

The Focariæ, above alluded to, were forbidden the license of the city of London in the year 1129,[14] and an imperial edict ordered their capture throughout the empire of Frederick II. a century later.[15] Domiciles for degraded women were, indeed, recognized as a necessity, equalling the demand for lodging houses and cafés. The strictest surveillance was maintained over these, and repeated regulations defined the basis on which the advantages of their vocation were accorded within municipal limits.

One of these enacted a uniformity of attire. At the period when Froes, of Holland, farmed London Bordellos or bawdy houses, owned by the mayor, the inmates wore a distinctive vestment of red stripes and party colored head-dress.[16] They appear, however, anterior to such ordinances, to have arrayed themselves in garments well recognized as the costume of depraved females. In the year 1058, the appearance of one is thus described: "Seated on a jaded mule, her locks unloosed and falling upon her shoulders, holding a gilded rod in one hand, with which the listless animal was urged forward, and by means of her indiscreet clothing excited the travelers' attention in the highways."[17]

Streaming tresses appear to have characterized ancient Roman maidens of this class, while their Athenian sisters wore

---

[10] Pantegruel, Liv. III., chapit. 32.

[11] Lambert, Hersefeld Annales, sub v. 1066.

[12] Giselbert, Chronicon Hanoniense, sub an. 1184.

[13] Hemingberg, Chronic., sub an. 1198 and 1215.

[14] Wendover, Flor. Histor., Tom. II., p. 210.

[15] Ricard. de San Germano, Chronic., an. 1228.

[16] Stow, Survey of London, p. 553.

[17] Hemingberg, Chronicon, Tom. I., p. 500.

gaudy and highly ornate garments.[18] After the consort of Louis VII. of France, had by mistake kissed a prostitute, it was decreed such persons thereafter should be prohibited the chlamys or cape.[19]

Other peculiarities of dress distinguished the frequenters of the Roman Lupanaria, of which the bitter satires of Tacitus make repeated mention,[20] although this variation was rendered indispensable by cubicular exigencies.[21] In the city of London, as in other municipalities, their residence was contracted to certain streets, or the west part of Southwark, where such signs as a gun, castle, crane, cardinal's hat, the bell, or swan, made these resorts unmistakable.[22]

In Paris, these females were domiciled in a quarter ultimately designated Clapier, a name, as Lacroix urges, perpetuated to modern times.[23] Occasionally during the Middle Ages, the proprietress of bordellos was an abbess, who appeared greedier of terrestrial profit than the rewards of self-denial,[24] and sometimes the scandalous deportment of anchorites visiting such houses became a matter for the monastic chroniclers.[25] In the year 1321, an English cardinal purchased a Lupanar in London, as a profitable investment for sacerdotal funds.[26] A century later these houses of infamy in Naples were taxed, with their incontinent denizens, by the municipal authorities.[27] The object of secluding or aggre-

---

18 Panciroli, Rer. Memorabil, Deperdit., Tom. I., p. 205.

19 Bouquet, Receuil des Historiens Français, Tom. XVI., Præf. p. 26.

20 Annales, Lib. XIII., c. 25; and Lib. XV., c. 37.

21 Panciroli, op. cit., p. 168. Further on this subject, Tertullian, Ad Uxorem, cap. 3.

22 Stow, Survey of London, p. 7.

23 Lacroix, Prostitution au Moyen Age, fol. 11; cf. Du Cange, Glossar., sub v. Clapier.

24 Lacroix, op. cit., fol. 22.

25 Annales Corbeienses, sub an. 1113.

26 Rymer, Foedera, Tom. II., p. 880.

27 Lacroix, op. cit., fol. 14; and Du Cange, op. cit., sub v. Gabella. Taxed in the year 1283, Ibid., v. Putagium.

gating disreputable women within certain metropolitan limits, appears to have been the withdrawal from virtuous contemplation of the sight of a glorified vice, so that honest people might shun the dangers incident to a close vicinage.[28] Whenever an orderly citizen complained of their presence at Ravenna, a statute required them to instantly depart the neighborhood.[29]

Legislation of imperial Rome allowed such complaints, and usually transported the offending debauchées to licensed Lupanaria—sometimes expelling them beyond the city, or ordering them to the suburbs.[30] During the first crusade of Frederick I., emperor of Germany, a rigid decree was enforced subjecting the dissolute of both sexes to compulsory natation in cold running streams, perfectly divested of clothing, in winter or summer. The order curiously enacted that the bystanders should laugh at and otherwise deride the offenders.[31] Like statutory penalties were inflicted by an ordinance of Louis IX. of France, in the year 1269.[32]

In the year 1097, incontinent females were so numerous in the Crusading armies that they were forcibly driven out of camp.[33] Hemingberg asserts that in 1291 there were thirteen thousand loose women supported by the Templars[34]—an evil perpetually recurring among the Crusaders.[35] A house of disrepute appears to have been maintained by Saracens at Ahir in the twelfth century.[36] Towards the conclusion of the Mid-

---

28 Panciroł., Mem. Deperd., Tom. I., p. 204.

29 Von Raumer, Geschichte der Hohenstauffen., Th. VI., p. 513.

30 Panciroli, op. cit., p. 204.

31 Ansberti, De Expedit., p. 65; Arnold, Chronic. Slavor., Lib. IV., c. 8.

32 Ordonnances des Rois de France, Tom. I., p. 105, Art. 5.

33 Rog. Wendover, Chronicon, Tom. II., p. 95.

34 Chronicon, Tom. II., p. 24.

35 Otto Frising., Gesta Imp. Freder. I., Lib. III., cap. 26 and 46; and Lib. IV., cap. 76; and Giselberti, Chronicon Hanoniense, sub an. 1188.

36 "Nota apud Ahir publicum prostibulum meretricum." Arnold, Chronic. Slavor., Lib. VII., cap. 8.

dle Ages, a law of the municipality of Brunswick enacted that all prostitutes within the city should be under the direction of the public executioner. In order that all avocations, however infamous, might aid in accumulating funds for the city, it was also decreed that persons of this class should pay a fixed sum towards metropolitan service. Proprietresses of brothels were classified as debauchées, and subjected to the same tax.[37] In the interest of commercial travelers during those remote epochs, numerous statutes were promulgated by civil authorities, by which protection was provided against the rapacious and tyrannical spirit distinguishing these feminine sphinxes.

Many Italian cities forbade their presence within wine-houses, as unusually prejudicial to the immature morals of the young; but Northern municipalities afforded unusual facilities for the pursuit of this nefarious vocation. A Turin ordinance ordered their forcible removal from churches after nightfall.[38] While, indeed, the prostitute was by specific rescripts debarred from an inculpation of criminal force,[39] by a law of 1192, she was protected in judicial proceedings, but refused a hearing when an unjust accusation was made by her to extort money.[40]

Violence towards women, whether impure or chaste, was punishable in diverse localities with gradually increasing severity from the monetary compensation of older Teutonic legislation, to the barbarous punishment of entombing alive.[41] Frequently the heavier penalties of the punitory codes were

---

[37] Ordinarius Senat., Brunsvic, cap. 91.

[38] "Item, quod omnes meretrices in vigiliis nocturnis publice expellantur de ecclesiis." Monumenta Hist. Patr., Italiæ, Tom. I., p. 726.

[39] Decretum Leopoldi, sub an. 1220, in Wiener Yahrb, 1827, p. 18. Accusation of bastardy—"filii meretricis"—by this decree was punished by money fine, but failure to pay provoked scourging and flaying alive: "Verberetur et decutetur." Ibid., p. 19. The penalty in Mantua for vilifying a woman—"meretricem or coredissam"—was ten solidos, in the 13th century. Monumenta, cit., Tom. I., p. 67.

[40] Von Raumer, Geschichte der Hohenstauffen, Th. VI., p. 513.

[41] Lex Ripuariorum, Tit. XXXIV., lex. 1.

modified by marriage, if the parents assented,[42] otherwise the criminal was capitally dealt with.[43] Early Gothic statutes were especially severe in their repression of inciting girls or virgins to systematic incontinence, punishing both by death,[44] public scourging of the impenitent in the year 504,[45] and nose slitting, as late as the twelfth century.[46]

In the year 1254, a decree of Saint Louis directed, that men frequenting houses of ill-repute should be branded as infamous, and forever rendered incapable of testifying.[47] Unsuccessful crusading in the East made this monarch so highly sensitive upon this grievous stain in municipal government, that by his ordinances all women addicted to this nefarious system were declared outlaws; and as an attestation of an earnest determination to compel these abandoned creatures into a more salutary life, he ordered their personal goods, clothing, furs and tunics or linen chemises—pecium,[48] to be taken in custody, and by such as granted the usage of a domicile a year's leasehold of the property should be forfeited.[49]

As a result of this brutal legislation, troubadors complained that disconsolate maidens might be seen everywhere, followed by excellent citizens, victims of their amatory charms.[50] Whether, indeed, the ardent imagination of adolescent medi-

---

[42] "Lo stuprator d'una vergine era tenuto a sposarla si i parenti consentivano e s'ei n'era degno." Cibrario, Economia Politica del Medio Aevo, Tom. I., p. 193.

[43] Edicta Theodorici, cap. 39.

[44] Ibid.

[45] Lex Wisigothor., Lib. III., cap. 18.

[46] Constitutiones Regni Seculi, Tit. XLVIII.

[47] Ordonnances des Rois de France, Art. X., Tom. I., p. 79.

[48] Baluz., Concilia Narbon. I., p. 77; Du Cange, Gloss., sub v. Petium.

[49] Ordonnances des Rois, Tom. I., pp. 74, 104. Later statutes of the rulers of France conceded the right to municipalities of maintaining houses of resort for public women—"maison pour l'habitacion et residence des filles communes." Ibid., Tom. XX., p. 180.

[50] "Ainsi, on ne voyait partout que filles éplorées quittaient cités et les bons bourgeois qui les avaient aimées couraient après elles par amour ardent." Capefigue, Histoire de France, Tom. I., p. 266.

æval students of law and medicine rendered them more accessible to the susceptibilities of female society, it was universally accepted as a legal maxim that scholars, owing to indolent natures and luxurious habits, were particularly influenced by meretricious women.[51]

Municipal law of a rigorous character seems to have become indispensable in the French cities wherever universities were located, since immediately above apartments occupied by law or medical students, were the resorts of prostitutes,[52] and indeed, it was accepted as a rule of interpretation in certain causes involving judicial inquiry into these intimacies, that all women frequenting the abodes of scholars, should be regarded as public debauchées—especially was this the case in Italy.[53] A noted mediæval professor of medicine, sojourning in this country, narrates singular customs of Neapolitan women, who carried their virginal deceptions to the nuptial chamber;[54] but though the devices of the Florentine ladies for recalling recollections of their husbands and lovers during a prolonged absence may argue marvellous fidelity, the historian cannot reproduce the inculpation by Villannova of a more serious crime,[55] even in the unimpassioned enclosure of a dead language.

Doubtless, in unnumbered instances, natural modesty due the sex asserted itself and provoked kindly commendation, although the biting scandal of their licentious tongues demanded unmitigated censure.[56] Public females sometimes, in the fullness of remorse, assumed vows of future chastity under

---

51 Panciroli, Rer. Memor. Deperd., Tom. I., p. 205.

52 "In parte superiori magistri legebant, in inferiori meretrices inter se et cum Censonibus (sic. Qu. Lenonibus) litigabant." Bulaeus, Historia Universitatis Parisiensis, Tom. II., p. 687.

53 Panciroli, op. cit., p. 205.

54 Villannova, Breviarii, Lib. III., cap. 6, col. 1338.

55 Ibid., cap. 9, col. 1346.

56 "Prævalet in lingua qui non est fortis in armis;
Nullus in hoc pugna plus meretrice potest."

Abelardi, Opera, Tom. I., p. 346.

church sanction, and became an integral portion of nunneries, which action the annalists highly eulogized and gave the most extended notoriety, as an example to be followed by their associates.[57] As hitherto stated, sacerdotal authority afforded the most unyielding patience in sincerely struggling to reclaim these degraded personages, destructive alike to morals and health, and oftentimes individual exertions returned notable results.

Fulco, of Neuilly, intimately associated with the Crusades against Constantinople,[58] illustrated his talents as an evangelist among abandoned females. By well directed and industrious persistency he procured from the Parisian authorities an agreement by which the city should endow with a thousand livres, and the University students two hundred and fifty, each reclaimed prostitute upon her contracting honorable marriage.[59]

Reformatory movements among this class were organized on a munificent scale by famous mediæval preachers, who, under pontifical warrant, boldly proclaimed that the person accepting a stained creature in matrimony might justly claim the vast benefactions incident to saving a condemned soul from perdition.[60] Saint Louis coöperated to check the fearful tide of immorality, by erecting an eleemosynary establishment for the gratuitous distribution of bread to indigent, deserving girls, exposed to dissolute and dishonest lives.[61]

At the close of the tenth century, the punishment inflicted upon women of this class in Poland was terrible, and in the high-

[57] Chronicon Engelhusii, ap. Leib. III., p. 1037.

[58] Bulaeus, Hist. Universit. Parisiensis, Tom. II., p. 518 seq; and Albert Stadens, Chronicon, sub an. 1198.

[59] "Casum ex fragilitate timentes data eis in datem non modica pecunia legitimo connubio reformavit." Otto Fris., Continuat., San Blas, cap. 47.

[60] Bulaeus, op. cit., Tom. II., pp. 519 and 687.

[61] Vita et Conversio Sancti Ludovici, cap. 9; apud Duchesne, Tom. V., p. 452. Fulco had great success in this reform, and induced many women to cut their flowing tresses and enter penitential houses. San Blas Contin., cit., cap. 47; and Bulaeus, op. cit., Tom. II., p. 518.

est degree unnatural, while the male accomplice, wherever such action involved violence, was subjected to inhuman torture.[62] By their utter disregard of canonical regulations, monasteries aided in the corruption of morals and propagating of disease by disreputable females.

In the year 1129, a church synod authorized Henry I. of England to execute the laws against infraction of celibacy by the monks; but according to the inculpation of Wendover, this monarch accepted money from conventual brethren, and abandoned them their paramours.[63] In many abbeys the maintenance of concubines, perhaps wives, was so customary that the bishop of Constance forbade the Zurich municipality expelling this fragile sex, on the ground that such action was exclusively within episcopal jurisdiction.[64]

Oftentimes these uncanonical indulgences were not restricted to humble recluses—bishops themselves debauched the nuns,[65] and at a time when insignificant embraces were placed under the ban, a pontifical legate[66] was surprised flagrante delictu with a prostitute. In the year 1190, the Danish peasantry aggregated themselves in favor of the priests against the bishops exacting the expulsion of illicit concubines, in order that the priesthood, possessing their own consorts, would cease to abuse the wives and daughters of the peasantry.[67] Through the sordid avarice of prostitutes, independent of the transmission of disorders of most aggravated types,[68] degraded women inflicted upon convents enormous losses of treasure by the indiscreet generosity of their monastic lovers. During the dire-

---

[62] Dithmar, Mereseb. Chronicon, Lib. VIII., p. 248.

[63] Flores Historiarum, Tom. II., p. 210.

[64] Bluntschli, Geschichte des Zurich, p. 82.

[65] Hume, History of England, Vol. II., p. 48. Convents furnish Boccacio, Il Decamerone, with convenient sources for such scandals.

[66] Panciroli, Rer. Mem. Deperdit., Tom. I., p. 205.

[67] Von Raumer, Geschichte der Hohenstauffen, Th. VI., p. 180.

[68] Villannova, Breviarii, Lib. II., cap. 43, col. 1288. The embrace of such women was recommended by this great mediæval professor as a cure for insanity. Breviarium, Addit., Lib. I., cap. 18, col. 1096.

ful necessities besetting the Bremen episcopate in the first half of the eleventh century, entailing the squandering of its munificent accumulations of gold, silver, and sacred vessels embellished with valuable gems,[69] vast numbers of these precious stones were delibertely stolen by amorous inmates, and donated to rapacious debauchées.[70]

Deplorable consequences of warfare were aggravated by their presence in the armies, provoking contagious maladies, and sharing the booty of sacked cities. In the year 1084, after the capture of Augusta by means of false keys, the victors made an irruption into the cloister, and having fired its stipendiary appurtenances, proceeded deliberately to pollute with abandoned women, holy structures contiguous to the convent.[71] The annalist cited under the year 1092, affirms that the spirit of evil among the Scandinavians provoked a category of vices of such gigantic development that the most debasing crimes failed to excite attention.[72]

One of the sweeping charges made against Christian, archbishop of Mayence, in the year 1179, was, notwithstanding his vast erudition of Latin, Greek, Roman, Chaldaic, Apulian, and Langobardic languages, his prostitutes entailed upon him heavier expenditures than the charges of royal representation.[73] Although clerical magnates resisted encroachments on their liberties of concubinage, when a certain count in the thirteenth century abandoned his legitimate spouse to follow the fortunes of a meretricious female, the prelate of the Archiepiscopal See quickly excommunicated him. This extraordinary remedy does not appear to have alarmed the erring couple; on the contrary, the concubine opened a lodging-house or hostelry opposite the monastic portals, and the illustrious but dishon-

[69] Adam Bremen, Gesta Hammab. Pontific. Lib. III., c. 3.

[70] "Gemmæ autem distractæ quibusdam meretriculis donatæ sunt." Albert Stadens, Chronicon, sub an. 1066.

[71] Chronica Augustensis, sub an. 1084.

[72] Ibid., sub an. 1098.

[73] Chronica Bremensis, sub an. 1179.

ored Westphalian, as landlord, attended the guests who honored the inn with their patronage. The chronicler, however, declares they ended in squalor their existence, because such goods as they possessed were wasted in riotous excesses, after the manner of actors—histrionico more.[74] Jewish women appear to have shared the frailties of their Christian sisters, according to a formal incrimination by Berthold, abbot of Saint Gall, in this century, against an anchorite of this cloister, whom he accused of thieving and having deserted the monastic habit to live licentiously for several years with an incontinent Jewess.[75] In the year 1295, a monk of Corbeil, singular to state, procured a dispensation from the pope releasing him from monastic vows, and married; the conventual historian doubted the possibility of happiness emanating from this marriage, and intimates his opinion of the woman.[76]

---

[74] Chronicon Rastendense, ap. Meib., Tom. I., p. 106.

[75] "Vixit luxuriose cum quadam Judæa." Goldast., Alemannicor. Antiquitat., cap. 98, p. 57.

[76] Annales Corbeienses, sub an. 1295.

CHAPTER XXIII.

Pestilences and Epidemics in the Middle Ages—These Oftentimes Predicted—Defects in Sanitary Arrangements—Municipal Authorities Endeavor to Repress Pestilence—The Death Penalty Passed upon Blundering Physicians—The Yellow Plague in England—Terrible Ravages—Causes of Epidemics Accurately Traced—Frequently Charged to Diabolical or Stellar Influences—Awful Malady of 1348—Great Mortality at Marseilles—Its Route along the Water Courses—Medical Skill Fails to Arrest It—Jews Charged with Poisoning the Water—Female Surgeons, etc.—Order of Flagellants—Dancing Pestilence—Its Infects Abhor Red Colors.

PESTILENTIAL diseases, from the decline of Rome to the termination of the Middle Ages, in whatever form they appeared, were usually preceded by such natural phenomena as attracted notice of contemporaneous annalists, who in many cases made a permanent record of these strange occurences. Earthquakes, falling mines, inundations, comets, and stains on clothing, houses and utensils, which after the most careful ablution reappeared more vividly than before, belonged to these miraculous events appurtenant to each specific epoch, preceding the approach of epidemics, spreading fear and consternation among all nations.

As possible precursors of epidemics, the habits of animals, according to high medical philosophers,[1] should be closely observed as an indication of future diseases, it being urged that serpents shunned their usual places, and birds, instead of flying by day, went in flocks at night, on account of atmospheric corruption.[2] During the thirteenth century, the nature

[1] Villannova particularly, whose unusual judgment, for the thirteenth century, may be ascribed to his notable acquaintanceship with Arabic writings, which he acquired by sojourning in Spain. Vita Villannova, cap. 2.

[2] Villannova, Breviarium, Lib. IV., cap. 32.

of comets was sufficiently understood to be described as a "blazing star or incendiary cloud,"[3] and they performed an important function in prognosticating pestilences or other phenomenal disorders, which were predicted upon a minute astrological scheme to the first years of the fourteenth century.[4]

It was usual for astrologists by a series of complicated stellar and mathematical calculations to prophesy the certainty of epidemic maladies, and forward copies of their prognostications to all leading monasteries of Europe. Rycard San Germain reproduced one under the year 1229, drawn up and issued by a Toledo savan.[5] Disregard of sanitary rules, woolen clothing[6] perhaps, and a limited supply of linen vestments worn by the mediæval populace, prelates and beggars, dwellings of defective construction, doubtless aided in propagating the frightful calamities of pestilence. A more malignant cause was the arrangement of private houses and public structures, alike erected upon the principle of resisting armed aggression and successfully defending them through prolonged sieges. In these, contiguous to the principal edifice and part of it, were immense reservoirs constantly filled with water and magazines stored with provisions. This fluid, after the lapse of time under confinement, reached absolute putrefaction; and when the germs of disease began to spread among the countries of Europe, its progress was accelerated by such filth, which developed these seeds into pestilential bloom.

Under the stress of defective regulations, it was impossible systematically to bury the rapidly increasing dead, or prevent infection. In the sixth century, when a frightful pustular malady racked with mortality the metropolis of the Eastern Empire, destroying nearly ten thousand citizens daily, none

---

[3] "Quem quidam dicunt ignitum sidus, quidam nubam ascensam." Annales Capit. Cracoviensis, sub an. 1264.

[4] Ricobaldi, Compilat. Chronolog., sub an. 1312.

[5] Cronica, sub an., cit., p. 980; Fl. Wig., Flor. Hist., Tom. II., p. 156.

[6] Ricobaldi, Histor. Pontif. Roman., sub an. 1230†.

could be found willing to inhume or cremate decaying cadavera.

Municipal authority superintended these burials, and when cemeteries were gorged with the dead, the roofs of several large turrets were removed to receive the bodies, and after being filled to repletion, the covering was replaced. These singular sepulchres became sources of propagating a disease which a scholastic annalist affirmed so pernicious that the human race nearly succumbed;[7] the contents were therefore subsequently shipped to sea, on transports and there sunk.[8] At a somewhat later epoch, the entire Roman empire was subject to a pestilence, preceded by the usual signs, and apparently provoked by the heterogenous admixture of foreign nationalities, with enervating depravity of Italian cities. The most celebrated victims of this epidemic, in the year 582, were the bishop of Nantes and the duchess of Burgundy, Austregild. A curious circumstance renders her death of especial significance in this inquiry, as attesting the enforcement of the ancient Teutonic law, authorizing surviving kinsmen to pass judgment upon the medical attendant of a defunct.

Prior to her death, the Burgundian queen accused the physicians of administering potions intended to deprive her of life, and entreated the king to avenge the crime. After the solemn obsequies were performed, the sorrowing consort, oppressed by the weight of the oath freely given to the deceased princess, satisfied the posthumous desire of the dead by slaying her surgeons.[9]

Charlemagne's expedition against the Huns in 791, resulting in the total extinction of their empire, was grievously embar-

---

[7] "Exitalis pernicies generi humano incumbebat." Evagrius, Scholast. Histor. Ecclesiast, Lib. IV., cap. 29.

[8] Procopius, De Bello Persico, Lib. II., c. 22.

[9] "Rex vero peracto ex more exsequio, oppressus ingenuæ conjugæ juramenta, implevit præceptam iniquitatis; nam duos medicos qui ei studium adhibuerant, gladeo ferire præcipit." Gregor. Turon., Historia Francorum, Lib. V., c. 35; and Ibid., Hist. Franc. Epitomata, cap., 82; also, Baronius, Annales, sub an. 582, Tom. X., § 27.

rassed by a malignant pestilence, which ravaged almost the entire force of his army horses, so much so, indeed, that the metrical annalist of the time dilates grandly upon the destructive energy of this disease, and asserts that of all the vast legions of cavalry, barely a tenth part of the quadrupeds escaped.[10]

At intervals during the Middle Ages, with greater or less frequency, maladies of mortal infection suddenly appeared, against which medical and sanitary knowledge of the time was utterly impotent. In the year 1093, an epidemical disease devastated large portions of Germany, succeeded by singular phenomena. The principal event appears to have been a flaming fire moving throughout the entire universe,[11] and may be taken as an equivocal description of a lurid comet.

Blood-marks, with which the dread approach of destroying maladies was announced, oftentimes presaged the death of prelates or pontifical magnates; which occurred in the year 1130, when Bertold, bishop of Hildisheim, and Honorius, the pope, died.[12] In the latter part of the seventh century, the yellow plague, which almost denuded England and Ireland of its population for a period of twenty years, was preceded by an awful eclipse on the first of May.[13] This pestilence was particularly severe in the Northumbrian district. The number of victims that fell before its raging advance is incalculable, while its death-list was swelled from the ranks of the most exalted and humblest monks. A more excessive destruction seems to have raged among the Irish, of whom two-thirds at least perished.[14]

Twenty-one years later, this destroying malady yet lurked among the Anglo-Saxons in an unusually malignant form. Great peers of the church were swept away by the pestilental

---

10 Anon., Annalista, Carolimagni, Lib. II., indic. 14.

11 Chronicon Stadense, sub an. 1093; ap. Meib. I., p. 452.

12 Ibid., sub an. 1130.

13 Flor. Wigiorn., Chronicon, Tom. I., p. 25 seq. Symeon Dunelh., Histor Ecclesiæ, Lib. I., cap. 5.

14 Beda, Eccles., Histor. Septent., Lib. III., c. 27.

storm, which continued to scourge the whole of Britain.[15] Paganistic Danes, according to the annalist of 897, preceded the terrible malady, which added to the inexpressible vexations and sufferings of the English people, and destroyed prelatial magnates and royal ministers, together with others equally distinguished.[16]

Early in the ninth century the mortality in many parts of Germany was so great that in the convents religious services were abandoned.[17] Towards the close of this era a plague was traced with unusual discrimination to the putrefaction of untold millions of dead locusts.[18] Pestilences in the Germanic empire appear to have raged with so remarkable virulence in the year 995, as to depopulate entire towns and cities,[19] and sometimes confined their destructive energies to the male sex, while women possessed almost total immunity.[20] The epidemic at Rome, in the year 1167, by its mortality among men, necessitated widows and other ladies seeking husbands from adjacent Italian cities.[21] These infectious diseases were generally ascribed to astrological or diabolical provocation,[22] but that of the year just designated, by the attestation of a contemporary, arose from malaria or impure air.[23]

It would seem that some of the great mediæval epidemics were of eastern origin, and through inefficient quarantine by the Venetians, imported in the ordinary course of commercial transport, or by the return of their disorganized and diseased armies from the Levant. By the latter agency, in 1172, an

[15] Fl. Wigiorn., Chronicon, Tom. I., p. 38.

[16] Ibid., Tom. I., p. 115.

[17] Annalista Saxo, sub an. 807.

[18] "Ex earum autem fœtore atque putredine aër corruptus diram pestem finitimis generavit." Ibid., sub an. 884.

[19] Ibid., sub an. 995.

[20] Altahens. Maj. Annales, sub an. 1059.

[21] Otto Frising., Gesta Frederic. Imp., Appendix, Lib. IV., an. 1168.

[22] Ricobaldi, Compilatio Chronologia, sub an. 1312.

[23] Helmoldi, Chronicon, sub. an. 1167.

awful pestiferous disorder was introduced into Venice. On the cowardly retreat of the republican forces from the isle of Scio, where this plague had revealed itself, before their arrival at the shores of Italy, the soldiery on board the transports were decimated almost to annihilation. Upon its introduction at Venice, this pestilence made frightful ravages among the immense populace, as it had done two centuries previous.[24]

For a prolonged period thousands of citizens perished daily.[25] Frequently the accurate judgment of medical philosophers was able to predict the approach of dread diseases on account of the atmosphere indicating an unusual impurity, as happened in the year 1191, when the emperor of Germany, as early as the fourteenth of April, withdrew his forces into the mountains for sanitary safety.[26] From the Justinian pestilence throughout the Middle Ages, no infectious malady excited greater terror or caused such terrible destruction of human life, as that which appeared in the provinces of Northern Italy late in the year 1347.[27]

In Venice its approach was announced by a series of earthquakes, commencing on the 25th of January ensuing. For a period of fifteen days repeated shocks overturned numerous public edifices, shattered into fragments three enormous bell-towers, and inspired unutterable consternation among the inhabitants. To these calamities succeeded the plague of 1348, originally introduced through the close commercial relations between the Genovese and the Ottoman empire. From the shores of the Black sea it was carried in trading vessels to Sicily, and thence spread in a most malignant form to the Tuscan countries—notably Florence.[28]

In this city, according to the vivid discription of Boccaccio, an eye-witness to its fury, more than a hundred thousand per-

[24] Daru, Histoire de Venise, Tom. I., p. 27.

[25] Ibid., Tom. I., p. 28.

[26] Hugonis, Chronicon, Continuat. Weingart, sub an. 1195.

[27] Daru, op. cit., Tom. I., p. 124.

[28] Boccacio, Il Decamerone, Prefazione.

sons perished during the height of this epidemic.[29] Naples lost sixty thousand of its inhabitants, Sienna eighty thousand, and Genoa forty thousand.

It has been asserted that at this epoch Europe was decimated to three-fifths of its population.[30] Annalists of the time dilate with horror upon the unmitigated severity of this destructive pestilence, and such of them as survived it apostrophized its malignant energy, at one time, as threatening the complete extinction of the human race. Indeed, in many localities the proportion of the living to the victims was infinitely less than the conjecture of the chroniclers, which Daru inclines to doubt.[31] The annals are nearly unanimous in stating its origin to be traceable among pagan Mussulmans beyond the sea; and so grievous were its ravages in many localities, towns and cities, that the country for a thousand paces in every direction was depopulated of every human being.[32] The route of this mortal malady, whether originally by sinister approaches emitted from the densely populated Chinese empire,[33] or directly originating with the Ottomen, followed with an irregular, irrational serpentine movement, in the general direction of water courses—so much so in fact that its progress and virulent forces were usually confined to seaport cities, and thence along inland streams to larger provincial towns and hamlets.

Especially was such the pathway relentlessly pursued by this awful destroying agent throughtout Italy,[34] in the Venetian country, and in Provence. At this epoch, the Romish hierarchy occupied the city of Avignon, and during three days preceding Lenten Sabbath, more than fourteen hundred dead bodies were entombed. But the most sinister statement of the contemporaneous chronicler whom we follow, is his decla-

---

[29] Daru, Histoire de Venise, Tom. I., p. 124.

[30] Ibid.

[31] Ibid.

[32] Rebdorf, Annales, sub an. 1347.

[33] Chronicon Oldenburg, Archi-Comit., sub an. 1350.

[34] Rebdorf, op. cit., sub an. 1347.

ration, that in the municipality of Marseilles so many men perished as to leave the city actually uninhabited![35]

Its subsequent route was across the Alps, passing these high altitudes without mitigating the infectious malignancy, into Hungary, ravaging the whole of Germany, thence into France, where, as in Ireland, a third portion only of the inhabitants survived its calamitous attacks.[36] Immediately after the brief but decisive campaign against the Poles, anterior to the year 1350, the pestilence began to reveal itself in the more obscure places of the Germanic empire. In these regions, the approaching appearance was heralded by the most sombre and unnatural phenomena, such as incredible famine, forcing humanity to eat herbs similar to beasts, inundation of many cities and towns, while, indeed, in the same year a marvellous drought was followed by storms of such deluging rainfall as to sweep away entire villages.[37]

Medical skill receded before the inroads of this unprecedented malady, which maintained a destructive virulence in some provinces for a whole year,[38] in others extending to three.[39] It was generally accepted at this epoch that the malady originated in the Oriental Indies, transmitted by extreme filth, and creeping by stealthy marches as far as the British Isles,[40] where it entered England at the principal maritime ports of Southampton and Bristol, during the year 1348.[41] Strange to narrate, notwithstanding the philosophical sagacity touching the origin and development of this dreaded disease,

---

[35] "Imo dicebatur, quod in civitate Marsiliensi ex hoc pestilentia tot homines moribantur, quod locus quasi inhabitabilis remansit." Rebdorf, Annales, sub an. 1347.

[36] Ibid.

[37] Chronica Oldenburgensium, sub an. 1350.

[38] Rebdorf, op. cit., sub an. 1347.

[39] Chronic. Oldenburg., sub an. 1350.

[40] "Pestis lugubris et miserima," etc., "quæ primo in Asia, apud Indios, ob quasdam bestiolas incipiens." Ibid., sub an. 1350; and Chronic. Oldenberg., sub an. 1350.

[41] Knyghton, De Eventibus Angliæ, Lib. IV.; ap. X. Script., p. 2598 seq.

popular frenzy seized upon the horrible suggestion, that the Jews were chargeable with its propagation by means of poisonous philters.[42] Such clamorous inculpation was sufficient to arouse the insensate fury of a degraded and terrified populace.

Everywhere these inoffensive citizens were slaughtered, as a chronicler of the time ingenuously writes, after the manner of cattle—more pecudum.[43] Impartial criticism must decide that superior sanitary precautions by the Israelites enabled them materially in escaping the destructive energies of this disease, which apparent exemption stirred the envious rage of their Christian enemies. In a single province of Germany, during the triennial devastation of the plague, over five thousand hermit friars perished, according to the annals of this order.[44] Substantially identical indications of that sensitive, nervous excitability related by the historian of the Justinian pest,[45] were reproduced in the year 1348.

Men, frightened to the very verge of insanity, abandoned their domicils, and wandered aimlessly in woods and forests; vineyards and fields were deserted, nor was the voice of a human being to be heard. In the dreadful silence of night, and the more appalling tranquillity of the noonday, sounds as of a tumultuous crowd were distinctly perceptible, and at times the suppressed repercussion of an advancing army struck the sensitive ear, but in no direction were their footsteps visible.[46] To the excited vision of many, two angels typifying the malevolent and beneficent principles were presented sweeping through cities in the awful gloom of night: the malignant spirit, with hunting-spear in hand, by permission of the good angel, struck the portals of certain abodes—on the following day, all the occupants were dead.[47] The pestilence arrived in

---

[42] Chronicon Oldenburgens., sub an. 1350.

[43] Chronicon Schawenburgen, sub an. 1348.

[44] Chronica Oldenb., sub an. 1350.

[45] Procopius, De Bello Persico, Lib. II., cap. 22.

[46] Chr. Oldenburg., sub an. 1350.

[47] "Tunc visibiliter multis hominibus videntibus apparuerunt duo angeli, unus

England preceded by unusual events, which, in this instance, was incessant rain for three or four months.

At the very beginning its ravages were terrible, especially in the north and on the eastern shores, where the mortality was slightly over a half. From the trustworthy attestation of Murimuth's continuator, living at the time of this epidemic, an excellent notion of its awful malignity may be gathered. He states in many religious houses, out of twenty inmates, oftentimes there were barely two persons surviving its destructive energies.[48] According to the information evidently obtained by the chronicler from reliable sources, in numerous localities a tenth part of the inhabitants only escaped. As an aggrandizement of so deplorable calamity, a pestiferous infection suddenly fell upon domestic animals, which prevented annual returns of the soil; and then, as he gloomily narrates, the land formerly thrifty with culture, became a solitude, abandoned by the peasantry, and remained untilled.

So great was the misery that it was feared these provinces would never be restored to their previous condition.[49] The plague of 1355, in England, evidently the propagation of the earlier, was expressly ascribed to malevolent spirits.[50] This disorder seems to have caused partial insanity, which forced the infects to wander like frenzied imbeciles and demoniacs, howling through city and hamlet, in the street and on the public highways, everywhere throughout the realm.[51] The third and last of the great pestilences, which for an intermittent period of twenty years had scourged the people of

---

bonus alter malus transeuntes per urbem nocturno tempore: malus tenebat venabulum in manu," etc. Chr. Oldenburg., sub an. 1350.

48 "In quibus vero religiosis domibus, de viginti non superant nisi duo." Ad. Murimuth, Chronic. Continuator, sub an. 1348, p. 178.

49 Ibid.

50 "Temptatione malorum spiritorum." Knyghton, De Eventibus Angliæ, Lib. IV., p. 2598 seq. "And the fendes was seen in mannes lykenesse, and spake unto men as they traveled by the way." Fabian's Chronicle, p. 474, Ellis. Ed. Not in Ed. of 1559.

51 Demons seen in 1100. Fl. Wigior., Chronic., Tom. II., p. 46.

England, began in the year 1369, presaged by incessant inundations and almost total destruction of the grain crops, so that in the ensuing year a measure of flour sold at three solidi.

Mortality of man and beast, at this period, was enormous. One victim was Edward III's. queen Phillipa, among a multitude of eminent spiritual and secular noblemen.[52] The pestilence of 1348 was carried up the Rhone by two fishermen, who communicated it to their spouses. The chronist adds that every human being in the hamlet died with the disease,[53] and during the height of the plague along the shores of this stream, unnumbered dead of towns and cities were thrown at night into the river.[54] An attempt was made in Paris, to enforce a system of sanitary precaution, by forbidding barbers to furnish baths, and surgeons, both male and female, were interdicted throwing blood of pestifers in the streets and alleys of the city.[55] With few exceptions all the monarchies of Western Europe were swept by this fearful malady, everywhere revealing itself with dreadful and uniform symptoms. Ulcerated suppuration[56] was the earliest form of the disorder, whose progress after the few first hours advanced to more serious manifestations. With men, and this sex appears to have been originally more liable to inoculation, the disease appeared in the form of glandular ulcers beneath the armpits and upon the genitalia or elsewhere.[57] In many localities it was adolescent males who perished, either through excruciating physical agony, in six or eight days, or by excretion of sanguinary

---

[52] Ad. Murimuth, Chronicon Continuator, p. 195 seq; and Fabian's Chronicle, p. 245.

[53] "Duo piscatores per Rodanum de partibus inferioribus cum piscibus ascendentes Lugdunum—Lyons—subintrant, et continues vicus ubi hospitabantur inficebatur, et mulieres simul illorum duorum piscatorum pestifera contagione morientes." Herman Corneri, Chronicon, sub an. 1348; and Vitorudani, Chronicon, sub an. 1348.

[54] Ordonnances, Rois de France de la Trois. Race, Tom. II., p. 383.

[55] Ibid.

[56] Boccacio, Il Decamerone, Prefaz., p. 5.

[57] Rebdorf, Annales, sub an. 1348, Freher. I., p. 630.

exudation. Such diseased spots were denominated emunctoria by physicians, because the secretions or subtle perspiration were the more readily emitted by nature through these parts.[58] Throughout Germany this epidemic raged with undiminished virulence for five or six years, and had not altogether disappeared long afterwards.

Popular notions touching the poisoning of wells and springs by Jews, largely aided in propagating the curious order of Flagellants, or a religious order of scourgers, without an acknowleged head.[59] The advent of this singular mania or malady is chronicled as early as the year 1248, when for the first time they appeared in Bohemia.[60] A record is made of their sad procession in Poland twelve years later,[61] and at the same time they are alluded to in Italy, as a novelty.[62] Usually they traveled in troops of seventy or eighty, armed with a knotted scourge, and by force of fervid enthusiasm, induced multitudes to join their intrepid ranks.[63]

In the year 1260, urged by the necessity of counteracting the consternation which rendered the encroachment of epidemics of comparative ease, this system of public penance spread so rapidly through many provinces, that it was everywhere received and hailed as miraculous.[64] Their first appearance in Southern Europe was assigned to a slender procession from Perugia[65] to Florence, enlarging by the accession of noblemen and merchants in the beginning, and afterwards by rustics and vagrants.

This mode of penitential suffering, according to contempor-

---

58 Rebdorf, Annales, sub an. 1348.

59 Chronicon Schawenburg., sub an. 1348.

60 "Flagellatores iverunt primii, incipientes in Bohemia et post per mundum." Chronicon Engelhusii, sub an. 1248; Leibnitz II., p. 1119.

61 Annales Capit. Cracoviensis, an. 1260.

62 "Quæ fertur Perusii recipisse exordium." Ibid.

63 Rebdorf, Annales, sub an. 1349.

64 Chronicon Australis, sub an. 1261, Freher. I., p. 461.

65 Annales Capituli Cracoviensis, sub an. 1260.

aneous writers and ocular witnesses, was harsh, horrible and pitiable to behold. The immediate object of such organized system of corporeal flagellation was the invocation of the curative powers of divine angelic hosts through self-inflicted pain, in order that this potential sacrifice of personality might provoke a restoration of the infirm to health, and preserve the robust against the destroying force of pestilential maladies, produced by malignant spirits. Entirely nude from the navel upwards, a vestment of close texture falling to the feet covering the lower body, they marched with head and face concealed, in order that their identity might remain a mystery.[66]

Slowly advancing in pairs or triplets, oftentimes clerics with a banner or crucifix displayed attending, they scourged themselves twice each day during thirty-three days, in commenmoration of Christ's Passion, wherever their ambulatory movements found them, constantly chanting certain songs drawn from the Passionale, with distinct movement by twos or threes in a solemn whirl, or completed the melancholy intonation in sacred edifices; sometimes falling insensible to the earth, or rising in genuflections, elevated their naked arms imploringly to heaven, alike indifferent to mud or snow, the heat of summer and the frigidity of winter.[67]

In Italy, as they passed along the highways, the monotonous cry of "Peace! peace!" was sounded, while the women flagellants moving in troops partially disrobed, regarded those non-conforming to these usages as sacrilegious.[68] In the year 1261, so rapid was the increase that they were numbered by thousands among all nations.[69] Pontifical and secular contempt of this popular frenzy gradually tempered the excessive zeal into a corporation, denuded of its exciting displays.[70]

During the stretch of time over which the ardent fanaticism

---

[66] Chronicon Augustalis, sub an. 1260.

[67] Ibid., sub an. 1260

[68] Ricobaldi, Historia Imperatorum, an. 1260.

[69] Chronica S. Aegidii, sub an. 1261.

[70] Chronicon Augustalis, sub an. 1261, Freher. I., p. 534.

of their original enthusiasm glowed with undimished passion, in Germany as early it would seem as 1349, near the festival of the Lord's Ascension, a body of Flagellants in proceeding through a town in the diocess of Bamberg, where were domiciled great numbers of Jews, were most unexpectedly assailed by the disgusted Hebrews, who deliberately assassinated fourteen of these inoffensive penitents, and as a fitting termination to so valorous a deed of inglorious murder, fired the citadel and destroyed several citizens.[71]

In the same year, however, the scourgers, under the puissant exhortation of a German nobleman, seized an opportunity to slaughter all the Jews at Cologne,[72] perhaps by way of retaliatory vengeance. Thus advancing from city to village, through towns and hamlets, with blood-stained scourges and burning tapers in hand, they recruited immense crowds to their penitential ranks.[73]

Prophetic voices quickly developed among the Flagellants, which announced the forth-coming antipope.[74] It is stated in the trustworthy chronicles of the time, when this sect had exhibited its vigorous vitality for several months, the women began to assume this repugnant system of mortfication in vast multitudes, denuded to the waist, and scourging themselves severely. The exorbitant assumption by this people of their superior sanctity, their omnipotent force to remit vice and crime, and their unblushing proclamation of sortilege, combined with defiant disregard of sacerdotal authority, finally armed the regular church with indignation, especially when it revealed the singular fact that the laity preponderated more to the nude penitents than to their spiritual advisers, and led to the extinction of one of the most curious orders of the Middle Ages.[75]

---

[71] Rebdorf, Annales, sub an. 1349, Freher. I., p. 630.

[72] "Tunc vero omnes Judæi in Colonia interfecti sunt sub occasione dicta." Chronica de Marka, sub an. 1349; ap. Meib. I., p. 405.

[73] Chronicon Augustalis, sub an. 1260.

[74] Chronicon Schawenburg., sub an. 1348.

[75] Rebdorf, op. cit., sub an. 1348.

The last of the several epidemics described, had barely disappeared beneath the relentless power of the Romish Church, when a malady, the most remarkable perhaps ever chronicled in the history of the human race, suddenly manifested itself by an uncontrollable impulse to saltimbulation or dancing, either singly or in groups.

This disease may with justice be regarded as the very culmination of that excitability and exasperation of the nervous organism, so frequently revealing its direful virulence amid the strange eventualities of mediæval times. Doubtless the frightful calamities survived in the pestilential ravages of the fourteenth century, together with excitations attending the sombre sadness of the sanguinary Flagellants, precipitated the dancing frenzy at the close of the same era. In addition to these elements jointly or operating individually, the superstitious faith of those ages attests to what calamitous solstices the human mind may swing.

Vulgar traditions and unreliable legends, repeated nightly around the blazing fires of each domestic hearth, or gravely narrated to awe-struck multitudes at fairs, public markets and on great church festival days, assisted in maintaining an unreasonable spiritual activity. For centuries preceding the actual outbreak of the dancing infirmity, the mediæval mind was held to an abnormal strain by the impossible narrations written in monastic annals. A few of these will portray the condition of such superstitious faith. In the year 1200, popular tradition propagated the notion that a man by the name of Nicolanus Piscis, actually lived in the sea, and could not survive out of water—a domicil enforced upon him by maternal malediction.[76]

Towards the close of this century, it was everywhere believed that Authonica, an Italian woman, was delivered of forty-two children prior to her fortieth year, of whom several sets were twins, others quadruplets.[77] But another annalist

---

[76] Ricobaldi, Compilatio Chronologia, sub an. 1200.

[77] Ricobaldi, Historia Imperatorum, sub an. 1274. Human flesh eaten in the

does not hesitate to affirm the birth of three hundred sons in one parturition.[78] The same legend in Poland, ascribed only thirty-six at once to the noble lady, in the year 1270.[79] Famine was so severe in the year 1315, that women ate their own offspring.[80] Tartaric invasions of the Greek empire in the thirteenth century, produced such distressing misery that human beings were slaughtered like beeves, and their flesh exposed for sale as a vendible commodity in public markets.[81] During the great plague of 1348, deaths were so numerous as to preclude the possibility of burying them, and in the terror, both living and dead were carried to the cemeteries for burial.

From 1350 to 1383, inclusively, this saltatory pestilence devastated many places in Germany every seven years. The historian of the time from whom the foregoing is extracted, unequivocally affirms this malady at Paderborn was not entirely extinct in the year 1418, when he completed the Cosmodrome.[82] Ardent fanaticism developed from abnormal religious frenzy or irrational social life, and aggravated mediæval superstitions, conjoined to extreme dread of swiftly destructive maladies, prepared the popular mind for the singular disease which swept through Germany in 1374. It was described by chroniclers as a wonderful and unheard-of disorder, first arising in Cologne and vicinity, and quickly transmitted to other cities along the Rhine.[83]

Groups of both sexes, driven with the fury of Bacchanalian devotees, leaped and jumped in choral dances, totally divested

year 1070. Fl. Wigior., Chronicon, Tom. II., p. 4. A Polish annalist in the thirteenth century discusses the probability of green children. Annales Polonior., sub an. 1270.

[78] Chronica Osnabergens, sub an. 1270; ap. Meib. II., p. 217.

[79] Annales Poloniorum, sub an. 1270.

[80] Graystones, Historia Dunelmensis, cap. 36.

[81] " Interea fames horribilis et inaudita invasit terram Ungariæ, et plures perierunt famæ, quam antea a paganis, canes edebant et cattes et hominis, humana caro publice vendebatur in mundinis." Chronica Australis, sub an. 1242.

[82] Gobel., Person. Cosmodromii, Aetas VI., c. 59.

[83] Chronicon Engelhusii, sub an. 1374.

of personal volition, incited to involuntary muscular tremor and spasmodic movement by the resistless force of this singular malady.[84] In troops, they continued with feverish frenzy their morbid dancing upon the public thoroughfares, through churches, or in private houses, and suddenly, as though demented, would fall singly or in pairs to the ground.[85] A heavy girth or swaddling band encircled the abdomen, apparently to guard against the eruptive force of humid secretions, and, in case the cord attaching this girdle happened to become loose, the infects drew it tightly to its place; but even this did not appear to satisfy these maniacal invalids, who repeatedly demanded by-standers to tread their feet upon their stomachs while they reclined on the ground; consequently when one tumbled over he oftentimes raised two or three persons thus treading him by the distended elasticity of his abdominal muscles.

A curious characteristic of this disease was the abhorrence of red cloth and roseate shoes, which they held in mortal dread. The progressive increase of this malady may be readily inferred when it is stated, on first sight, these suffering and distorted dancers inspired spectators with a feeling of horror, which was gradually transformed into a species of fascination, provoking them to join their ranks. Although the sight of purple garments and pink shoes filled this stricken people with consternation, some were demonstrated to be deceived in colors, whose alarm was therefore fallacious.[87]

The annalist whom we have followed was an eye-witness to the painful antics of these diseased contortionists, and in the year 1418, when he completed his chronicle,[88] the disorder had

---

[84] Ibid.

[85] Chronicon Engelhusii, sub an. 1374.

[86] Gobelin Personæ, Cosmodromii, Aetas VI., cap. 59.

[87] "Pannum rubeum, et calceos rostrates se dixierunt abominari." Chr. Engelhusii, sub an. 1374. Municipal authorities interdicted the use of such apparel, on account of its exciting the possessed to frenzy. Hecker, Die Tanzwuth, p. 4.

[88] Gobel. Person., op. cit., Aet. VI., cap. 69.

appeared in Strassburg, where it was known as Saint Vitus' dance by reason of invalids frequenting his chapel for its medicinal property.[89] At all events, the visible manifestations of a painful malady were too evident for denial, although enlightened minds of the age were in doubt whether this singular pestilence should be classed as a physical disease, or attributed to besetment and possession by impure demons.[90]

Attempts have been essayed frequently to institute a possible similitude between the choral saltimbulations of the Middle Ages and the convulsive leaping of modern religious sectarians.[91] No doubt the external revelation of muscular action assimilates with that of their mediæval precursors, but the causes inciting such nervous exasperation were of such antagonistic character as to make the analogy only apparent, and not grounded in reality. Music was used with admirable results as a cure of this malady,[92] and may be taken as a correct exponent of the more ancient incantation, or song remedies in healing disorders.[93]

---

[89] Hecker, op. cit., p. 8.

[90] Gobelin Personæ, Cosmodromii, Aetas VI., cap. 69.

[91] Hecker, Die Tanzwuth, p. 79.

[92] Ibid., p. 42.

[93] "Si autem his conveniens adjungitur medicina," etc., "cum medicina corpus, incantatione anima adjuvetur." Constans African., De Incantat. et Adjurat., Epistol., p. 318.

CHAPTER XXIV.

Mediæval Universities for Medical Study—Parisian Schools—Great Excellence of Italian Colleges—Favorable Regulations for Students—Great Numbers Flock to Italy—Have their own Laws—Monetary Value of a Celebrated Professor—Colleges Confer Knighthood—Large Fees to Surgeons—Female Physicians—Public Surgery—Beneficial Ordinances for Medical Culture—Medical Books Translated Direct from Arabic—Text-books on Comparative Anatomy—Regulations of Frederick II. for the Study and Practice of Medicine—Schedule of Medical Fees.

THE ardent zeal displayed by Charlemagne upon his acquisition of the imperial crown to lay a solid foundation for the culture of letters throughout his vast empire, is sufficiently attested by diversified legislation, whose specific object was a mandatory regulation for the monasteries to organize schools of instruction in the famous liberal arts and sciences. The beneficial effects of these laws, entrusted to the administration of clerical authority, were fully revealed in the Middle Ages by the tenacity with which cloisters and convents adhered to their scholastic institutions, which, under discreet and judicious management, developed into the great Universities of Law and Medicine, the embellishment of mediæval Europe.

In the tenth century, Adam of Bremen referred with laudable pride to the flourishing schools of that church under the excellent direction of Tiadelhmus.[1] Early in the ensuing age, Odinkar, a nephew of the king of Sleswig, was converted from the worship of Thor and Odin, and after receiving Christian baptism was educated for an evangelical mission in the Bremen school.[2]

---

[1] Ad. Brem., De Gest. Pontif., Hammab., Lib. II., c. 10; and Albert Stad., Chronic., sub an. 961.

[2] Adam Bremen., Gesta Pontific. Hammab., Lib. II., cap. 34.

Educational establishments in the Gallic abbeys were famed in the time of the Anglo-Saxons, who sent their youth thither in large numbers for instruction,[3] a custom followed by the Danish Cnut, whose sons were entrusted to the French schools for scholastic culture.[4] The Scandinavians sent their children to Paris in the twelfth century, to be taught not only theology but secular sciences.[5] Some monastic schools excelled others in the diversity and thoroughness of tuition in divinity or theological readings, and also in mathematics, astronomy, geometry, music, and versification, according to the Hirsau annals,[6] and in the more intricate knowledge of the medicinal or curative art.

One of the most illustrious scholars of the tenth century, whose culture was obtained in the convent designated,[7] was Witchind, of Corbey, who signalized a sojourn at Hirsau by his solidity of erudition, and the vast number of disciples whom he left behind him. His successor, preceptor of Tiadelhmus of Bremen, likewise equally distinguished himself. In the early part of the eleventh century the schools of France had acquired extended repute, and were frequented by students from abroad in quest of advanced instruction in arts and sciences.[8] English rulers, perhaps from the time of national conversion to Christianity, were accustomed to defraying the current expenses of a school for their countrymen at the chief city of Christendom. The edifice erected in Rome by Offa, the Anglo-Saxon king, for the accommodation of students from England, was destroyed in 837 by a great conflagration.[9]

[3] Montalembert, Les Moines d'Occident, Tom. V., p. 265 seq. Famed in the seventh century. Hen., Huntingd. Historiar., Lib. III., p. 332.

[4] Gesta Cnutonis, Lib. II., cap. 18.

[5] "Nobiliores terræ filios suos non solum ad clerum promovendum, verum etiam secularibus rebus instituendos Parisius mittunt." Arnold, Chronicon Slavor., Lib. III., cap. 5.

[6] Chronicon Hirsaug., sub an. 890.

[7] Ibid., sub an. 952–4.

[8] Albert Stad., Chronicon, sub an. 1033.

[9] Wm. Malmsb., De Gestis Reg. Anglor., Lib. II., c. 2.

In general, conventual scholastic institutions were organized upon a dwarfed scheme, although educational facilities provided in the departments of Salerno and elsewhere, under exclusive control of the Romish hierarchy, more enlarged instruction.

Anterior to the twelfth century, however, scientific corporations, expanded to the dimensions required by the succeeding ages, certainly had no existence, such at least as presented in the era alluded to. The name universitas signified an association or organization in the sense assigned by civil law,[10] gradually developed by intercommunication of tutors to disciples of the selected subject of tuition, while the words studium generale had reference to the prerogative of each foreign or native student to procure this culture, involving the doctorate, and constituted the exclusive possession of these well equipped schools. Notwithstanding Italian universities, at their origin,[11] were independent of abject royal or pontifical control, the necessities entailed upon teachers by the fluctuating compensatory collections from their disciples forced them at a later epoch, in escaping this servile dependency, to accept sacerdotal jurisdiction; so that the thirteenth century witnessed this supremacy over the scholastic institutions, the chiefs of which were spiritual guides recruited from the ranks of the church.

In order that the department of theology might be suitably filled, the popes finally assumed the right of preferment; and indeed such official sanction was eagerly desired, as especially favorable to the popularity of the university.[12] In the contest to subject the students attending the Bolognese colleges in 1216, when the citizens sought to extend jurisdiction over them, Honorius arrayed himself with the scholars, and ordered the immediate repeal of laws affecting their freedom in that municipality.[13] In the preceding century, aided by royal and

---

[10] Savigny, Geschichte des Rœmischen Rechts, Th. III., p. 152.

[11] Ibid., p. 155.

[12] Von Raumer, Geschichte der Hohenstauffen, Th. VI., p. 341.

[13] Von Raumer, Geschichte der Hohenstauffen, Th. VI., p. 341.

pontifical sufferance, or important dotations, three schools, as early as 1158, had a reputation which extended throughout the whole of Europe: Paris for theological studies, Bologna for Roman or civil law, and Salerno as the chief medical school of the west. The Bologna University in the year cited obtained valuable immunities from Frederick I., emperor of Germany, at the diet of Roncaglia, in the month of November.

One of the priceless results of this legislation, intended perhaps exclusively for Bologna, was its ultimate interpretation so as to extend its beneficent franchises to all foreign students seeking information and higher education, whether of law or medicine, in the pontifical colleges. Stranger students, who exposed themselves to greater inconveniences in attending the Bolognese University, were conceded particular immunities. They were at entire liberty to travel to their destination unhindered, and any interference with these ambulatory prerogatives was interdicted by the severest penalties, nor were they liable to be arrested and held to answer for delinquencies of their compatriots. By a canon of the provincial synod held in Montpelier in the year 1195, all scholars, whether natives or otherwise, were to be protected in going or returning to France.[14]

But the ordinances of the Hohenstauffen monarch proceeded further, and directed when students were accused of crime, or required to appear in a civil action, the invaluable privilege was accorded of trial by a specially constituted tribunal. The phraseology of the code would seem to warrant the inference that this judicial function was to be performed by professors or bishops of the city.[15] Such franchises were certainly claimed and exercised by the scholars in the Medical Universities of Southern Italy at this epoch, by virtue of an application which the ordinance itself seemed to admit, although, as we shall presently see, specific regulations of equally exact and important character were promulgated by Frederick II., in the exclusive

[14] Concilium Monpeliense, cap. 7; apud Baluz., Concilia, Tom. I., p. 31.

[15] Codex IV., Titulus 13, lex. 5.

interest of medical culture. The profound concern manifested by the emperor at the Roncevaux Congress for the development of arts and sciences, appears from the rescript quoted. He says: "We consider it indispensable, as all good men merit our praise and protection, therefore those whose science and erudition are to enlighten the whole world shall be protected with unwavering carefulness against oppression."[16]

By gradual pressure entailed through necessity, and by interest of municipalities where these theological, law, or medical institutions were situated, a salutary eagerness began to display itself, to procure such professors whose extensive reputation and vast learning would add wealth and prosperity to the cities by the affluence of multitudes of scholars attracted thither by professorial fame. In many places—Bologna, Ferrara, etc.—these savans, or doctors, were relieved of public taxes and other civil burdens; oftentimes important grants sufficient to guarantee them a comfortable livelihood were cheerfully donated.[17]

Such arrangements were of vital necessity, inasmuch as the departure of a celebrated professor would cause the city to be nearly deserted by its students, who generally followed their tutor to his new professorship, a possible event sought to be avoïded by compelling the teacher to enter into a contract.[18] It was occasionally stipulated that the scientific lecturer thus provided by the municipal government should at his convenience publicly read for the exclusive benefit of native citizens; an agreement which, it would seem, was freely acquiesced in by the erudite doctors ambitious for local distinction.[19]

That assemblage of scholars, specially convoked by their rectors, was designated Universitas, or University, where the sense of the convocation was taken by a vote with white and black beans, and before which each matriculate must appear at

[16] Codex IV., Tit. 13, lex. 5; and Constitut., §§ 8–10.

[17] Tiraboschi, Storia della Litteratura Italiana, Tom. IV., p. 64.

[18] Petr. de Vineis, Epistolæ, Lib. VI., cap. 11.

[19] Tiraboschi, Storia della Litteratura, Tom. IV., pp. 56, 257.

least thrice a year to entitle himself to municipal immunities.[20] In order to render the ordinances of Frederick I. of useful efficiency, the provosts of these schools were at length conceded original jurisdiction over all students, excepting Germans regularly entered at the educational institutions.[21] As a further inducement for preserving the dignity of the Bolognese University unblemished, the prerogative of conferring the knightly orders was awarded it towards the close of the Middle Ages, which, however, seems to have partaken largely of the nature of a financial transaction.[22]

In the creation and incumbency of professorial offices, early in the thirteenth century, due regard was had, even in schools of less distinction, to elaborate culture of medical knowledge, inasmuch as two surgeons, confessedly engaged for educational services, conjoined with teachers of civil law, grammarians and two dialecticians, equipped the new institute at Vercelli.[23] Independent of these, municipal authorities employed several copyists, whose functions consisted in furnishing scholars with transcripts of books according to rates prescribed by the rectors. The Paduan University, from its location, enjoyed unusual advantages for obtaining a large clientage of students, and in the year 1262, added to other tutors three professors of natural sciences[24]—an incontestible indication of a growing demand in this cognate branch of medicine.

Later, this scholastic establishment passed into the custody of the Venetian Republic, whether to its advantage does not appear.[25] Great care was taken to obtain suitable occupants of University professorships, and oftentimes the applicants for them were subjected to a most rigid examination before a body duly commissioned. In the thirteenth century a statute

---

[20] Savigny, Geschichte des Rœmischen Rechts, Th. III., p. 182.

[21] Ibid., p. 194.

[22] Ibid., p. 235.

[23] Tiraboschi, op. cit., Tom. IV., p. 53.

[24] Muratori, Antiquitat. Italiæ, Tom. III., p. 910.

[25] Daru, Histoire de Venise, Tom. I., p. 183.

of Turin prescribed such inquiry into the qualifications of any strange physician, before receiving municipal sanction to practice medicine in this city.[26]

Fees of juristic or medicinal lecturers aggregated such large sums—carefully collected before proceeding with their readings—that not unfrequently these professors attained great affluence.[27] Public surgeons, engaged by the civil authorities of Milan, in this age, for gratuitous services to the poor,[28] received a salary from the city treasury amounting to fifty libros a year, in consideration of which they should care without reward for the sick in the municipal hospitals and prisons.[29] In this century, when a woman obtained the doctorate, it was deemed of so unusual occurrence as to receive specific mention. In the year 1236, Vitisia Gozzodini held public lectures in Bologna, on the Institutes of Justinian, and usually appeared in male costume.[30] The publicity of her readings, however, was confined to her own house.[31] Female professors of medicine, following the seclusive system of Vitisia, lectured during the twelfth and thirteenth centuries in Salerno, on medicine.[32]

Many women in England, shortly after the Conquest, as nuns in the wealthy monasteries, were occupied with the study of this art, and composed remedies, which they offered gratuitously to the indigent.[33] No monarch, from the time of Alfred

---

[26] "Item si quis extraneus medicus phisicus veniat in Thaurino ad habitandum examinetur a phisicis et clericis." Statuta Taurini, ap. Mon. Histor. Ital., Tom. I., p. 726.

[27] Sarti, De Profess. Boniensis, Pars I., p. 4, § 4 seq.

[28] "Unus medicus cirorgie, qui apelletur medicus pauperum, eligatur." Mon., Hist. Ital., cap. 160, Tom. II., p. 1038.

[29] "Et debeant medicane gratis infirmos hospitalium medioloni et carcerum." Ibid.

[30] Ghirardaeci, Historia di Bologna, Tom. I., p. 159.

[31] "Betesia figliuola e infina all'anno duodecimo di sua eta," etc., "in casa sua lesse la Instituta à piu di trenta scholari." Ibid.

[32] Haeser, Geschichte der Medezin, p. 198.

[33] "Beaucoup de femmes, dans les riches monastères, s'occupaient alors à etudiér la médicine, et à composer des remèdes qu'elles offraient gratuitement aux

the Great and Charlemagne, wielded the vast forces of a colossal empire in the interest of art and science, despite calamities by sea and land,[34] comparable to the Hohenstauffen emperor Frederick II., to whom medical culture of that age was deeply indebted for individual laws promulgated for its development, together with the reaffirmation of the ordinances of Roger of Sicily, directly contemplating this subject.

Although the medical institutes of Salerno and Monte Cassino were limited to the dwarfed influences of locality during the entire course of the preceding century, the rescripts of this illustrious ruler, combined with the lucid preparations of predecessors, enlarged the perspective of future usefulness to gigantic proportions. As a monarch of exquisite judgment, in view of the singular circumstance that Neapolitans used the Grecian dialect in defiance of the change of ages, he, similar to an earlier Sicilian conqueror,[35] directed the laws having especial reference to this people should be drawn up in this idiom.[36]

Great stress has been placed upon the uncritical assertion, that at this epoch such knowledge of Greek writers, medical and otherwise, as came to Western Europe, was derived from impoverished Latinized versions of Arabic translations, at a time indeed when the German emperor numbered his Saracen subjects in Sicily and on the peninsula by thousands.[37] In the age of Roger of Italy, an archbishop, Roboald, of Amalfi, was deeply skilled in Greek, Latin, and Hebrew[38]—a knowledge eclipsed by the Dalmatian cleric above mentioned.[39]

Hadrian's Greek attainments are made the subject of pane-

pauvres." Thierry, Histoire de la Conquête de L'Angleterre par les Normands, Tom. IV., p. 86.

[34] Tageoni, Descript. Exped. Asiaticæ; ap. Freher. I., p. 416.

[35] Bazincourt, Histoire de la Sicilie sous les Normands, Tom. II., p. 76.

[36] Von Raumer, Geschichte der Hohenstauffen, Th. III., p. 276.

[37] Tiraboschi, Storia della Litteratura, Tom. IV., p. 318.

[38] Muratori, Antiquitat. Ital., Tom. III., p. 918.

[39] Supra., p. 259.

gyrical praise by Bede in the eighth century.[40] Saracens in the twelfth century educated their children from infancy to readily interpret this language, with Latin and the Roman, or vulgar Italian idiom.[41] In the year 968, when Liutprand, the Othonian envoy to Byzantium, proceeded with his diplomatic mission, he was able to converse with tolerable fluency with the Grecian emperor,[42] sometimes having recourse to an interpreter.[43] A Corbey monk, forty years anterior to this period, read Greek at sight in the presence of King Conrad.[44] In the ensuing century, a practical use of this language was vigorously maintained,[45] so much so, indeed, that circular letters for elementary instruction were issued to certain monasteries in Germany.[46] In the year 1146, Burgundio, a Parisian, translated the writings of John of Damascus from original Greek into Latin.[47]

Reference has been made hitherto touching the translations of medical text-books by Constans Afer, in the eleventh century. Doubtless the writings of Grecian authors on this subject were freely reproduced by scientists of the Hohenstauffen era, and particularly in the fourteenth century, from their venerable dialect into mediæval Latinity. The burning desire of Frederick II. to accumulate scientific and literary material, revealed itself during the expedition of this ruler into Syria, by his enormous aggregation of Greek and Arabic manuscripts, of immense value to the monasteries of the West.[48] The emperor was deeply versed in natural history, and indeed, in

---

[40] Beda, Histor. Eccles., Lib. V., c. 33; and Sym. Dunelhm., Hist. Ecclesiæ, Lib. I., c. 14.

[41] Arnold, Chronicon Slavorum, Lib. VII., cap. 8.

[42] Liutprand, Legatio, cap. 51.

[43] Liutprand, Antapodosis, Lib. VI., cap. 9.

[44] Annalista Saxo, sub an. 948.

[45] Badonis, Syntagma; ap. Meib. II., p. 494.

[46] Udalric, Babenberg. Codex, Lib. II., cap. 4.

[47] Herman. Corneri, Chronicon, sub an. 1146; Muratori, Antiquitat. Italiæ, Tom. III., p. 918; and Chronicon Epp. Verden., cap. 36.

[48] Tiraboschi, Storia della Litteratura, Tom. IV., p. 75.

this department of medical analogy, he may be regarded as master. His treatise on falconry attests the profoundest acquaintanceship with the economy and anatomy of birds, and especially falcons, vindicating a claim to meritorious consideration divested of imperial authorship.[49]

A curious feature of this work is the careful and judicious treatment of maladies incident to birds of chase, and practical suggestions of admirable curatives, as well as sanitary rules whose adoption was designed to render them robust and spirited. Eichhorn alleges this compendium to be the earliest production in the nature of comparative anatomy.[50] It is evident, however, that works on such subjects were extant prior to Frederick II's. time, and necessarily traversing identical ground, and particularly since Albert Magnus himself avows large excerpts from the book of William, falconer to Roger, king of Italy.[51] But the most commendatory panegyric of the imperial treatise is the unstinted admission by this erudite pontiff, that his twenty-four chapters on falconry are a compilation principally prepared from the work of his patron, adding but little from personal resources.[52] Royal favor urged the court astrologer, Michel Scot, to translate Aristotle's natural history of animals,[53] although Latin versions of the Stagyrite's writings were made by order of the emperor, about the year 1220, drawn partly from Greek and partly from Arabic sources.[54]

The learned Scot appears to have shared the substantial patronage of Edward I. of England, who granted him a pen-

[49] Legrand d'Aussy, Histoire de la Vie Privée des Français, Tom. II., p. 5.

[50] "Der erste schriftsteller in der anatomia comparativa." Geschichte der Litteratur und Beredsamkeit, Th. II., p. 95.

[51] Albert. Magni, De Falconibus Asturib., cap. 18, p. 190.

[52] "Pauca de nostris adjicientes." Ibid., cap. 19.

[53] "Quem secundo loco compilavit a ejus precis." Muratori, Antiq. Ital., Tom. III., p. 945.

[54] "Circa 1220 jussu Frederici II., imperatoris, partim e Graecis, partim e Arabico sermone composita est per viros lectos in utriusque linguæ prolatione peritos." Fabricius, Biblioth. Græca, Tom. III., p. 205.

sion in the year 1291 for services rendered this sovereign.[55] Jordanus Rufus, who occupied the honored office of commander of the studdery, was largely aided and advised by the emperor in composing a work on veterinary surgery.[56] Owing to rare advantages of intimate intercouse with Oriental princes, the German monarch procured, as his predecessor before him, the transhipment of elephants, camels, giraffes, lions, leopards, tigers, etc., to both Germany and Italy, where, to the excited glee of the people, they were perambulated through provincial towns as instructive exhibitions.[57] Such animals, of value for the study of comparative anatomy, as lions, camels, apes, and ostriches, were utterly unknown to Northern Europe, or the West, anterior to gifts sent imperial Otho in the middle of the tenth century.[58] Before the close of this era, a camel was donated to Otho III. by a popish magnate.[59] Six camels and two leopards given to Henry, emperor of Germany, in the year 1172, were regarded as a munificent present, and altogether worthy of an Eastern soldan.[60] It is worthy of note in the time of Frederick II., that the people of Spain appear to have kept zoölogical gardens, inasmuch as a great number of lions, ostriches, parrots, etc., were sent this hero by Genovese legates, selected among spoils captured at the sacking of Almeria and Lisbon.[61]

Half a century prior to the Roncevaux ordinances of the First Hohenstauffen, which established literature and science on a solid basis throughout Italy, Roger, king of the Sicilies, a descendant of William the Norman, observing the expansion

---

[55] Rymer, Foedera, Tom. II., p. 533.

[56] Tiraboschi, Storia della Litteratura, Tom. IV., p. 213.

[57] Rycardus San Germano, Chronica, sub an. 1228; and Wilkins, Crusades, Vol. VI., p. 510.

[58] Annalista Saxo, sub an. 955.

[59] Annalista Saxo, sub an. 986.

[60] Arnoldi, Chronic. Slavorum, Lib. I., cap. 9. Touching gifts of curious animals to Frederick I., vide Ibid., Lib. IV., cap. 8.

[61] Otto Frising., Gesta Frederici Imper., Lib. IV., cap. 13^{b}.

of medical studies within his limited kingdom, and especially at Salerno, by the advice of spiritual and secular peers of the realm, issued an edict requiring each person desirous of engaging in the healing art to present himself for an examination before royal officials, who should pass judgment upon his qualifications.[62] If the board of examiners refused a certificate of ability in the practice of medicine, and in defiance of such adjudication he presumed to attend invalids as professional adviser, for such temerity he was punished by imprisonment and confiscation of his goods and chattels.[63]

Necessity evidently compelled the enactment and rigid administration of this law, at least the inference is unequivocal from the concluding sentence of the rescript, that this legal ordinance was enforced as a guard for his subjects against dangers incident to the mendacious practitioners of medicine.[64] Although the law here referred to is the earliest known European regulation by competent authority, touching the professional use of this science preceded by judicial examination, at Jerusalem in the year 1090, a standing rule in the code of this kingdom prescribed formal investigation into the possible acquaintanceship of any person, whether "from beyond the sea," or Saracen,[65] before proceeding to cure maladies.[66] The examiners were selected by the archbishop, who scrutinized the applicant's abilities under the pontifical presidency, and, having satisfied themselves as to his learning, gave him a license—evidently written—to practice medicine "in land and town," subject to archiepiscopal jurisdiction.[67]

---

[62] Constitutiones Regni Siculi, Titulus XXXIV., De Probabili Experientia Medicorum, Lex I.

[63] Ibid., Lex IV.

[64] "Hoc enim prospectum est, ne in regno nostro subjecti periclitentur ex imperitia medicorum." Ibid., Lex I.

[65] "Similemente nessun medico extraneo, che venisse d'oltra mar ò di li infideli non deve medicar de urina nessun." Le Assisse del Reaume de Hyerusalem, cap. 218.

[66] "Fin che non sia provato da li miglior medici de la terra." Ibid.

[67] "Medicar li deva esser data licentia de medicare per la terra dove val per la città di quae Vescovo." Ibid., p. 529.

If it appeared that he lacked sufficient knowledge of the art, the pontiff and authorities notified him either to leave the city at once, or remaining, to abandon the profession absolutely. In case he disobeyed, he was scourged publicly and driven out of the municipal limits.[68] When Frederick II., in the year 1224, founded in Naples a new university, he granted access to all subjects of his immense empire,[69] and endowed it with the most celebrated professors of the age.[70] To such students as applied for matriculation especial immunities were conceded, and the solemn sanction of the ordinance stipulated entire freedom of person and independence of goods from municipal assessments.

In order to concentrate local scholars within the precincts of their own university, he directed all pupils attending distant institutions to immediately return to Naples under a penalty, neither should any depart the Sicilian kingdom for scholastic purposes. In publishing this statute, apparently monopolizing the educational interests of Southern Italy, he suggested the amenities of the location, plentitude of provision, and its unalterable tranquillity.[71] Notwithstanding the ponderous weight of state affairs at home and abroad, resting heavily upon the Hohenstauffen ruler, his constant attention, when temporarily relieved of the emergencies of imperial government, was devoted to developing polite letters and the cultivation of scientific studies. Some of his rescripts at this period warrant the conclusion that no one was permitted to instruct or give readings in grammatical art to any but children, excepting in the Neapolitan domains.[72]

Of the decrees challenging unstinted eulogy and respect, promulgated by the emperor for the progress of sound science

---

[68] "Et farlo frustrar per la terra." Ibid., p. 529.

[69] Peter. de Vineis, Epistolæ, Lib. III., cap. 10. Especially as a place for liberal arts: "doceri artis cujusque professionis." Ibid., cap. 13.

[70] Ibid., Lib. IV., cap. 7.

[71] Gobelin, Personæ Cosmodromi, Aetas VI., cap. 54; De Vineis, Epistolæ, Lib. III., cap. 13.

[72] Gobelin, Person., op. cit., Aetas VI., c. 54.

and maintenance of sanitary conditions, those relating to medical qualifications are pre-eminently superior for the age. The sale of diseased meats, particularly unhealthy pork and deleterious bread, was forbidden under severe punishment.[73] Accurate notions of sanitative requirements were well understood and practiced in the Middle Ages in the interest of good health. In the twelfth century, it was a usage of the nobility to take up their residence in mountainous regions to escape the intense heat of summer, and purely for sanitary benefit.[74] Lady Margaretta was conveyed thither under medical advice, in order to derive the advantages of pure air, which was vital in her depreciated physical state.[75] A city ordinance of Turin forbade householders throwing waste or excremental matter over balustrades or out of the windows, into the public streets.[76]

By the mandatory directions of the Neapolitan constitution, no person could be admitted as a student of medicine, unless previously for three years he had familiarized himself with logical science; neither must he teach in a school, nor exercise the craft of curing diseases without an examination by medical scientists at Naples or Salerno, who should make inquiry into the sufficiency of his knowledge of medicine and surgery. In order that public sanction might attest, as far as possible, the abilities of the postulant, his credentials were to be presented to the royal officers, who thereupon issued letters patent, authorizing him to practice medical and surgical art,[77] drawn as follows: Noster N. ad curiam nostram accedeus examinatus fidelis et de genere fidelium artus, et sufficiens ad

---

[73] Rycard, San Germano, Chronica, sub an. 1232.

[74] Geiselberti, Chronicon Hanoniense, sub an. 1194.

[75] "Propter salutatem æris advehi fecit." Ibid., an. cit. Further, Ibid., sub an. 1195.

[76] "Item quod nemo ejiciat vel effundat urinam, vel aliquid putredinem, vel quid aliud horribile de lobia, vel fenestras." Statuta Taurin.; ap. Monument, Histor. Ital., Tom. I., p. 726.

[77] Constitutiones Regni Siculi, Titulus XXXIV., Lex 3.

artem medicinæ exercendam extitit, per nostram curiam approbatur.[78]

It is evident from the regulation compelling legal attestation of Salernite professors, that this school yet maintained its ancient reputation, notwithstanding the founding of a new University in Naples. In the ordinary course of study at regular medical institutes, when the matriculate had devoted himself with assiduity to mastering Galen and Hippocrates, together with surgical operations, presupposing a certain knowledge of anatomy, during a continuous period of five years, he was entitled by the law of the land to an examination before the proper board.[79] To a diploma thus signed and sealed, granting unimpeded exercise of the profession, the imperial chancellor, illustrious Peter de Vigne, makes allusion in a letter from which we have quoted.[80]

Minute and specific rules were prescribed for professional guidance of youthful physicians, and to whose observance they were solemnly sworn,[81] requiring gratuitous attendance upon indigent invalids who, with others, should receive at least two visits daily, and, if summoned, once at night. Whenever a physician suspected pharmacists or compounders of medicaments, as failing to prepare medicines in strict accordance with prescriptions, it was his imperative duty to report such delinquents to civil authority for punishment.

Practitioners were prohibited a price beyond an amount fixed by law for medical visitations, and cautioned against secret association with druggists to defraud patients by illegal additions to the legal cost of compounding remedies, which prohibition naturally rendered it essential for physicians to

---

[78] Petrus de Vineis, Epistolæ, Lib. V., cap. 24.

[79] "Libros authenticos, tam Hippocraticos quam Galeni, in scholis doceant tam in theorica quam in practica medicinæ, et præsertim anatomiam humanorum corporum," etc. Constitut. Reg. Lic., cit., Lex 3.

[80] Epistol., Lib. IV., c. 24.

[81] "Iste medicus jurabat servare formam curiæ, hoctenus, observatem." Ibid., Lex 3.

complain of unjust pharmaceutical charges, and to make payment for medicines upon the schedule of prices established by advice and consent of a medical faculty sanctioned by statute.[82] Large cities at that distant period alone possessed public pharmacies, exclusive of the monasteries, whose function was preparing medicaments subject to supervision of the profession, the number of whom was not limited in this inquiry, only in conformity to specific regulations. Ancient statutes holding these compounders responsible for negligence were rigidly enforced during the Middle Ages, the penalty for which uniformly extended to loss of personal goods—oftentimes to capital punishment.

Sales of deadly poisons for other than recognized legitimate uses were repressed by the ignominious death by hanging. Apothecaries were allowed excellent but regular profits upon their wares, in just proportion to the diminishing stock of commodities and scant supply, or the possible inactivity of certain but necessary unvendible stuffs: into this calculation a fair proportion of money invested also entered.[83] As an admirable sanitative precaution, no flax or hemp was permitted to be fired within a quarter of a mile of an inhabitable place.[84] Whether the frequent epidemics ravaging mediæval cities, accessible to vessels laden with pestilential germs from the Levant, forced a higher grade of sanitary ordinances touching inhumations, this emperor ordered that dead bodies of men or animals should be buried in remote localities, or shipped to sea and carefully sunk. A pestilence arising in the year 1231 from numbers of locusts in Apulia, the emperor decreed that sworn emissaries should take and burn a certain measure of these insects each morning before sunrise.[85]

Sepulchral preparations throughout mediæval times were of

---

[82] Constitutiones Regni Siculi, Titulus XXXIV., Lex 4.

[83] Ibid., Lex 4.

[84] Rycardus San Germano, Chronica, sub an. 1232, reproduces the decrees published under the Constitutions, Lib. III., Tit. XLVII–LXXXII.

[85] Rycardus, op. cit., p. 105.

simple character. After clothing with suitable vestments, the cadavera, even of royalty, were enrolled in bull's hide for burial,[86] or girthed with ropes.[87] According to a writer of the early thirteenth century, the dead were transported on inland streams, drawn through the water, with a coin securely fastened in the mouth.[88]

---

[86] Rog. Wendover, Flor. Historiar., Tom. IV., p. 134.

[87] Flor. Wigiorn., Chronicon, sub an. 1141, Tom. II., p. 134.

[88] Gervasii Tilburniens, Otia Imperialia, Dist. III., cap. 90. It may be added here, as remotely connected with the subject, that bodies of the drowned were in pagan times carried immediately to the temple of Thor or Odin—perhaps for divine resuscitation. Vita S. Swiberti, cap. 12.

CHAPTER XXV.

Public Physicians Salaried by Municipalities—Translations from Arabic—Hyperbolical Panegyric of Eminent Professors—Guild of Physicians in Milan, Thirteenth Century—Corporation of Apothecaries—Union of Pharmacists and Medicists Forbidden by Law—Distinction of Bologne's Medical Schools—High Salaries of Professors—Culture of Botany—Thaddeus, Master of Villannova—His Commentaries of Hippocrates and Galen—Anatomy—Physicians not Allowed to Marry till A. D. 1451.

THE example of the illustrious Hohenstauffen emperor, in honoring the Neapolitan University with his amity and protection, was strictly followed by Charles I., his successor, who called thither, in the interest of medicine, Philip da Castilenio, to whom an annual stipend for professional services, of twelve ounces of gold—Tarrene[1]—were given, a sum of considerable magnitude for a person of whom nothing is known.[2] Evidently the introduction of Arabic methods in preparing medicaments, and a better system of cures, either through Constans Afer or Gerard of Cremorn, who was, according to Sarti, the first to translate Saracen medical text-books into the Vulgate,[3] after the famous Carthaginian, found an early entrance and fervid welcome in the schools of Salerno. At all events, under munificent patronage, the medical universities of Sicily advanced, from the close of the twelfth century, to the apex of justly-earned celebrity.

With heroic rhythm, in the year 1198, Ægidus Corbeilens lauds the Salernite school in panegyrical terms, and declares the city anciently sacred to Phœbus, and nurse of Minerva, was then "the fountain of physic, the athlete of cures, and

[1] Du Cange, Glossar., sub v. Tarreni Salerniti.

[2] Tiraboschi, Storia della Litteratura, Tom. IV., p. 209.

[3] De Professorib. Bononiensis, Tom. I., p. 511.

the very gardener of medicine,"[4] and attained untarnished celebrity for the restorative properties of its medications. With burning enthusiasm he chants the transcendant excellence of pharmaceutical compounds, the notoriety of which, it seems, had expanded throughout the universe—per orbem—causing great affluence to Salerno. Saracen mixtures were well known to Ægidus, and in eulogizing Salernite medicaments, he refers to compositions wholly made up of Arabic drugs.[5] In the opening stanzas the versifier pays a glowing tribute to medical professors of this venerable institution, whose names do not appear in the erudite collection of Fabricius, although according to the learned historian of Italian letters, they were distinguished in their day, and left to posterity certain treatises upon subjects highly important in the treatment and cure of diseases, by the subtle preparation of food and drink for invalids.[6]

The first of these Petras Musadinus, Ægidius affirms to be the culmination of glory to Salerno, and like the dazzling rays of a cloudless sun must gild its other fame for all time;[7] the second Maurus, who had received the vigor and intellectual strength of the former, so that medicine lost nothing by the death of Musadinus. Among noted medical celebrities of the age alluded to in this poem are Matthew Plateus, the medicinal remedies of whom the spirited author reduces to verse, and Orsus, a Salernite physician, famed for conversational powers.[8] Johannes was equally lauded for his poesies by Ægidus, and to Romoaldus is awarded the commendation of

---

[4] "Urbo Phoebes sacrata, Minervæ sedula nutrix,
Fons Physiciæ, pugil encrasiæ, cultrix medicinæ."

Libri Quator de Virtutibus et Laudibus Composit. Medicorum, Lib. III., v. 467, p. 502.

[5] "Trifera Saracenica," Ibid., p. 661; and "Cum rheubarbicis data Saracenica dragmiis et mirobolanis," etc., "mixtis." Ibid., v. 742 seq.

[6] Tiraboschi, Storia della Litteratura, Tom. IV., p. 211.

[7] "Musandinus apex, quo tanquam sole et nitet et nituit illustris fama Salerni." Aegid. Corb., op. cit., Lib. I., v. 91.

[8] Ibid., vv. 112 and 120.

profound acquaintanceship with civil and canon law, but final and transcendant excellence as a professor of the curative art, to whom he gives the cognomen of "medical president."[9] Rumoald's distinction as an author of physic—auctorem physiciæ, or successful practitioner—obtained for him the position of official medical adviser to the pope.[10] During the thirteenth century there was rapid increase throughout Italy in the number of medical schools.

Physicians in Milan, in the year 1288, were so numerous that they aggregated over two hundred, and were, perhaps, organized in a guildic corporation.[11] The Ferrara College of Medicine at this epoch, in conformity to statutory regulations, prescribed the conditions under which entrants into the profession should be privileged to practice. It was enacted that each practitioner should possess a horse upon which his patients were to be visited, and whenever a certain number of troops under orders from this city, or the Est Marches, were called into active service two surgeons must accompany them.[12] At Brescia, the medical profession in its collegiate form obtained from episcopal authority a confirmation of these valued immunities and prerogatives conceded them by imperial patronage.[13]

About this time physicians and apothecaries instituted themselves into a guild at Florence, similar to other trades.[14] In the same century, a municipal law of Nice interdicted absolutely such union of medical professors and pharmacists,[15] and elsewhere conjurations for other than legitimate traffic were

---

9 Aegid. Corb., Libri Quator de Virtutib. Medic., Lib. I., v. 131 seq.

10 Muratori, Scriptores Rerum Italiæ, Tom. VII., p. 206.

11 Ibid., Tom. XI., p. 712.

12 "Et teneatur quilibet ipsorum medicorum habere suam equum proprium, super quo equitare debeat et possit per civitatem visitando infirmos." Borsetti, De Gymnas. Ferrar., Lib. I., c. 1, p. 11.

13 "Hic privilegia immunitatis medicorum—largissima manu confirmavit." Malv., Chronicon, cap. 124; ap. Murator., op. cit., Tom. XIV., p. 962.

14 Ungewitter, Geschichte der Hændel, p. 234.

15 Monum., Hist. Patr., Tom. I., p. 97 seq.

placed under the ban.[16] The Paduan University does not appear to have devoted much attention to the curative art, inasmuch as instruction in medicine there was by private, unprivileged tutors. Bologna, during the course of the thirteenth century acquired universal fame for the eminence of its medical and law schools,[17] and in the preceding age the honorary title of Master of Medicine was freely assumed by the profession there, of whom one, mentioned in Sarti's able biographies of Bolognese professors as the first, was Jacobus Bitinarius, who, in the year 1199, entered into orders among the regular canonicals of Saint John the Martyr. In Sarti's Nectrologium he is designated: "Dompnus Jacobus Medicus Canonicus." By testamentary disposition, his library went to the church of Saint Victor.[18] Towards the middle of the thirteenth century, a custom appears fully established to crown with laurel such devotees of the Æsculapian art as attained high distinction in the Universities, or were designated by the popular applaudits as worthy of this great honor.[19]

A lively emulation arose between the legists and medicists of Bologna in the nature of an unusual zeal to comment and elucidate the writings of venerable predecessors; consequently a body of medical commentators or scholiasts originated and remained separate from University departments. For a prolonged period, as hitherto stated, both public lectures on law and medicine had depended upon the generally scant and uncertain fees of disciples. The earliest celebrated professor of the Bolognese medical school to receive a municipal stipend was Johannes of Parma, in the year 1304.[20]

The civil authorities of Bologna, perhaps instigated by the older Sicilian ordinances, as early as 1214 regulated a definitive compensation for medical attendance upon indigent infirm

---

[16] Statuta Taurinini, ap. Mon., Hist., cit., p. 724.

[17] Savigny, Geschichte des Roem. Rechts, Th. III., p. 183.

[18] Sarti, De Professorib. Bononiensis, Tom. I., Pars 1, p. 441.

[19] Ibid., p. 434 seq.

[20] Ibid., p. 435.

within limits of the municipality. The salary awarded the Lucchese professor, thus called to a foreign city to practice gratuitously his vocation, was fixed at six hundred Bolognese liri.[21] At a somewhat later period, a Bergamese physician, designated as a Master of Medicine by the argumentative persuasion of an annual pay of high figure, was induced to migrate thither to occupy a domicile specially erected for him, which it was agreed should thenceforth remain his permanent abode.[22] The vast number of practitioners existing by the intelligent skill of this profession in Bologna at this period, may be gathered from the fact, that this art was already subdivided into diverse parts, such as doctors of physic, barber medicastres, physicians for the eyes and various parts of the body.[23] This state of surgery, in the fourteenth century, caused Philip the Fair, king of France, to enact a law which compelled the male and female surgeons of Paris to be licensed.[24]

Notwithstanding the possible degradation of surgical art in the great centres of medical culture, in the scientific examination of the human frame upon anatomical principles and a systematic endeavor to supply rational medication chemically compounded, it is demonstrable that at this epoch Italian universities were so far equipped with such appliances as to necessitate the employment of professors of botany and chemistry, whose specific functions were the suitable preparation of pharmaceutical compounds.[25] For this purpose botanical gardens were most assidulously cultivated.[26] The accepted union of astrology and alchemy with mediæval medical art, even at an age when particular attention was given to the perusal and study of great Arabic writers on the latter science at Bologna,[27]

---

[21] Ibid., p. 444. Further on this subject, Monument, Histor. Patr. Italiæ, Tom. II., p. 1038.

[22] Tiraboschi, Storia della Litteratura, Tom. IV., p. 216.

[23] Sarti, De Profess. Bonon., Tom. I., p. 434 seqq.

[24] Ordonnances des Rois de France, Tom. I., p. 491 seq.

[25] Sarti, op. cit., p. 437 seq.

[26] Ibid.

[27] Ibid., Tom. I., p. 435.

was reaffirmed in the personal profession of two famous scholars devoted to these sciences—Franciscus Asculanum and Petrus Albana, the former of whom taught astrological medicine to Bologna students for thirteen years.[28]

In the contract reproduced by Sarti, binding Hugo[29] of Lucca to attend the impoverished sick of Bologna gratuitously, the agreement stipulated that, in case of severe maladies treated by him among citizens of mediocre means, he should have the legal right to demand and receive a load of wood, and from affluent invalids, twenty solidi, or a measure of hay.[30] It was made imperative upon the Lucchese surgeon whenever demanded, to accompany the municipal troops in their predatory campaigns. In the year 1218, he was regularly enrolled in a professional capacity, and attended a regimental body of Crusaders of Bologna, in an expedition to Palestine, where he remained for three years, and returned to this city for permanent residence.[31]

This famous physician acquired great distinction by the successful application of vinous potions, as a cure for aggravated wounds, which he appears to have been the earliest to adopt as a standing remedy. To his medical knowledge he added an excellent understanding of the principles of chemistry, and doubtless secured, during the sojourn in Syria, like other pilgrim surgeons of high professional culture, many valuable notions hitherto exclusively the property of Saracen physicians. Bologna's wide-spread repute for its medical schools in this age attracted students and professors not only from Italy, but as far north as England, rivaling indeed the exalted celebrity of Salerno.

Nicholas of Farnham, an Englishman, formerly professor of

---

[28] "Franciscum Asculanum, vulgo Ciccuni appellatum,, non minus doctrina quam vitæ suæ casibus, qui extremis hujus sæculi XIII. annis astrologiam Boniæ docuit scholaribus electus." Ibid.

[29] Master of Villannova, Breviarium, Lib. I., cap. 14; Additiones, col. 1086.

[30] Sarti, De Professor. Bonon., Tom. I., Pars. II., p. 146.

[31] Ibid., Tom. I., Pars I., pp. 448, 457.

philosophy in the Paris University, domiciled himself in the above metropolis, where he both studied and taught medicine, with which he appears to have had a renowned familiarity as then practiced.[32] The Sicilian provinces were frequented by eminent English physicians in the century preceding, whither they came seeking the munificent patronage of Roger.[33] Nicholas remained at Bologna, until the year 1241, previously directing his attention to sacred studies, at which period, accepting the suffrages of an election to the Durham Episcopate, where his accession was signalized by miracles and general gayety of the monks. Seven years later, however, the erudite pontiff being accused of simony, at the pressing instigation of the archbishop of York the see was declared vacant, and another selected in his stead.[34]

Among the most distinguished Bolognese professors of medicine at this epoch, the Florentine Thaddeus, master of Arnold Villannova—Brevarium, lib. I., c. 14, Addit. col., 1086—may be classed as preëminent, although the discreditable legends touching his dullard youth and somnolent temperament have been seriously questioned by Tiraboschi.[35] His biographer recites that until thirty years of age, Thaddeus was noted for an invincible stupidity, and employed the time listlessly by the sale of trivial tokens,[36] apparently dwarfed by those natural impediments to mental development which frighten parental affection, and chill the interest of unindulgent tutors. Similar to undeveloped intellects of juvenile years, suddenly the energy of genius stimulated the sluggish inactivity of the Tuscan into rapid and marvellous fruition.

Having obtained profound insight into the entire range of liberal arts and sciences, the basis of an accomplished scholar, he abandoned himself thoroughly, with a robust mind, to the

---

[32] Ibid., Tom. I., p. 448. In the year 1229.

[33] Gervasii Tilburniensis, Otia Imperialia, Dist. III., cap. 112.

[34] Robert de Graystones, Historia Dunelhmensis Ecclesiæ, cap. 5, p. 41 seq.

[35] Tiraboschi, Storia della Litteratura, Tom. IV., p. 418 seq.

[36] Sarti, De Professoribus Bononiensis, Tom. I., p. 467.

painful acquisition of medicine, and in the year 1260 opened a scholastic professorship in this art at Bologna. To this illustrious scientist the commendation is due of having made a practical introduction of Arabic sciences to the medical schools of Italy.[37] Notwithstanding many of Thaddeus' commentaries on Hippocrates and Galen would be at the present time rejected with derision, he was the first known mediæval writer who essayed in good faith, and with excellent judgment, to unite the philosophy of the age with rational medicine. As a further claim to grateful distinction, it should be stated that much of valuable lore appended to his treatise on the great precursors of the curative art was translated directly from Saracen sources.[38] In his day, this professor obtained the honors of oracular celebrity. As the earliest author and lecturer to reveal the most sacred and recondite signification of works commented by him, he quickly acquired the same confidence in medical exegesis as was accorded to the Florentine Accorso, a learned expounder of civil law, his contemporary.[39]

A commentator of Dante's Commedia, in the year 1262, apostrophises Thaddeus as a famed physician, and declares him to be equal to Hippocrates in originality.[40] A Ferrarese writer, with unmeasured panegyric, designates him as the most skilled medicist of the age[41]—a phraseology exactly reproduced by an annalist in the year 1295, the date of the erudite scientist's death.[42] Consequently, the unusual exemptions and franchises granted him by the civil authorities of Bologna appear to be in harmony with the ranking eminence reflected upon the University. It was decreed that Thaddeus and his heirs should

---

[37] Ibid.

[38] Sarti, De Profess. Bonon., Tom. I., p. 467.

[39] "Chiosatore e illuminatore di ragione civile." Villani, Vite d'Illustr. Fiorentini, p. 32.

[40] Dante, Paradisio, Canto XII., "e a Taddeo," Comment., Benevenuti Imolensis; ap. Murator., Antiq. Ital., Tom. I., p. 1262.

[41] "Medicorum magister peritissimus." Murator., Scrip. Ital. Rer., Tom. IX., pp. 143, 253.

[42] Ricobaldi, Historia Imperatorum, sub an. 1295.

be privileged to purchase or inherit property wherever they elected, while such scholars as frequented his medical lectures were entitled to immunities identical with those allowed the students of civil and canon law. This ordinance, ipso facto, elevated medicine to the same grade as other studies.[43]

His vast renown caused him to be summoned to Athens professionally, by the magnates of secular and ecclesiastical society, from whom he received munificent compensation. In the year 1285, upon accepting a call to render medical services to an Italian nobleman, he demanded a solemn assurance from the elaborate escort conducting him before the suffering aristocrat, that during the voyage to Bologna he should be subjected to no damage, and afterwards be returned uninjured in person and goods. No restraint was to be used to detain him in Modena against his wishes, and in case of any or all of these articles being contravened, the procurators mentioned should indemnify him in the sum of three thousand Bolognese liri.[44] Similar guarantee was obtained from the invalid peer, who agreed to pay him the above amount of money for his personal attendance, upon restoring to health the illustrious patient. Whether this excessive charge represents the measure of value for medical services or simply a contingent payment, it is manifest the profession at this period boldly demanded and received large sums in the ordinary exercise of the practice of medicine.[45] Dante, however, at nearly the same epoch, states that a cavalier should give a scudi for each visit by a physician.[46] Thaddeus' heavy bequests attest the immense accumulation of wealth by this professor, who directed two thousand five hundred lire to be permanently invested as a fund for deserving indigents of Bologna, and a further sum

---

[43] Sarti, op. cit., Tom. I., Pars II., p. 227, subtitulo, Rubr. III., De Privilegiis Mag., Thadei Doctores Fixice. Further, p. 155.

[44] Sarti, De Profess. Bonon., Tom. I., Pars I., p. 469.

[45] Ibid., p. 434; and Muratori, Scriptor. Rer. Ital., Tom. XX., p. 54.

[46] Dante, Convivium, Tom. I., p. 23.

sufficient to defray the collegiate expenses of a Minorite monk in studying theology at Paris.[47]

Among excellent results from his career as professor and educator, his translation of Aristotle's ethics, commended by Dante,[48] and the famous comments upon the Aphorisms and Prognostications of Hippocrates and Galen, are worthy of specific mention.[49] William of Brescia attained high distinction on account of his erudite science and the several treatises composed by him on medicine. After directing the studies at Padua for many years, attracted by the reputation of Thaddeus, he placed himself under the Florentine's instruction, and finally reached to so great eminence as to obtain a laurel crown and be advanced to the honorable office of personal physician to the pope.[50] In addition to other sacerdotal dignity, he became an archdeacon at Bologna.[51] A favorite subject for treatment by eminent physicians at that remote period, seems to have been the preparation of treatises on preserving health.

Thaddeus, himself, was author of a work involving this subject still extant in the Vatican library, and William of Bresicia enlarged his own dissertation so as to include remedies for all maladies, concluding it by designating himself as "aggregator," on account of selecting diversified curatives or rescripts from numerous medical authors. These efforts appear to have obtained especial commendation, and were much used by medicists of the ensuing age. One of Thaddeus' pupils arose to eminence as a rival to his master, and by reason of successfully adapting his science to curing distinguished personages.

From a nobleman of Este, to whom he was called pro-

---

47 "Pro expensis unicus fratris de ordine Minorum de provincia Bononiensis, qui stare debeat in studiis Parisiensi." Ibid., Tom. I., Pars II., p. 156 seq.

48 Dante, op. cit., Tom. I., pp. 29, 33.

49 Known as "Thaddei Expositiones Operum Hippocratis;" vide Sarti, op. cit., Tom. I., p. 472.

50 Pezii, Thesaurus Anecdot., Tom. I., p. 430.

51 Sarti, De Profess. Bonon., Tom. I., p. 436; and Pezii, Thesaur. Anecdot., Tom. I., p. 430.

fessionally, he obtained a sum of money equal to two hundred and sixty gold florins.[52] Simon of Genoa, by some asserted to be a monk, was the last of medical professors in the thirteenth century to receive the honors of his science. Tiraboschi attributes to him the authorship of an excellent treatise on the clue to health, entitled clavis sanationis.[53] About the middle of this era, Roger, of Parma, a city celebrated for the excellence of its grammar school so early as the eleventh century,[54] by personal experiments and such as were drawn from Arabic sources, drew up several treatises touching upon anatomical science.[55] This original anatomist and compiler appears to have occupied the office of Chancellor in the University of Medicine, at Montpelier, which evidently owed much of its scientific origin to Spanish Jews, because a century anterior to the period under notice it was visited by the traveler, Benjamin, who declared the city was only known as a place favorably situated for commercial traffic.[56]

Guy di Chauliac, with other eulogistic references to Roger as the first anatomist of the Middle Ages,[57] distinctly states, according to the admissions of Roland of Parma, also famous for surgical and anatomical skill, that he had followed almost servilely both the sense and letter of the erudite manuscript prepared by his predecessor.[58] A heated discussion, verging upon fanaticism, suddenly arose touching a claim by this able dissector to have cured a pulmonic malady by the excision of a lung. Enthusiastic partisans asserted such surgery to have been performed by Roland, others equally confident attributed it to Villannova's master, Hugo of Lucca. Sarti inclines to the

---

[52] Sarti, op. cit., Tom. I., p. 486.

[53] Tiraboschi, Storia della Litteratura, Tom. IV., p. 226.

[54] "Urbs Parma, quæ grammatica manet alta." Vita Mathildæ Ducatricis, cap. 11, v. 6, etc.

[55] Fabricius, Bibliotheca Latinit., Tom. VI., p. 119.

[56] Benjam. Tudelensis, Itinerarium, p. 15.

[57] "Quorum primus fuit Rogerius." Chauliac, Capitulam Universali, Præfat.

[58] Ibid.

belief that both were successful in restoring to health a person abandoned in the last stages of pulmonary disintegration, and by this equivocal suggestion seeks to reconcile the contradictory statements emanating from admirers of these rival surgeons.[59]

Several treatises of the Parma anatomist are still extant in the British Museum under the title: "Flossula seu Apparatus quator Magistrorum super Chirurgium Rolandi."[60] In addition to these, he published a pamphlet on the best method of curing pestilential diseases,[61] and another on Physionomia, or "Rolandi Physionomia in sex libros divisa."[62] A leading surgical operator in this century, Jamerius, appears to have obtained the repulsive appellation of "Brutal in Dissection," for the same reason as applied to Archogathus, while Bruno is placed by Guy di Chauliac in honorary conjunction with Roger and Rolandus. Bruno's chief excellence in this branch of medical economy was collating and admirably commenting on the writings of Galen, Avicenna, and Albucazi, and in this interesting occupation he labored under the great disadvantage of lacking an entire translation of the Galenic books—all of which at this epoch had not been reproduced in a Latin version.[63]

It has been alleged this surgeon enjoyed the amity of the illustrious Petrarch, thus transporting his existence to the ensuing century, a notion which the erudite Tiraboschi utterly disproves.[64] Notwithstanding the inculpation against Theodorick of Lucca, that he boldly appropriated the most valuable parts of his system of curatives from Bruno, adding to it such elements filched from his compatriot master, Hugo, he

---

[59] Sarti, De Professor. Bonon., Tom. I., Pars I., p. 449. Patristic biographers fondly dwell on such exercise of divine power exhibited through saintly physicians. Petrus Emerit., De Vita Patrum Emeritens, cap. 4.

[60] Catalog., MSS. Angl. et Hib., Tom., I., p. 169, Codex 350.

[61] Fabricius, Biblioth. Med. et Infin., Latinit., Tom. VII., p. 122.

[62] Tiraboschi, Storia della Litteratura, Tom. IV., p. 230.

[63] Chauliac, Capitulum Universali. Praef.

[64] Storia della Litteratura, Tom. IV., p. 231.

was nevertheless one of the most skilled and successful anatomists who applied indifferently vinous lotions as a standing remedy for serious wounds.[65] This eminent dissector and medicist of the thirteenth century arrived at Bologna when the University was at the apex of professional glory, accompanying the famous Hugo, his tutor, under whose direction for a prolonged period he pursued the practice of this science.

Finally, influenced by an aspiration for closer relations with the church, he assumed monastic vows in the Order of Preacher Monks, but continued to practice medicine, although the canons forbid its exercise professionally—consequently such uninterrupted pursuit may have been limited to the conventual infirmaries, or these ecclesiastical edicts were not vigorously enforced until a later epoch.[66] Pontifical favor followed the labors of Theodorick, being elevated in the year 1262 to the episcopal mitre of Bironti, and finally to that of Cervia, whose incumbency he accepted the year of his death, in 1298. His residence appears to have been permanent at Bologna, where he faithfully prosecuted the curative art, and aggregated large sums of money. Among specific inventions applicable to the cure of aggravated diseases and wounds, first made during the Middle Ages by the Lucchese surgeon with beneficial results, was the use of mercurial ointments,[67] although Freind declares similar ungents to have been known to Aetius.[68]

Anterior to this century, it is uncertain whether these valuable remedies were of extensive application, but at the period before us, or later, Chauliac urgently recommended them as possessing remarkable sanitative properties.[69] Unprofessional writers advised the preparation of unguents, presumably magical, according to a gossiping chronicler of the thirteenth century, beneath the bright glances of a virgin's eyes, in order to

---

[65] Ibid., Tom. IV., p. 233.

[66] Sarti, De Professorib. Bononiensis, Tom. I., Pars I., p. 460.

[67] Freind, Historia Medicinæ, p. 575.

[68] Ibid., p. 393.

[69] Tractat. I., Doctrina I., de Anatomia, cap. 5, p. 10.

render them efficacious.[70] Influenced by charitable impulse, doubtless, the episcopal surgeon wrote an elaborate treatise, still in manuscript, touching the maladies of horses and their proper remedies.[71] Some of his dissertations and compilations, of great utility at the time, were translated into the Catalan dialect by the Bishop of Valencia, to whom he dedicated them.[72]

Preceding the close of this age, two medicists attained wide spread fame by their successful practice and the publication of important anatomical works, which in those days appear to have captivated attention more readily than treatises especially of maladies. One of the physicians, designated William of Piacenza, was equally expert in medicine and surgery, whose abstruse system, as then understood and taught, he illustrated by admirable works on both subjects.[73] In defiance of canonical interdicts against ecclesiastical profession of medical science, sarcerdotal authority manifested praiseworthy interest in the composition of text-books. It was indeed in deference to the urgent request of a Piacenza abbot, that the erudite surgeon alluded to prepared a treatise on the conservation and care of health. His other surgical writings were completed in the year 1275, in Verona, whither he was called by the municipality, and regularly salaried as medical adviser to the city. Prior to his advent there he was a resident of Bologna for many years.[74]

Medical and surgical attendance at this epoch appears to have been engaged with the same intricate formality as other contracts, sanctioned by law and attested with legal solemnity. Thus for example William, the surgeon, entered into bonds drawn up by a notary, regularly signed and sealed, with a German student matriculated in the University, by which he

[70] Gervais. Tilburn., Otia Imperialia, Lib. I., cap. 17.

[71] Sarti, op. cit., p. 460.

[72] Tiraboschi, Storia della Litteratura, Tom. IV., p. 235.

[73] Chauliac, Capit. Univers., sub fin.

[74] Tiraboschi, Storia della Littèratura, Tom. IV., p. 236.

agreed to cure him of a distressing disorder, specifically and in detail set forth, designated "Fleume sarse," within two years from date of the obligation. In case of restoration to perfect health, the invalid bound himself likewise to pay thirty-six Bolognese liri.[75] This erudite physician, together with Lanfranc, secured a numerous patronage on account of the remarkably soothing nature of unguents and emplastra for grievous wounds.[76]

Perhaps the most famous medical and surgical practitioner of his age was the Lanfranc alluded to. Notwithstanding the superior excellence of Italian scholastic institutes, the Milanese scientist passed into France, where he quickly ascended to the dazzling apex of celebrity. In the preface of a work of surgery, composed in honor of Philip, the French monarch, it is stated he was constrained to abandon his native country, on account of persecution by Matthew Viconti, Duke of Milan. His first domicil was at Lyons, where he remained long enough to write a compend of anatomy for practical use, and when otherwise disengaged from professional duties, directed the education of his sons.[77] This is a singular fact when it is considered that physicians were enforced celibates and not allowed to marry during the Middle Ages—it being assumed that sanctity must largely coöperate in producing favorable results as an adjunct to medicaments. The members and professors were all clerics and unmarried, which was the logical deduction of that transcendent worth which religion ascribed to the state of chastity.[78]

Ecclesiastical sanction was not given to the nuptials of physicians until the year 1451.[79] High dignities in the Parisian

[75] Sarti, De Professorib. Bononiensis, Tom. I., Pars I., p, 460 seq.

[76] Chauliac, Capitulum Universale, sub fin.; and Tractat. I., Doctrina. I., de Anatomia, cap. 5, p. 10.

[77] Tiraboschi, Storia della Litteratura Italiana, Tom. IV., p. 238.

[78] "Les membres et professeurs des universités fussent tous clerco ou célibitaires: suite de la haute estime que la religion attachoit a l'état de virginité." Notices et Extraites des MSS., du Bibl. Roi., Tom. V., p. 492.

[79] "C'est qu'en 1451 que les medecins obtinerent d'etre maries." Ibid.

University were filled by unmarried professors of medicine until 1542, when these were conceded the right of matrimony by pontifical allocution, conveyed thither by an ablegate specially dispatched.[80] On Lanfranc's arrival at Paris, he shortly aggregated so great a number of disciples that other medical professors urged him to promulgate in book form a complete treatise on surgery and medicine, which he at length completed in 1296. In this work, the author admits his Milanese nativity, and the former usage of the curative art while living there.

He also recites a remarkable cure effected by him of a diseased canonical affiliate of the Order of Saint Augustine, who while riding horseback narrowly escaped death by a fall. To him doubtless surgical science owed its most decided progress towards an enlightened system based upon anatomy. While it should be admitted with unreserved candor that at this period medicine and surgery were taught at the Italian Universities by the most skilled tutors of the age, it must be confessed likwise that original research and invention were practically unknown.

In nearly every instance a professor of these arts arose to eminence and just distinction through servile imitation or abject translation of Greek and Arabic authors—a subserviency admitted by Chauliac, who refers to his Saracen predecessors,[81] and contemned with bitter sarcasm, as we shall hereafter observe, by Petrarch.[82] As a consequence, while medical science of the Arabs, and its cognate departments were far advanced, Italian scientists still slumbered over Latinized versions of Moslem authorities, contented indeed to rest inert and slothful before the surprising accumulations by infidel scholars of valuable contributions to a profession evidently used in Western Europe as a means of gain. Nevertheless, the free adoption

---

[80] "Car et permisit per privilege especial aux docteurs en medecine de pouvoir estre mariés." Pasquier, Recherches sur l'Histoire de France, p. 244.

[81] Chauliac, Capitulum Universale.

[82] Petrarca, Senil., Lib. XII., Ep. 2.

of such writings aided in resurrecting medicine from the tomb of ignorance and superstition, where it had rested for centuries, and provoked the well-directed enthusiasm for the science in Italy throughout the fourteenth century.

CHAPTER XXVI.

Students and Student Life in the Middle Ages—Great Numbers at the Medical Schools of Salerno and Bologna—Ordinances of Church Synods—Montpelier—Mature Age of Mediæval Students—Their Apartments Designated as Hospicia—Feuds between these and Civilians—Ecclesiastical Authorities Interfere—Seditions—Popes Invariably Favor Students—Freebooter Scholars—Rates of Lodgings Specified to Prevent Exactions—Straw Bales used by Students for Seats—Examination of Graduates—Books and Libraries for Consultation—Copyists—Great Prices of Manuscripts—Books not Dutiable—Standard Text-books Maintained by Municipalities for Accurate Transcripts.

FAVORABLE legislation by the Hohenstauffen emperors, involving as we have seen especial franchises and immunities to professors and scholars, attracted large numbers of eager students to the Universities of Italy during the twelfth and thirteenth centuries. The great reputation of these theological schools at Paris caused an immense affluence of pupils at the same epoch that the law and medical colleges of Bologna and Salerno drew students of these sciences into Southern Europe. Scholars returning to their homes, after engaging in the studies selected at foreign Universities, were frequently welcomed publicly by admiring compatriots.[1] Excepting unimportant educational establishments of slightly more elevated gradation in Italian cities, the only preparatory tuition was to be found within the monasteries, or located elsewhere under exclusive sacerdotal direction.

Frequent pontifical allocutions and synodal canons prescribed certain studies as mandatory in conventual schools, generally classified under the denomination of studium generale, in order to prepare aspiring disciples for the elaborate University instruction. While Bologna and Salerno were approaching the full development of their scholastic greatness,

[1] Comitum de Schawenburg; apud Meiborn, Tom. II., p. 513.

other Italian cities gradually realized the absolute necessity for intermediate schools, which, without rivaling the expansive colleges, so closely assimilated to them as to admit of easy and natural transition to the higher educational institutions. Reggio, Parma, Trevisio, and other important towns, maintained at public expense grammarians or philosophical teachers accessible to the people, and also theological instructors for clerical pupils.[2]

Succeeding church synods repeated the original mandate, that suitable persons should be appointed to impart knowledge to the monks without compensation, that each cathedral should provide a professor of polite letters, and the metropolitan see should be equipped with a theological tutor.[3] Five years were fixed for the study of logic and philosophy, and four for theology,[4] although students oftentimes pursued a seven years' course, as attested by the statement of Petrarch, concerning his sojourn at Montpelier.[5]

By a decree of the Turonese council convened in the year 1236, it was ordained that no person should be honored with a judicial appointment, or be privileged to appear to the bar as an advocate, unless he had previously studied civil and canon law consecutively for the period of three years.[6] It will readily appear from the prolongation of such prescribed study in these scholastic institutions, that the number of students at times must have been enormous, especially in Paris[7] and Bologna. In the latter city, about the year 1260, there were over ten thousand.[8]

---

[2] Tiraboschi, Storia della Litteratura, Tom. IV., p. 74.

[3] Von Raumer, Geschichte der Hohenstauffen, Th. VI., p. 343.

[4] "Deinde post quinquennium audivi." Pezii, Thesaur. Anecdot., Tom. I., p. 430.

[5] Petrarca., Rerum Senil., Lib. X., Ep. 2, p. 868.

[6] "Nisi per triennium jura audierint." De Avocatis, Concilia Turonesis, cap. 2; Labbe, Tom. XXIII., sub an. 1236.

[7] Alberici, Chronicon, p. 451.

[8] Odofredus: "Vidi ego Bononiæ, aderant eo tempore ferme decem millia scholarium." Muratori, Antiq. Ital., Tom. III., p. 899.

26

A century later the roll of regular pupils at the University of Oxford reached the almost incredible figure of thirty thousand.[9] As early as the year 1209, there were about three thousand scholars at this illustrious institution.[10] Independent of favoring state and municipal regulations, which alike adjusted the price of commodities and lodging for the scholars, in order to bring the same within the possibilities of indigent students, at Montpelier the praiseworthy ordinance was enacted directing the selection of four Bachelors, to whom the specific duty was assigned of assisting matriculates in their studies. For that purpose they were authorized to propose certain treatises to the medical professors, best adapted to that end.

Minute statutes were published establishing the particulars of attire and weapons to be borne by scholars, and also distinctly forbidding any such hilarious sports as breaking into private houses on fête nights, or disturbing the tranquillity of the lecture rooms.[11] It was not essential that pupils should subject themselves to graded lectures, since these were arranged upon a scheme permitting the youngest and oldest alike to be appreciative auditors.

Scholars in attendance upon these public readings of law and medicine, were of far more advanced age than the matriculates in modern universities. This was rendered necessary by the distant location of the schools, the routes to which, in the Middle Ages, were attended with considerable peril and great inconvenience. Doubtless the native students were of less mature years. Petrarch began the study of civil law before attaining the age of fifteen,[12] and Andrea, an Italian, so young indeed as to designate himself puerulus—a small boy.[13] In general, when these scholars arrived at the University from

---

[9] Turner, Hist. of England, Vol. II., p. 583.

[10] Rog. Wendov., Flor. Historiar., Tom. III., p. 228.

[11] Savigny, Geschichte des Römischen Rechts, Tom. III., p. 399.

[12] Rerum Senil., Lib. X., Ep. 2., p. 868.

[13] Sarti, De Profess. Bonon., Tom. I., Pars. I., p. 372.

abroad, there are excellent reasons to suppose their ages ranged between twenty and thirty, or older. According to the tendency of the times, students organized themselves into clubs or guilds for mutual protection, associations which papal authority was impotent to destroy.[14]

It would seem in the thirteenth century, as in more recent times, immediately after having arranged for the fees with the law and medical professors, as allowed by the statutes of 1220 and 1242,[15] they incorporated themselves into these unions, whose history, especially at Oxford, where this form of aggregation assumed the shape of aiding the indigent pupil,[16] shows the character of the period, in the struggle between rival guilds, in which many members were killed.[17] In nearly all universities, the medical and law professors maintained an official styled Banquierus, who superintended the audience-room, carried the manuscript rolls for consultation or reference, and of right demanded and received from each auditor twelve deniers for such services. The tutors gradually obtained the statutory rights requiring payment of stated compensation from their disciples. Usually this was a minimum of five sous, although night lectures commanded double price.[18]

Apartments occupied by students were, for the most part, congregated in particular localities, and in England were denominated hospicia.[19] More direful, indeed, than internal feuds, was the embittered hatred between them and citizens of the municipalities where the universities were situated. In

---

[14] Von Raumer, Geschichte der Hohenstauffen, Th. V., p. 344.

[15] Savigny, Gesch. des Römisch. Rechts, Th. III., p. 396. Frederick II. of Germany established the salary system, so that learning might be obtained by impoverished pupils. Gesta Frederici II., etc.; ap. Eccard. I., p. 1026.

[16] De Chambre, Histor. Dunelh. Eccles., p. 138.

[17] Matthew Paris, Histor., sub an. 1258.

[18] Savigny, op. cit., Th. III., p. 397.

[19] Fortescutus, De Landib., Legg. Angl., cap. 49; and Flor. Wigior., Histor., Tom. II., p. 174.

the year 1200, the servant of a German divinity student at Paris, by order of his master, sought a tavern or wine-house, to procure wine. During the purchase, he was set upon and so badly beaten that in the melée the pitcher which he brought with him was broken. The theological scholars of the same nationality, hearing the affray, assembled and entered the saloon, where they in turn savagely assaulted and wounded the host, whom they left half dead. A great riot ensued among the populace, who were led by the Provost of the city himself, and attacking the quarters of the students' hospicia, assassinated the offending German, together with several of his companions.

The University authorities appealed to the king, who ordered the apprehension and incarceration of the Provost and accomplices. On account of the French monarch's fear that these pupils would abandon the city and go elsewhere, they obtained more enlarged and valuable concessions, in the interest of permanent peace and tranquillity. The incriminated official, upon being informed of the royal indignation, attempted to evade the scourging demanded as his punishment by escaping from confinement, but gliding down a fragile rope, it broke and instantly killed him.[20] In the middle of the next age, an immense sedition arose between the Oxford scholars and the townsmen. The citizens, with the assistance of the peasantry from the surrounding country, assaulted in great numbers their aggressors, with such atrocity as to wound many and kill some. After having destroyed their property, the assailants were forced to flee.

Ecclesiastical interposition produced a temporary armistice by means of a sacerdotal interdict. By this compact it was agreed that the laity of Oxford, as offenders in the riot, should thereafter perpetually abstain from maliciously or wantonly injuring the scholars, or inciting them to anger. The civil authorities gave to the University as damages two hundred

---

20 Roger. Hoveden, Annales, p. 803 seq.; and Fl. Wigiorn., Chronic. Continuat., Tom. II., p. 164.

and fifty pounds sterling, saving the right of indemnity to aggrieved individuals.[21] Three years later the excommunication against the city was removed. It is stated by the annalist that the sedition was caused by citizens violently assaulting several clerics residing at Oxford as students, and for this contempt of priestly vestments the malediction was laid upon the municipality.[22]

In the year 1229, at Paris, a vengeful tumult of the laity again broke forth with dangerous violence, in which many consecrated scholars were murdered. The origin of this seditious trouble appears to have originated in the unjust and indelicate accusation against Blanche, queen of France.[23] Large numbers at a later date abandoned the Parisian University, and scattered to celebrated schools in the provinces, or entered as matriculates at Anjou to complete their studies.[24] About the middle of the same era a conflict suddenly originated in the mutual hatred between members of the great French University and the mendicant friars, which even terrible loss of life was unable to terminate.

Results identical with those above described followed the sanguinary struggle. So many students deserted the city that royal and papal interference was necessary to secure tranquility, and their return,[25] under the express stipulation of full indemnification, out of the government exchequer, of personal losses.[26] In utter defiance of carefully digested statutes of the Bologna University, it was oftentimes difficult to preserve public peace, frequently broken by slothful or hilarious students; so much so indeed that an illustrious writer of the age com-

---

[21] Adam Murimuth, Chronicon Continuat., sub an. 1354.

[22] Adam Murimuth, Chronicon Continuat., sub an. 1354.

[23] Matthew Paris, Historia, sub an. 1226.

[24] "Ita ut studium in Andegaviam transferrentur." Albert Stadens, Chronicon, sub an. 1279.

[25] "Egressi per diversas provincias sunt dispersi." Gesta Ludovici, Lib. IX., p. 597.

[26] Herman Corneri, Chronicon, sub an. 1234.

plained that the University authorities failed to mete out justice sufficient to secure repression of these scholastic wrangles.[27] In the repeated collisions between citizens of Bologna and the scholars, its law schools were in danger repeatedly of total extinction. Sometimes the matriculates in a body abandoned the city, driven to such extremity in vindication of their valuable rights, and solemnly pledged themselves under mutual oath never to return again, When, therefore, a truce had been agreed to, it became indispensable for pontifical power to absolve the obligated disciples of law and medicine, in order that they might renew their studies without perjury.[28]

Usually such adjustments were signalized by a confirmation of old immunities, or by the concession of new ones.[29] In the year 1237, or according to the Cottonian manuscript of Hemingburg's chronicle in 1238, Otho, a lateran legate, was sent to England, where he arrived in July, invested with plenary authority to correct excessive dissipation of both clerics and people. On arriving at Oxford, the cardinal and his suite were received by masters and students with utmost gayety.[30] Inasmuch as the scholars were more readily inclined to the delectations of disreputable women,[31] one of the earliest attempts of the papal emissary was the repression of scholastic debauchery.[32]

When the tutors and scholars in the University became acquainted with the immediate object of the legate's visit, they were highly incensed. Having aggregated their members into formidable array, they made an irruption upon the messenger's retainers, killing three and wounding many. The papal plenipotentiary himself fled, and took refuge in the sewers of

---

[27] Tiraboschi, Storia della Litteratura Italiana, Tom. III., 396.

[28] Sarti, De Professor. Bonon., Tom. I., Pars II., p. 106 seq.

[29] Ibid.; and Herman Corneri, Chronicon, sub an. 1234.

[30] Matthew Paris, Histor., sub an. 1238, p. 317.

[31] Panciroli, Rerum Memorabil. Perdit., Tom. I., p. 206; and Bulæus, Histor. Universit. Parisiensis, Tom. II., p. 687.

[32] Hemingb., Chronicon, sub an. 1237.

Ossenay, until the burning wrath of the Oxford students and professors had subsided. The seditious fury becoming at length allayed, he placed the entire town under an ecclesiastical ban, while the king ordered the arrest and punishment of the principals in the outrage, directing them to be sent to London for trial.

The chronicler thus sneeringly concludes his narration of this event: "When the cardinal had loaded himself with money, and promulgated certain edicts, he returned to Rome."[33]. At a later date the Oxford students exhibited their hate of Israelites, into whose avaricious hands they had evidently fallen for usurious pledges and advanced funds, by stirring up sedition against them. It is not stated, however, what crime was charged to their account—perhaps the practice of sortilege with Talmudical books, which were ordered burned in the year 1255, by the Gallic Synod, as furnishing the magic for such prognostications.[34]

Notwithstanding the assassination of many Jews at Oxford, during the affray referred to, lawful proof was not produced to convict the parties accused. The presence of vast multitudes of scholars in constant attendance upon college lectures in the cities of Europe during mediæval times, was as stated, the source of inexhaustible wealth to citizens. In order to conciliate and retain them, municipalities where medical and other schools were located granted franchises of the most valuable character, to the universities and their matriculates. These were, however, at times, insufficient to restrain the ungovernable impulses of adolescent literates from abandoning the city, subjecting them to such indignities as to provoke sanguinary resistance. To place these oft-repeated migrations under the restrictive obstacle of a religious obligation, Bolognese students were formally sworn not to desert the city, either individually or with their professors.

In all civil annoyances imposed upon foreign pupils and

---

[33] Ibid.

[34] Baluzius, Concilia Narbonne, Tom. I., p. 76.

tutors, the ponderous influence of the Popes appears to have been unreservedly in favor of equitable adjustment of the difficulties.[35] Annals of this part of the thirteenth century show most unmistakably that about the year 1222, Bologna scholars transferred their studies from that municipality to Padua.[36] Frederick II. when in collision with Bologna, endeavored to destroy the usefulness of the University by annulling its privileges; but the causes provoking an armed struggle ceasing, the enlightened but irritable monarch hastened to withdraw his obnoxious rescript. During the conflict with Austria, students of that nation were banished from Universities situated on territory of the German empire.[37]

Indolent or sluggish matriculates, more ardent in pursuing pleasure and worldly gratification than the substantial happiness of letters and science, organized themselves somewhat upon the scheme of condoterii, and in this incorporated shape wandered as well-armed vagrants throughout the different provinces of Europe, forcing themselves, in defiance to clerical resistance, upon the hospitality of convents and cloisters, or perhaps nunneries, and sought the companionship of listless patrons of wine-houses, which naturally conducted to the bordellos of prostitutes. Both civil and canon law were invoked, and severely applied, to crush out this manifestation of scholastic vagrancy, and punished such vagabonds by imprisonment and deprivation of all ecclesiastical immunities.[38] Indigent students of fair repute, compelled by their impoverishment to join these ambulatory outlaws, were not only urgently recommended by frequent synods to indulgent citizens and affluent cloisters as objects deserving of generosity, but provision was made by the emperor Frederick II., for their support by private and public funds.[39]

[35] Herman. Corner., Chronicon, sub an. 1234; and Tiraboschi, Storia della Litteratura, Tom. IV., p. 45.

[36] Muratori, Scriptor. Rerum Italiæ, Tom. VIII., pp. 372, 421–59 and 736.

[37] Pezii, Thesaurus Anecdot., Tom. I., p. 430.

[38] Ibid., Tom. II., p. 526.

[39] Gesta Frederici II., Imperator.; ap. Eccard., Tom. I., p. 1026.

Notwithstanding minute regulations, published by municipal authority where Universities were established, touching lodgings, dress and food for students, there were complaints to the officials of Paris in this age, that the price of apartments had gradually advanced until it was excessive.[40] Attached to all mediæval colleges were numerous halls, devoted either in whole or part to lecture auditoriums, under the management of the faculty, or used by specific branches of culture connected with the regular course of study.[41] The slender appointments of these rooms, otherwise commodious, may be inferred from the fact that students attending the University lectures there during the Middle Ages used a bundle of straw to sit on, which they brought with them.[42]

In the bloody affrays so often precipitated between clerical scholars and their natural antagonists—the laymen—rivals for the affections of incontinent women, these bundles of straw became dangerous allies in firing the woodwork of resisting domiciles opened for secular refugees. It may be stated here, that the magnificent abodes of nobility at this epoch were plentifully strewn with straw instead of carpets, and the same stuff provided in winter to render the cold less sensible to the feet on festival days in large churches and cathedrals. There was a street in Paris where it was sold for the purpose of exclusive use by students attending medical and other instruction in the cheerless audience-rooms of the University. For centuries this custom of vending straw to the matriculates furnished a name for the street, which was denominated Rue du Fouare.

Philosophic licentiates were obliged to provide the Chancellor of the University with this material, each of them paying for that purpose the sum of twenty-five sous.[43] After the medical or law student had completed the time specified for faithful study of these sciences, he was entitled to an examin-

---

[40] Pezii, op. cit., Tom. VI., cap. 151, p. 427.

[41] Savigny, Geschichte des Römisch. Rechts, Th. III., p. 374.

[42] Legrand d'Aussy, Histoire de la Vie Privèe des Français, Tom. III., p. 160.

[43] Ibid., Tom. III., pp. 154–161.

ation for promotion, which involved the stately reception of the honorary and profitable title of Doctor. As early as the year 1158, such doctorates of laws are mentioned by a contemporaneous writer present at an important Imperial Diet in Italy, who further adds, they were conferred by Bologna.[44] In the ensuing century, medical students passing stipulated examinations were honored with the gradation of Doctors of Medicine or Physic—doctores medicinæ, or fixicæ.[45] In the year 1267, a Polish student, upon returning to his native land from Bologna, brought with him a doctorate, which was esteemed of sufficient importance to be permanently recorded in the annals of Poland.[46]

This advance or promotion brought the newly created doctor the privllege of professing his law or medicine without hindrance, and gave him jurisdiction over his disciples, including the right of participation in the examining conclave.[47] In the thirteenth century the doctoral presentation was attended with signal splendor, and performed at cathedral churches, in the presence of a convention or judicial faculty. Here the licentiate who had passed the private and public examinations, and obtained the title of licentiarius, read an argumentation upon a subject cognate with his profession, which was afterwards opened to the scholars for discussion. When this disputation had terminated, the arch-dean of the university, with a suitable address, endowed him with the doctorate, the insignia of whose dignity consisted of a book or manuscript volume, a doctor's hat and ring, while at the same time his proper seat in the Minster was assigned him. The procession then left the sacred edifice with pomp equal to the ceremony with which it entered.[48]

---

[44] "Viros disertos, religiosos et in lege doctissimos, legumque in civitate Bononiensi doctores et multorum auditorum præceptores." Otton. Frising, Gesta Frederici Imperatoris, Lib. IV., cap. 5.

[45] Sarti, De Professor. Bonon., Tom. I., Pars I., p. 434; and Pars II., p. 227.

[46] Annales Polonorum, sub an. 1267.

[47] Savigny, Geschichte des Römisch. Rechts, Th. III., p. 206.

[48] Ibid., p. 214.

Monasteries from their institution endeavored to assemble, in an apartment specially dedicated for the purpose, such books, whether relating to profane or sacred letters, as were procurable by purchase or transcription. Charlemagne himself took great pride in the collection of a library tolerably complete for his age. This aggregation, including many volumes gradually gathered, he directed by his testament should be disposed of at appraised prices, whose proceeds were donated to paupers.[49]

Oftentimes books of certain kinds were carried about by their owners in sacks.[50] To these indeed, or isolated parcels, such as the poems of Saint Columba, preservative powers were ascribed, and likewise borne as amulets in the din of sanguinary battles.[51] The gift of elaborately illuminated volumes was highly prized as the most suitable expression of personal esteem. When, therefore, in the year 844, Hraban Maurus, of the Fuldane cloister, presented to His Holiness the Roman Pontiff a metrical treatise, De Laude Sanctæ Crucis Christi, illuminated with symbolic types and figures, it was deemed a public event worthy to be enrolled in the cloister annals.[52] As early as Bede's day the nobility were accustomed to seeking access to monastic libraries for purposes of reading.[53] The prior of Lauresheim, in the tenth century, was highly praised for numerous treatises which he had composed and donated to the monastery; the bindings and ornamentation of ivory and inwrought silver were admirable to behold;[54] and when, several ages later, the convent was rifled of its literary treasures, three volumes of this lot appear to have consti-

[49] Eginhardi, Vita Carolimagni, cap. 33; vide Mabillon, Annales Benedicti, Tom., II. p. 335.

[50] Ekkehard, jun., De Casibus Monaster. S. Galli, cap. 1.

[51] Montalembert, Les Moines d'Occident, Tom. III., pp. 124, 138.

[52] Annales Francor., Fuldens, sub an. 844; Histor. Monast. S. Emer., Ratisponæ, sub an. 888.

[53] Beda, Histor. Ecclesiar., Lib. III., c. 27.

[54] Chronic. Laureshamensis, sub an. 970; vide Freher., Tom. I., p. 128.

tuted the chief element of chagrin.[55] Oftentimes these inestimable collections were stolen by cloister officials, for sale or other disposition.[56]

Penitential offerings were esteemed of greater potential efficacy if these included manuscript dissertations on sacred or profane subjects,[57] and the aggregation of such objects constituted frequently the principal panegyric of a defunct bishop.[58] The King of Germany, in 1052, stirred with charitable pity for the undeserved catastrophes which had overwhelmed the Bremen episcopate, contributed among other holy furniture a number of books to the monastic library.[59] Dissipation of these collections by fierce conflagrations provided the mediæval annalist with suitable subjects of lamentation, in whose devouring element oftentimes the most prized appointments of a beloved abbey vanished before affrighted monks,[60] or the peaceful inmates of a tranquil cloister would awake in the silence of midnight to see the appalling spectacle of their library fired by the lurid flames of the Norman Viking's torches.[61]

Siward, abbot of Rastedense monastery, possessed a great number of well assorted volumes for the twelfth century. Towards the end of his pontificate, he formally presented to the cloister his entire aggregation of books, collected by purchase or copies, during a long and active life. Among these were diverse works on episcopal ordination, a missal and matutinale in one volume, together with a graduale, one collectorum, excerpts of canons, four evangelists, by himself, a herbarium and lapidarium, bound together; the Gemmam, or speculum of the soul; one elucidarum; penitential Baptistery; Chron-

[55] Chronic. Lauresh., sub an. 1125.

[56] Ekkehard, jun., op. cit., cap. 15.

[57] Dithmar, Chronicon, Lib. II., p. 37.

[58] Ibid., Lib. VI., pp. 160, 183.

[59] Albert Stadens, Chronic., sub an. 1052.

[60] Gobelin, Personæ. Cosmodromii, Ætas VI., cap. 50.

[61] Adam Bremen, Gesta Hammab., Pontif., Lib. I., cap. 23.

icles; Isidore's Highest Good; the regula of Benedictus, a martylogum, in one volume; a divine officio, penitentia, and a philology in one volume; the life of Saint Mary of Egypt; orators, Juvencus, Sedula, and Prosperus, bound in one; six books on the virtues of medicine; Plato's Timaeus, Prosper Regula de Visibus, Theodolun, Cato, and Ivorum, the Pandects, Horace, and Boethius,[62] and a work on the signification of episcopal vestments.[63]

In this list, which is specially reproduced as an exhibition of a well-filled monastic library in the Middle Ages, some treatises on medicine certainly appear. It is also probable that the herbarium of Abbe Siward was the work of Dioscorides. Several centuries subsequently, a prior of this cloister presented the archbishop of Bremen with a Decretalium, the Summam Raymundi, and Johannus de Ascula.[64] Lay scholars of that distant era were certainly versed in the classic remains of Roman poets and historians. In the year 1295, a high secular functionary of a province in Germany died, whose celebrity was mainly attributable to his vast knowledge of ancient authors, acquired during student life, at the University of Paris.[65] In the register of books published by the Oldenburg annalist, the price of a scant number of volumes was estimated, about the middle of the fourteenth century, at the enormous value of two hundred florins.[66]

The eagerness with which monastic students sought to obtain transcripts of Roman writers, may be inferred from the readiness of Gallic monks to exhange in the ninth century a portion of their saint's body for a correct copy of Cicero.[67] Manuscript copying during mediæval times constituted, ex-

---

[62] Ratperti,.De Orig. et Divers. Casib. S. Galli, cap. 10.

[63] Chronicon Rastedense, sub an. 1134.

[64] Ibid., sub an. 1374.

[65] "Oratorum ac Poëtarum et Historicarum familiaritate, dum esset in Universitate Parisiensi." Chronicon Oldenburgens., sub an. 1295.

[66] Ibid., sub an. 1295.

[67] Depping, Histoire des Expeditiones des Normands, p. 146.

clusive of conventual scribes, an important element of successful livelihood.[68] In all monasteries, apartments set aside for shelving books[69] were under the care of a custos or chantre, who was compelled to exercise vigilant attention over his literary aggregation, and was restricted from loaning or selling the works without equivalent value. The mental vision of this high dignity was sometimes clouded either by abstinence or excess, which evoked invisible spirits, as happened to Becelinus in the year 1095, who beheld a spectre in the library.[70]

On the establishment of English abbeys, it was apparently a uniform custom to request through letters patent of neighboring religious houses such contributions of manuscripts as they felt at liberty to donate, which when thus given were certified for authenticity and accuracy.[71] In order to render these collections tolerably complete, whether consisting of sacred letters, including decretals and canons, or the writings of ancient medical sages, Hippocrates, Galen,[72] Dioskorides,[73] Soranus, Isidore,[74] and others, it was a general usage to import from foreign sources duplicates and triplicates of original text books, of such for instance as the Justinian Pandects.[75] As early as the time of Benedict Biscop, the monastery library of Weremouth in the seventh century was largely enriched by literary additions of this monk, to whom England owed the introduction of stone churches and glass windows.[76]

Among other gifts to the convent were three copies of the Pandects denominated. However, when in advanced age this

[68] "Scribendo videlicet libros, quos vendidi et in id redegi, quomodi potui,' etc. Opusculum Reinhardi, an. 1100; ap. Leibnitz I., p. 705.

[69] Chronic., Epp. Hildesham, cap. 21.

[70] Annales Corbiensis, sub an. 1095.

[71] Dugdale, Monastic. Anglicon., Tom. I., p. 924.

[72] Richerius, Historiarum, Lib. IV., c. 50.

[73] Roberti Swaphami, Cœnobii Burgens, Historia, circ. 1194, p. 99.

[74] Ekkehard, jun., De Casib. Monast. S. Galli, cap. 10.

[75] Du Cange, Glossar., sub v. Pandectæ.

[76] Wm. Malmsbur., Gesta Regum Angliæ, Lib. II., c. 2.

ecclesiastic took one of them, evidently in lieu of finances to defray expenses of returning to Rome, he expressly abandoned the remaining pair to the monastic library.[77] Compared with the sombre and gloomy apartments where mediæval monks congregated their manuscripts, the libraries of the Roman empire were of startling magnificence. The most notable of their vellum books arranged in rolls were oftentimes studded with gold and silver, frequently with polished brass embellishments.[78] Illuminated manuscripts still extant attest the frequent use of wooden chests for storing conventual volumes.[79]

The libraries of the monasteries were in general, before the eleventh century, of trifling utility and limited numbers.[80] During the Gothic campaigns in Italy, the monasteries enrolled their parchment books, and hid them in the most secret resorts.[81] Of this early period, a copyist of manuscripts at Novalla was celebrated for the correctness and velocity of his transcriptions.[82] The principal cause of the elaborate assemblage of books owned by the Corby monastery was a regulation by Prior Machevart, in the eleventh century, requiring each novice upon entering this convent on the day of his profession, to present the library with a volume of prescribed utility and value. At the same time he issued an order to all abbots whose cloisters were subject to his jurisdiction, directing them to proceed at once to have the annals of their monasteries drawn up in writing, of which copies were to be sent to him.[83] In the year 1060, Albert de Hambeore, or Hamburg, enriched the Corby collection with many books.[84]

Urged on by their ardent enthusiasm to accumulate valuable

---

77 Beda, Hist. Wirem., c. 15.

78 Panciroli, Rerum Memorabil. Deperdit., Tom. I., p. 64.

79 Du Cange, op. cit., sub v. Libellare.

80 Tiraboschi, Storia della Litteratura, Tom. II., Lib. I., c. 4.

81 "Libros atque membranas." Chronicon Novaliciense, Lib. II., c. 19.

82 Ibid., Lib. III., cap. 20.

83 Annales Corbienses, sub an. 1097.

84 Ibid., sub an. 1060.

works on theology or medicine with which noted abbeys abounded, patrons of noble birth frequently donated as much as a hundred pieces of gold for the purchase of such manuscripts.[85] Mendicant friars in the fourteenth century manifested an inordinate greed for treatises on theology, canon law and physics, and sought to rival clerical antagonists in England by aggregating the largest libraries. At the time mendicant convents became famous for enlarging collections of theological and medical volumes, their inmates endeavored to entice aristocratic pupils to their schools. In the year 1357, the archbishop of Armeagh, in a sermon before the Pope at Avignon, accused these beggar monks of sometimes discharging disciples from educational establishments on account of failing to procure them, "oon gude bible, nather othere convenable bookes."[86] The great prices, perhaps exaggerated,[87] which transcripts or original manuscripts, whether vellum, parchment[88] or paper—the latter was used in the fourteenth century[89]—readily commanded, necessitated such ordinances by municipal authorities where universities of medicine, etc., were established, as to bring the use or acquisition of text-books within the compass of individual finances of attending students. In some places books for professors and scholars were admitted within the city free of duty.[90] By an ancient regulation, the university officials of Paris were privileged to attend the great fairs along the Seine for the purpose of selecting by right of priority such vellum or parchment, together with such other utensils, as were requisite for transcripts or original compositions.[91]

---

[85] Ibid., sub an. 1233. The records of this abbey state a curious fact, that in the year 1306 a peasant was accidentally shot through the body with a *leaden* bullet by a hunter in the excitement of the chase. Ibid., sub an. 1306.

[86] Turner, History of England, Vol. II., p. 583, No. 28.

[87] Savigny, Geschichte des Röm. Rechts, Theil III., p. 594 seq.

[88] Tiraboschi, Storia della Litteratura, Tom. IV., p. 75; and Hallam's Literature, Vol. I., p. 142.

[89] Toulman Smith, English Guilds, p. 133.

[90] In Padua, Faccioloti, Fast. Gymnas., Tom. II., p. 10.

[91] Histoire d'une Feuille du Papier, p. 87.

All principal universities maintained a functionary to whom this duty was especially delegated as a regular occupation, classified as stationarius, nearly equivalent to the English vocable stationer. A law of the Parisian school, in the year 1275, made it compulsory for the incumbent of this honorable and profitable office to solemnly obligate himself to faithfully perform the functions of this avocation, adhering to such usages and statutes regulating the traffic of receiving, keeping, exposing and selling vendible books.[92] The Alfonsine laws prescribed the duties of a stationarius to be the constant supply of books of pure and reliable text and glosses, which they were required to loan scholars at regular rates for transcription, or emending older copies.[93] Although the statute arranging the duty of the Parisian librarian evidently contemplated the purchase and sale of books as a proper element of his profession, the Bolognese ordinances specifically interdicted such commercial traffic under heavy penalty,[94] while the attributes of the office were distinctly defined to be, similar to the Spanish rules, the procuration of expurgated text-books for loan at fair prices to students, for copying or correction of transcripts. Law professors appear to have leagued with the stationarii of Bologna, to enhance the compensation of circulating volumes, and to exclude certain glosses in the interest of those which both found financially more profitable.[95] Consequently the more enlightened arrangements facilitated the acquisition by medical and other students of those treatises absolutely indispensable for the successful and intelligent study of their professions. In numerous cities of Italy, anterior to the establishment of important educational institutions, municipal

92 "Corporeale præbeant juramentum qui vulgo Librarii appellantur, quod libros recipiendo vænales, custodiendo, esponendo, venendo eosdem," etc., "fideliter et legitimi se habebant." Bulæus, Histor. Universit. Parisiensis, Tom. III., p. 419.

93 Du Cange, Glossarium, sub v. Stationarius.

94 Savigny, Geschichte der Röm. Rechts, Th. III., p. 588.

95 Sarti, De Profess. Bonon., Tom. I., Pars II., Rubr. II., p. 224.

authorities would agree to procure at their own expense and maintain one or more revised copies of desired text-books or works of reference, for the sole purpose of copies.

By a statute of Nice, in the thirteenth century, a public copyist was hired at the city's cost, apparently to facilitate the procuring of accurate and reliable transcripts from authoritative manuscripts.[96] It will readily occur to the reader that the possession of such volumes of acknowledged value and purity as to text and gloss, whether of Hippocrates and Galen, or the Digests and Pandects, was equivalent in many cases to the increased affluence of the university or municipality controlling them, and their custody became the object of especial concern. Therefore, peremptory statutes made it a criminal offense to sell these, particularly to foreign universities[97]. Touching the medical works of Arabic authors, although the frequent reference by writers of this age to Saracen treatises not yet translated into mediæval Latinity, attests an extensive familiarity with Oriental languages during the twelfth and thirteenth centuries, such compends prepared by Arabs on medicine were generally accessible to the student through Latin versions.

Gerard of Cremorne sojourned nearly ten years at Toledo, in the twelfth century, among the Spanish Arabs, where he went for the expressed purpose of acquiring their dialect and to translate authoritative medical text-books for use in Southern Europe, of which there was great dearth.[98] Arnold of Villannova studied the Arabic language among the Saracens of Spain.

This illustrious scientist was equally skilled in a thorough knowledge of Hebrew and Greek;[99] and, similar to his great

---

[96] Statuta Niciæ; ap. Monum. Hist. Patr. Ital., Tom. I., p. 718.

[97] Savigny, Geschichte des Röm. Rechts, Th. III., p. 588.

[98] "Hic diu in Hispania cum inter Arabos versatus esset, primos aliqua Medicorum Arabum opera in Lingua Latina convertit,+1130-40." Sarti, De Profess. Bonon., Tom. I., p. 511; and Muratori, Antiq. Ital., Tom. III., p. 936.

[99] Vita Villannovae, cap. 2.

predecessor in this service, he devoted many years to the careful compiling of Arabic medical writings, to be used exclusively as text books in Western Europe. Among many others, he translated the famous Avicenna's: De Viribus Cordis.[100] Simon of Genoa was also serviceable in reproducing the medical treatises of the great Arab scientists into the Vulgate. An Italian library still possesses in manuscript such a translation of a suppositious work of Hippocrates on diseases of horses, made by Magister Moyses de Palermo,[101] evidently a Jew.

---

[100] Ibid.; and Freind, Historia Medicinæ, p. 543.

[101] Tiraboschi, Storia della Litteratura Italiana, Tom. IV., p. 342.

CHAPTER XXVII.

Medicine in the Fourteenth Century—Progress in Chemistry, Pharmacy and Anatomy—Petrarch's Aversion of Physicians—Charges them with Mendacity—Their Greed—Pomposity and Elaborate Costume—The Poet's Satires—Physicians go in State—Carry Medical Books with them —Decline of the Salernite School—Commentators of Arabic Books of Medicine—Public Lectures—Illustrious Patients Forced to Pledge Jewels for Medical Attendance—Celebrated Italian Professors—Medicine as part of General Education—Authority of Arabic Writers Diminishes —Junction of Astrology and Medicine—Great Stipends Paid Medicists —Treatment of Eye Maladies—Digest of Pharmacy—Style of Graduates—Early Knowledge of Oriental Languages.

MEDICAL science in the fourteenth century was exposed to the same implacable enmity of illustrious scholars which had characterized the incipient practice in the ages of Cato and Pliny. It is true the curative art during the era immediately preceding the one before us, had made rapid advance from the scrutinizing investigations of Rolandus the anatomist, Thaddeus the professor of medicine, and Villannova the practical chemist, in the mystic domains of dissection, pharmacy, and pathology, although the embittered hatred of Petrarch, as the most renowned and influential savan of the period, in a measure delayed the progress of this science. This impassioned hate was directed equally against the system and its practitioners.

In one of his epistles to Franciscus di Sieno, a famous physician of this epoch, the Florentine poet, with infinite complacency, relates an incident with spiteful jocundity against medicists. Clement VII., the Roman Pontiff, being seriously ill of a malady which excited grave apprehension touching the possible restoration to health of this aged prelate, Petrarch, sufficiently intimate with the pope, wrote him to guard himself especially against medical treatment, which, in the hands even of the most eminent physicians of the times, was synonmous with certain death.

At the same time he called his attention to a witty inscription on a tombstone: "The multitude of physicians has killed me!" and charges the profession with mendacity in parading a slender stock of medical knowledge.[1] The surgical advisers of His Holiness, upon reading this severe letter, ridiculing in the most withering paragraphs the science of which the pontifical physician was a principal practitioner, replied in bitter and indignant Latin. Resulting from this inimical correspondence was a treatise by Petrarch entitled: Invectivarum contra Medicium quendam,[2] or Invectives against Medicists, in four books, in which, divested of philosophical moderation of language, the avocation of medicine is held up to scorn and contempt. In another epistle he deliberately declares that medical consultation is utterly useless.[3] Nothwithstanding frequent protestations that the work was designed to distinguish the false from the good, it sweeps remorselessly, like an unrestrained hurricane, all, even the pure, before its tempestuous inculpation. Allusion has been made to the nature of vestments incident to conferring the doctorate upon aspiring scholars; but a letter from the satirical and erudite laureate to the equally famous Bocaccio furnishes a valuable insight into this usage touching the dress and habits of the medical guild in that age. It was customary for physicians to appear in public with all the splendor and magnificence which social gradation and affluence could provoke. Their attire consisted of royal scarlet, plenteously embellished with priceless gems or rings, finished with gilded spurs. Petrarch gibes the profession by saying its members lacked little of the honors of a triumphal procession, with its most solemn adjuncts, since they could and did rightfully boast of having slaughtered at

[1] "Mendacia vero medicorum, sed eorum qui falsi medici volunt odi fateor." Petrarca, Rerum Senil., Lib. XV., Ep. 3. Cf. Xiphil., vit. Hadriani, p. 296.

[2] Editio Baslæ, A. D., 1554.

[3] "Nihil adjuvat Medicos consulere." Petrarca, op. cit., Lib. XIII., Ep. 8.

least five thousand men; but the only element wanting in such munificent tribute to murderous genius, obscured behind the scalpel[4] and monumental pile of drugs, was the trifling difference of circumstances under which the assassinations occurred. Wreaths of laurel and mural crowns were justly due to him who slew many enemies with a gauntlet of steel, while in the case of medical murders it was compatriots ruthlessly destroyed by an unarmed person dressed in the toga.[5] From several physicians to whom he propounded questions, the answers were confirmatory of the contempt in which practitioners of the age should be held, one of these appears to have obtained the honors of special laudation on account of an injurious confession made by him that he was not so impious as to use an art to captivitate the mind, when he knew it to be fallacious.[6] The anecdote related by the satirist touching a venerable medicist will fully reveal the social gradation of the profession in Italy at this era. Summoned to attend Galeazzo Visconti, the celebrated Lombardic autocrat, it was agreed the professor should receive for curing the ducal patient the sum of three thousand five hundred scudi, besides expenditures entailed by the journey, at the end of which a magnificent reception awaited him.

Petrarch affirms he was in Milan the day of this surgeon's arrival. Upon entering the city he dispatched a messenger to the Duke, notifying him of his presence in the municipality; whereupon Galeazzo, awakened from a sound slumber, directed that the pompous medicastre should be formally received, as was the usage, with splendor and gayety. Servants, a detachment of cavalry and courtiers, escorting a steed gentle as a lamb and white as unstained snow, for the illustrious physician, advanced to meet this mighty representative of a legalized corporation of assassins, sacred within purple robes and its ornamentation of glittering jewels.

---

[4] Du Cange, Glossar., sub v. Spatula.

[5] Petrarca, Rerum Senil., Lib. V., Ep. 4.

[6] Ibid.

This fêted practitioner, apparently of Teutonic nationality, by the haughtiness of his deportment, inspired the populace with a belief that so much pompousness must equal divine puissance, and could resurrect the very dead. Upon entering the ducal palace, the German Hippocrates ordered fresh eggs and a certain preparation of flour concocted into a beverage. The result of this magnificent visitation was the rapid increase of Galeazzo's malady, and the loss of the charlatan's impudence, who finally declared he must consult his magic books for an infallible remedy.[7] From so illustrious a personage, who had experienced the most disenchanting of all events, an actual trial of their skill, it is by no means surprising that the active mind of the amatory song-writer, and equally lucid satirist, should subject medical pretenders to the scorn of literary ridicule.

He proceeds to narrate in unrivalled beauty and impressiveness his experience, which exposed the entire profession to remorseless jocundity. In the month of May, 1370, a sudden attack of malarial fever prostrated him, and perhaps some years later concluded an existence of incalculable worth to letters and philosophy; at least the epistle constituting our guide expressly states at the time of its composition he was still troubled by recurring intermittent maladies.[8] Physicians hastened to offer gratuitous attendance with the same alacrity as in the epidemic of 1359,[9] under the impulse of benevolent affability towards the distinguished invalid, and the urgent demand of the son of Jacopo, his patron Francisco di Carrara.

After deliberating a long while, the only point, as the poet humorously writes, upon which they united was in asserting pretentiously Petrarch's death at midnight of the same day, the evening of which had already begun. Their only remedy proposed was a forcible restraint from sleep by the aid of exciting cordials, which would prolong his life until the following dawn.

[7] Petrarca, Rerum Senil., Lib. V., Ep. 4.

[8] An excellent resume of Petrarch's life is prefixed to the Didot Ed. of Le Rime di Petrarca, p. 23 seqq.

[9] Sade, Memoires de Petrarche, Tom. III., p. 523.

In accordance with his usual unmistakable commands to the servants, and passionate appeals to personal friends, that no physician should be permitted to approach him, the illustrious poet abstained from following the prescription of his medical advisers, but reposing the whole night in the sweet, tranquil slumber described by Virgil, the next morning, when the astute medicists arrived, as he says, to arrange funebral preparations, they found him pleasantly engaged in writing. They expressed their stupefaction by exclaiming: "He was a wonderful man!"[10]

Unswerving fidelity to the medicinal treatises of the Arabs, doubtless, retarded the rapid progress of medicine in Western Europe as an independent science during the fourteenth century. We have adverted to the extensive use of Saracen sciences and the servility of imitation, especially in Italy, where translations and perhaps original treatises were carefully preserved by the stationarii for professional consultation. This blind and irrational subserviency highly offended the inquisitive spirit of Petrarch, who seized an excellent opportunity in corresponding with a medical friend, to express with impassioned indignation his contempt for Arabic poesy, which he asserted to be effeminate and horribly obscene, and so far as scientific testimony was valuable, he hesitated not to declare[11] in distinctive terms his disapprobation of it.

Evidently a too rigid adherence to the system of these authorities undermined the beneficial expansion of the Salernite school, towards the close of this era. In his description of a journey to Palestine, alluding to the Neapolitan kingdom, the Florentine unequivocally sets forth the remarkable decline of this University of Medicine when he says: "Here Salerno may be seen, which formerly possessed fame as the source of the sciences, but now presents the decrepitude of dotage."[12]

[10] Petrarca, Rerum Senil., Lib. XIII., Ep. 8; and Lib. XIV., Ep. 14. Also, Vita de Petrarca, p. 34.

[11] "Seclusis Arabum mendaciis." Petrarca, op. cit., Lib. XII., Ep. 2.

[12] "In quo Salernum videbis. Fuisse hic medicinæ fontem fama est, sed nihil, quod non senis exarescet." Petrarca, Itinerarium Syriacum, Tom. I., p. 560.

Although original methods of tuition appear to have been maintained in the Italian universities, the Gallic schools rivalled these in the absorption of useful professional talent. The poet laureate himself, as we have seen, at an early age pursued a course of law studies at Montpelier, which apparently had overshadowed the traditional renown of Italy for general culture, and was certainly in high repute in the fourteenth century—so much so, indeed, as to induce Villannova to seek its medical and scholastic lectures.[13]

A singular confirmation of the decadence of Italian schools at this epoch may be gathered from the significant conduct of a Paduan nobleman, who selected with vigilant care twelve youth from families of his principality, and after fully equipping them with outfits and finances, sent them to the Parisian University, in order that there they might aquire a more profound and skilled knowledge of medical science than was taught in their own country.[14] Notwithstanding this evident tendency to send students abroad for such education, there were professors of this art still extant in Italian colleges whose eminence, perhaps exaggerated, and erudition, gained them almost divine honors. Of these, the Florentine Dino, after having for years obtained in Bologna the supreme glory for successful teaching of medicine, being forced to leave the city through that envy which is ever the repulsive portraiture of weak minds, continued elsewhere his public lectures and repeatedly declined to return to the celebrated university from which jealousy had driven him.[15]

So great was his reputation that during his sojourn at Bologna, his expanding celebrity drew multitudes of scholars from the most distant parts of the universe to the city.[16]

[13] Vita Villannovae, cap. 2; and Freind, Historia Medicinæ, p. 543.

[14] Vita Princip., Carrariensis; ap. Murator., Scriptor. Ital. Rer., Tom. XVI., p. 168.

[15] Villani, Vite d'Illustr. Fiorentine, p. 47.

[16] "Che di volontà di tutto l'universola studio fu promesso alla cathedra." Ib., p. 47.

While domiciled here, he commenced full commentaries on the writings of Avicenna, in universal renown at this time, perhaps through the admirable versions of Villannova,[17] proceeding, however, with his usual lectures, until deprived of this right by a municipal edict, as suggested above.

Whatever may have been the apparent causes of Dino's banishment from Bolonga, the subsequent career of this great scientist was adventurous, and seems to have consisted in emigrating from place to place, until the year 1319, when he completed his comments of Avicenna, at Florence. Whether Bolognese envy or national hatred compelled him to abandon the city in the first instance, or on account of a curious diatribe touching the bold plagiarisms of a defunct physician's compendium, which enhanced so greatly the professional celebrity of the persecuted Florentine as to provoke numerous demands from contiguous cities for his permanent residence among them,[18] cannot be certainly established, although the incontestible fame of Dino caused him, in companionship with an equally known physician, to be selected as professional advisers of a notorious Paduan statesman, dispatched to Florence on an embassy. In a metrical narrative of this journey to the Tuscan city, the invalid envoy describes his sudden malady and the general characteristics, moral and physical, of the attending surgeons. Subsequently, but prior to the year 1325, this famous professor retired to Sienna, in order to continue his medical readings. As an indication of a popular and apparently just celebrity, it is stated many Bolognese students followed him to his new professorship.

At the epoch of his final voyage to his native city, having completed the commentaries on Avicenna, he read them publicly in the cathedra or lecture dais—an event by no means unusual at this period of the Middle Ages in Italy, where

[17] Vita Villannovæ, cap. 2. This scientist was upon most intimate terms with the king of Aragon, and proceeded to Avignon in the year 1309 as envoy extraordinary to Pope Clement V., in order to negotiate a recognition for his patron of the title "King of Jerusalem." Freind, Historia Medicinæ, p. 543.

[18] Villani, op. cit., p. 52.

oftentimes expository lectures in the nature of textual comments were delivered in public upon Avicenna, Galen, and Hippocrates.[19] In the year 1327, the illustrious Florentine closed his earthly existence in this city, having obtained a just reputation as the chief medical scientist of the time.[20] Besides the Avicennian expository treatises, extending his renown in that age, Dino wrote a compendium of Hippocrates on obstetrical knowledge, some letters touching the sanitary property of supping and dining, and a book on surgery. To these should be added, as betraying talents of antagonistic description, a lucid explanation of a famous amatory chant by Guido Cavalcanti.[21] Careful analysis of this professor's character attests that at times he would ascend to ecstatic contemplation in the quiet seclusion of his private doorway, while the opinion—nearly unanimous—regarding his genius,[22] awarded him the noble commendation of readiness to attend gratuitously the diseased—a suitable appendix to that distinguished acumen by which his vast illustration was fairly earned.[23] Equally famed for the tuition of medicine and his lucubrations on this subject, was Torrgiano, also of Florence, and contemporary with Dino.[24] Having completed his professional studies at Bologna, he opened a school for the curative art at Paris. Touching his skill and profundity in medicine, he received the eulogy of transcending ordinary commentators, which laudatory title was conferred on account of an excellent analysis of the Galenic system, and under such designation this work was published.[25]

---

[19] "Hic in expositionem Avicennæ, Galeni et Hippocratis," etc., "præcipue codex ille nostræ Avicennæ." Muratori, Scriptor. Italiæ Rer., Tom. XXIV., p. 1165.

[20] Villani, Vite d'Illustr. Fiorentine, p. 46 seq.

[21] Fabricius, Biblioth. Latinit., Tom. II., p. 39.

[22] Petrarca, Rer. Memor., Lib. II., cc. 3 and 4.

[23] Villani, Vite d'Illustr. Fiorentine, p. 46 seqq.

[24] Ibid., p. 49 seqq.

[25] Fabricius, Biblioth. Latinit, Tom. II., p. 66.

Frequently medical professors attained to so great eminence during the Middle Ages that affluent invalids readily believed it impossible to escape death unless such attendance should be procured on terms dictated by the medicists themselves. Abuse of this morbid belief advanced these celebrated practitioners rapidly to enormous wealth and pomposity. In this age the great English surgeon Gaddesen,[26] and Nicholas Colnet, royal physician to Henry V., the latter of whom forced his patron to pledge certain jewels of the crown as a guarantee of annual salary,[27] may be referred to here as conclusive proof that the grade of the profession satirized by Petrarch was uniform outside of Italy, who accused its members with trifling with bodily ills in order to accumulate money.[28]

Panegyrical praise has been awarded Tomaseo, an Italian scientist of this century, whose vast ability doubtless justifies the hyperbolical encomium of Æsculapian similitude. In addition to wide-spread distinction and quickly-acquired riches, he was honored with the sincere amity of Petrarch, who has preserved in one of his letters an unequivocal attestation of the excellence and worth of the scientist. He unreservedly affirms, notwithstanding his well-known skepticism touching the science, that this medical professor was superior in deserving celebrity to all physicians of the age.[29] At the time of Tomaseo's visit to Viscount Galeazzo afflicted with gout, Petrarch asserts that in magnificent robustness of health, which was acknowledged to be the finest in the provinces, he resembled this great practitioner.[30]

An acquaintanceship with medicine was deemed essential

---

[26] Freind, Historia Medicinæ, p. 551.

[27] "Ferra le dit nostre Seigneur le Roy liverer an dit Nichol en gage joialx, queux par l'agreement se purront bien valoir la somme la quelle les ditz gages, pur icel quarter s'extendront." Rymer, Fœdera, Tom. IX., p. 235.

[28] "Medici, qui de malis hominium, ludum et mercemonium fecere." Petrarca, Rerum Senil, Lib. III., Ep. 4.

[29] Petrarca, Rer. Senil, Lib. XII., Ep. 1.

[30] Villani, Vite d'Illustr. Fiorentine, p. 49 seqq.

to the culture of an unprofessional scholar during the Middle Ages, developed as a proper sequence of ancient legislation by the Carlovingians, and canons of the church establishing the range of monastic education. As late as the year 1366, when a distinguished geometrician died in Italy, he directed by testamentary bequest his collection of medical books should be given to the modern rival of Æsculapius, the illustrious Tomaseo.[31] Villani relates a prediction, publicly announced by the great scientist, touching the day and manner of his own death, long in advance of the event, abundantly proving the profound conviction of mediæval medicists in the virtue of necromancy and astrological sortilege.

Persuaded of the near approach of the end of his earthly existence, he ordered an altar constructed in his domicile for the selemnizing of mass, importuning the clerical celebrant with utmost devoutness to consecrate the Corpus Christi, and while observing with steadfast gaze and awe-struck tenacity the transubstantiated material, expired at the prognosticated hour.[32] Among his published works are commentaries on the Galenic variations of fevers, and a treatise touching the most suitable mode of living during pestilences, evidently prepared for emergencies developed by the great plague in this century. His death alone prevented the compilation of the Summa Medicinæ.[33] A Florentine professor, Nicholas, arose to distinction in this age for the brilliancy of his medical knowledge, which celebrity was prolonged into the first year of the ensuing era. According to the energetic laudation of a panegyrist, this scientist's familiarity and skill in medicine were almost divine, combining a thorough culture of polite letters similar to scholars of the Middle Ages in Italy[34] and among the Spanish Arabs.[35]

---

[31] Tiraboschi, Storia della Litteratura, Tom. V., p. 253.

[32] Villani, op. cit., 49 seqq.

[33] Tiraboschi, op. cit., Tom. V., p. 254.

[34] Lanzi, Storica Pittorica della Italia, Tom. I., p. 13 seq.

[35] Leo Africanus, De Virib. Illustr. Arab., cap. 9, p. 268; and cap. 11, p. 273. Also, Freind, Historia Medicinæ, p. 504.

The writings of this accomplished professor were eagerly sought, and preserved their reputation unimpaired for curative methods, which engaged the attention of both practitioners and suffering infirm. From the adulatory encomiums of the writer referred to, it appears the medical profession of that time, after essaying the subtilities of the Arabian Avicenna, or the more ancient Hippocrates and Galen, abandoned the arbitrament of their authority and carried alone the works of Nicholas, which perfectly indicated what remedies controlled and vanquished the most obstinate diseases.[36]

So great indeed was the celebrity of this professor that a spurious antidotarium was attributed to him for several centuries.[37] Mediæval families whose members were distinguished for their knowledge of medicine similar to the medicists of remote antiquity,[38] transmitted the more recondite mysteries of the curative art to their posterity as an heirloom, and in this way the son of Bartholemew, William, the renowned Bologna doctor, obtained illustration as early as the year 1302.[39] His treatises on the cure of maladies have been carefully preserved, although the dedicatory letter prefacing the work betrays the undisguised frailty of vain scholasticism, and in the redundancy of phraseology utterly divested of signification, are certainly to be detected the traces of that constant tendency throughout the Middle Ages to inspire increased credulity by the collocation of mysterious words.

Notwithstanding this inculpation, his descendants were incumbents of professorial sittings at Bologna upon the highest compensation allowed in the year 1381, almost equalling the enormous salaries of the preceding era.[40] At this epoch, when the popular mind was still sunken into profound obscurity and ignorant superstition, when dedicatory prefaces to

[36] Mehus, ad Vit. Ambr., Præf., p. 29.

[37] Fabricius, Biblioth. Latinit, Tom. V., p. 111.

[38] Goujet, Origin des Arts et Sciences, Tom. I., p. 213.

[39] Sarti, De Professor. Bonon., Tom. I., Pars I., p. 483.

[40] Muratori, Scriptor. Rer. Ital., Tom. XX., pp. 54 and 940.

medical books sought to provoke unusual confidence, professors claimed the privilege of endowing themselves with the superbly ponderous title of Prince of Medicine.

So far as the panegyric of the Florentines designated above extended, doubtless there was abundant reason to assume the merit of this public honor, which oftentimes elevated the successful practitioner, in those distant ages, to transcendent grandeur, but when accorded unfitting personages, presents the appearance of unequivocal mendacity. At the close of the century under examination, Gentilis da Foligno, a medicist of trifling importance, was awarded, by vulgar acclamation, the colossal distinction, Divinus Gentilis Fulgiens nostræ et suæ ætatis Medicorum princeps—divine prince of physicians of his age.[41] To this adorable surgeon is to be attributed the determination of the Carrarese ruler to aggregate twelve Paduan boys, and after fully supplying them with liberal outfit and finances, to send them for medical instruction to the Parisian university.[42] Independent of his princely gradation in society, Gentilis is said to have been the personal physician to the Roman pontiff, John XXII., and that he died during the frightful pestilence of 1348, at Perugia.[43]

The predecessor of this pope in name was of profound skill in medical science, and wrote a work professedly for indigents, containing such directions as rendered the practice of the art possible, without having recourse to physicians.[44] The death of Gentilis seems to have been superinduced by the multiplicity of pestiferous patients, and prevented the publication of an elaborate treatise on the causes and remedy of the plague,[45] an effort, as hitherto stated, engaging the attention of other medical sages at this epoch.

[41] Ibid., Tom. XXIV., p. 1155.

[42] Ibid., Tom. XVI., p. 168.

[43] Fabricius, Biblioth. Latinit, Tom. III., p. 32.

[44] "Hic fuit magnus medicus, et scripsit librum in medicina qui Thesaurus pauperum vocatur: in aliis scientiis fuit generalis." Martini Fuldensis, Chronicon, sub an. 1276; ap. Eccord. I., p. 1715.

[45] Tiraboschi, Storia della Litteratura, Tom. V., p. 259.

Jacobus da Forli inspired so great affection in the people of Padua, on account of his vast science in medicine and its practice, that when he died early in the ensuing age,[46] the manifestations of grief were only equalled by those provoked by the death of Hippocrates.[47] During his life, this eminent practitioner attained the honorable distinction of Royal Divinity of Medicine, and was declared repeatedly by the famous Savonarola, also a physician, to be the first medicist of the time.[48] The accomplishments of Jacobus were of the most extended character, including public readings in natural and moral philosophy, logic, philology and medicine. After several years of exclusively philosophical lectures, otherwise the mediæval Quadrium and Trivium, he yielded himself up entirely to medical instruction in the Paduan University, where his system attained such high repute as to be prescribed by an authoritative decree as the order of examination—secundum questionem Jacobi Forlioiensis.[49] Greek authorities in medicine attracted earnest commentations from this erudite professor, of which the most celebrated were his exposition of Galen's Arte Medica, the aphorisms of Hippocrates, and the works of Avicenna.[50]

From the Sancta Sophia family descended a long and illustrious lineage of medical practitioners and instructors, whose fame spread beyond the limits of Christendom to barbarians—perhaps the civilized Ottoman and Spanish Saracens.[51] Of these, Marsiglius, according to the hyperbolical panegyric of enthusiastic Savonarola, describing "the magnificent ornamentations" of Padua, equalled divinity himself in ability to cure vexatious maladies, which procured for him the appella-

46 Facciolati, Fasti Gymnas. Pat., Pars II., p. 101.

47 Tiraboschi, op. cit., p. 261.

48 De Magnific. Ornament. Reg. Civ. Paduæ, Lib. I., cap. 3.

49 Tiraboschi, op. cit., Tom. V., p. 261.

50 Fabricius, Biblioth. Latinit., Tom. IV., p. 11.

51 De Magnif. Ornament., cit.; Lib. I., c. 3; Muratori, Scriptor., Tom. XXIV., p. 1163.

tion of prince and monarch of physicians, and entitled him to undivided honor from posterity. He narrates that Marsiglius obtained from all Italian Universities the erudition and science possible to be imparted, and having in turn lectured to them, communicated the redundant splendor of his brilliant science to less cultured ultramontane nations.

Visconti, the first duke of Milan, manifested especial interest in this professor. Consequently, when Marsiglius, confiding in his scholastic abilities, offered to attend university lectures at Paris, and to publicly dispute with its teachers any point of medicine or the liberal arts propounded for discussion, the ducal patron readily proffered to send the literary athlete thither at personal expense, an arrangement however which the sudden demise of Galeazzo rendered nugatory.[52] The immense stipend allowed the illustrious surgeon unequivocally proves the estimation in which he was held by Visconti. Under the denomination of physician ordinary to this prince, he received an annual salary or pension of one hundred and thirty liri, which for that epoch was an enormous sum of money.[53]

Professional treatment of the Milanese ruler by Marsiglius consisted of "solemn" liquids and famous medicaments compounded by the distinguished physician himself, which contemporary history affirms prolonged the august patient's life for several days. The annalist concludes the encomium by pronouncing him the best and most learned medicist of the universe.[54] This reputation obtained for him at the Bolognese university the signal distinction of reading his lectures on medicine in the morning—an honor usually restricted to

[52] Savonarol., De Magnific. Ornament. Paduæ, Lib. I., c. 3; ap. Murator., Tom. XXIV., p. 1163.

[53] Muratori, Scriptor. Rer. Ital., Tom. XX., p. 940. In the year 1342 Innocent, by decree, allowed astrologists reading at Placentia, the modest sum of thirteen lire. Ibid.

[54] "Reputato il migliore e piu sapiente medico del mondo." Istoria Padov.; ap. Murator., op. cit., Tom. XVII., p. 857.

native professors.[55] His brother also attained to eminence for the lucid expositions which he made of the works of Hippocrates, Galen and Avicenna, and for a commentary on a treatise by the Arabic scientist, commended for its remarkable excellencies.[56]

In the panegyrical inscription upon this professor's tomb in the Paduan cathedral, the ordinary exaggerations of such eulogies are far transcended, for he is declared "the most sublime monarch of medicine, and the very salvation of the city where reposes his sepulchre," and that "as the father of study he cured the maladies of the languishing." The versifier adds: "He extracted the inmost essence of Hippocrates, Aristotle and Galen, combining truest practice with the puissance of restoring health to the entire world, while his shining glory permeated the globe."[57] The Sancta Sophia family boasted with just pride of another famous medical professor, whose renown called him in extreme youth to the Austrian metropolis, where he publicly lectured on the science for many years; at the same time he was surgeon ordinary to the ducal magnates at a large stipend. Later in life he returns to his natal city with the moderate celebrity of "most famous."[58]

Italian colleges were singularly fortunate in possessing families whose medicinal culture, transmitted from more ancient progenitors, enabled many of their descendants to acquire great illustration and rare distinction for admirable works of medicine and surgery at the close of the fourteenth century, or early in the next. Prior to the year 1347, it is attested, the most famous Gallic surgeon of that era was a disciple of medicine, and perhaps anatomy, under a Bolognese professor. This tutor, named Bertuccius, is referred to by the celebrated Guido di Chauliac as his master—Bertuccius magister meus[59]—

---

[55] Ibid., Tom. XXIV., p. 1163 seqq.

[56] Muratori, Scriptor. Rer. Ital., Tom. XXIV., p. 1165.

[57] Tiraboschi, Storia della Litteratura, Tom. V., p. 265.

[58] Muratori, op. cit., p. 1165.

[59] Chauliac, Tractat. I., Doctr. I., De Anatomia, cap. 1, p. 3.

who fell before the destructive energy of the great pestilence.[60] A work in the nature of a compend of medicine by this anatomist is reproduced as a worthy monument by the erudite mediæval literary cyclopædist.[61] One of the numerous medical or surgical tutors of this epoch seems to have had such notable success in restoring health by means of unguents that he offered to cure Boniface VIII., the Roman pontiff, with them[62]—the medicinal property of which was largely increased by placing them upon the extremities.[63]

Other Italian professors of medicine, in addition to those already designated, have perhaps escaped oblivion through the pen of the illustrious Florentine, Petrarch. Albino de Canobia received from him a formal letter of acknowledgment of an invitation to accept the hospitality of the medical gentleman at his villa, and at the same time to receive professional attention.[64] To this courteous request the poet responded, and as a gracious concession to the polite offer of the scientific host, avowed, notwithstanding his enmity against the profession, that in trivial disorders it could be of slight utility. His epistles to Franciscus of Sienna, and William Rosen, both eminent surgeons and medical authorities, are charged with witty utterances at the expense of their avocation.[65] The former of these published at Avignon, in the year 1375, a work on the sanitary properties of the bath, which, it may be remarked, indicates extraordinary sagacity for the age, and another on the nature of poisons.

This author appears to have divided professional endowments between researches and lectures on the science of astrology in its remedial elements, and on medicine as a curative art. The extension of this popular credulity, touching the

[60] Muratori, Scriptor. Rer. Ital., Tom. XVIII., p. 402.

[61] "Collectorius artis Medicinæ." Fabricius, Biblioth. Latinit, Tom. I., p. 245.

[62] Chauliac, Tractat. I., Doctr. I., De Anatomia, cap. 6.

[63] "In extremitatibus Membrorum." Ibid., cap. 2, p. 10.

[64] Sade, Memoires de Petrarche, Tom. III., p. 523 seq.

[65] Petrarca, Rerum Senil, Lib. XV., Ep. 3; and Lib. III., cap. 4.

effective junction of these apparently disunited sciences, may be inferred from the fact that the erudite lecturer was personal surgeon to the pope, but such practice was the continuation of the earlier astrological system openly taught by Villannova and his predecessors, who claimed that certain elixirs must be prepared under lunar or planetary influences.[66]

Petrarch mentions John of Parma, in the most eulogistic terms, and in such warmth of laudation that its genuineness should not be questioned. He alludes to him as justly possessing a grand name, both at home and in the Roman court, then in the city of Avignon. Another curious statement clearly indicates the vastness of the number of medical adventurers in the pontifical capital. By way of suitable contrast, the poet-laureate asserts this reputation of the Parma professor would distinguish him amid the affluence of satraps and turbulent crowd of physicians at the papal court.[67] The celebrated historian of anatomy appears to have enjoyed an intimate acquaintanceship with the erudite scientist while in Avignon.[68]

The frequency of professional engagements in the leading universities of Italy, vindicates the solidity of his fame, while the magnitude of yearly stipends during his sojourn at Bologna and Brescia, demonstrates the importance of these lectures. At this period, as we shall presently discover, the practice and profession of medicine were restricted to the laity, and interdicted under severe penalties to clerics and regular monks. In defiance of such canons, Jacobus of Ferrara, early in this century—in the year 1311, incumbent of the episcopacy of Modena—had attained great distinction by preeminent medical knowledge, imparted in public readings and to schools of disciples.[69] Clement, the Roman pontiff, seems to have cherished medical talents.

---

[66] Rosarius Philosophorius, Lib. II., cap. 28.

[67] "Sed in Romana curia inter illos ingens medicorum turba." Petrarca, Rerum Senil, Lib. XII., Ep. 2.

[68] Chauliac, Capitulum Universale, Præf.

[69] Muratori, Script. Rer. Ital., Tom. XI., p. 58.

In the year 1307, Edward I. of England, addressed his Holiness a respectful petition asking for the return of Nicholas Tyngewick, royal surgeon, whom the Pope retained evidently as his own physician.[70] Villannova was also present about this period in Avignon, on political business for the king of Aragon.[71] Guido da Bagnolo, whom Petrarch honored with a sincere amity, freqently united with him during his sojourn at Venice, in supporting the philosophic argumentation of the Arabic sage, Averroes.[72]

Although possessed of sound learning and judicious intelligence, in the rapidity of discussion his ideas became confused, while at times the consciousness of his own mental superiority rendered him superb with pride and pomposity. Influenced by such weakness, Guido haughtily announced himself as physician to his majesty the King of Jerusalem and of Cyprus. The habits of this medical professor provoked luxurious indulgence during his residence at the Levantine Island, where he owned a slave by the name of Francesca. In the testamentary disposition of his personal property he directed that a daughter, offspring of the servile mistress, should be sent to Lombardy and placed under the tutelage of her paternal relatives. Upon arriving at marriageable maturity, she must be sought in matrimony only by a scholar matriculated at the Bologna University. He bequeathed his collection of medical books and treatises on art to the exclusive benefit of indigent students.[73]

The inscription on his sepulchral monument at Venice, with hyperbolical exaggeration, awards him the supreme praise in philosophy and medicine. It appears Guido drew up a chronicle in several volumes, containing notable acts of the Dukes of Reggio minutely narrated.[74]

---

70 Rymer, Fœdera, Tom. II., p. 1056.

71 Freind, Historia Medicinæ, p. 543.

72 Ibid., p. 504.

73 Faccioli, Memorie di Reggio, Tom. II., p. 251.

74 Prœm. ad Histor.; apud Muratori, Scriptor. Rer. Ital., Tom. XVIII., p. 1 seqq.

Towards the conclusion of this era a surgeon named Bartholomew, domiciled in Bologna, was celebrated for the remarkable success of his treatment of ocular maladies—so much so indeed as to be reputed miraculous for such diseases, and the preservation of sight. He received an annual salary from the municipal authorities of twenty florins, and quickly obtained satisfactory evidence of external fame beyond the place of his abode, where he was greatly esteemed.[75] Other departments of human physiology appear to have received especial study, and become objects of undivided practice, such for instance as removing calculus by surgical operation.

Several writings of this century, elucidating this important subject, were published, the titles of which we reproduce from Tiraboschi:[76] "Remedium adversus Lapidum efformationem in vesicis et Regimen ulceris vesicae." Increasing subdivision of medical science into its cognate branches entailed the necessity of preparing numerous compilations, designed doubtless for less celebrated and skilled practitioners of the curative art. Of these the Opus Pandectarum Medicinae appears to have been substantially an encyclopedia of alphabetical receipts for compounding medicaments, and a full explanation of medical terms, with their practical uses. This volume, of which many editions were subsequently published, has received the eulogy of Freind as presenting the most complete and satisfactory treatise on the curative properties of herbs extant in compendious form.[77]

From a statement contained in this pharmaceutical Pandect, it would seem that the compiler early in this century had been called to a professorship in the Salernite university.[78] Compared with the slender services by other European medical instructors of the age, the Italian writers, by no means ad-

---

[75] "Riputato uomo miracoloso per tutti i mali degli occhi, e per conservare la vista." Ghirardacci, Historia di Bologna, Tom. II., p. 455.

[76] Storia della Litteratura Italiana, Tom. V., p. 272 seq.

[77] Historia Medicinæ, p. 501.

[78] Pandect. Medicinar. Opus, p. 164.

vancing the science to its progressive perfection, were further in the van than their predecessors in elucidating obscure portions of human pathology; and for this reason the history of the economy of medicine as illustrated in the great schools of Southern Europe justly merits specific examination. Mondino's nativity, similar to the fate of the illustrious bard of Scio's isle, was claimed by five cities of Italy. Florence, Bologna and Venice, through distinguished scholars, assumed to prove the origin of the restorer of anatomical science in their several municipalities.[79]

Touching the Bolognese professor who appears to have particular claims to the individuality of the renowned anatomist, a document published by the careful biographer of the celebrated medical sages of that university, establishes Mundino's ancestry as parties to a contract with a famed tutor, thus solemnly obligated to instruct them in the details of this art upon the somewhat singular basis of a stipend in the nature of profit and loss.[80] According to the terms of this agreement, executed in the year 1270, the opening of pharmaceutical traffic was stipulated, which having continued for many years, was transmitted to this great scientist, whose highest encomium is contained in Sarti's brief phrase: " Mundinus anatomes restitutor—restorer of anatomy."[81] Thirty-six years after the institution of the drug trade, his uncle Lucian and one of the contracting parties to the bond, both apparently in full practice professionally, were elected to medical professorships in the university of Bologna.[82]

Ten years later, the son of Robert, King of Sicily, leaving the city under the propulsion of an insult, the teacher of medicine and his nephew, afterwards illustrious Mundinos, were dispatched with other principal citizens to offer suitable excuses

---

[79] Fabricius, Biblioth. Latinit., Tom. V., p. 90, calls him "Florentinus;" and Villani, Vite d'Illustr. Fiorentine, p. 55. Also, Freind, Histor. Medicinæ, p. 505.

[80] Sarti, De Professor. Bononiensis, Tom. I., Pars I., p. 463.

[81] Ibid.

[82] Ghirardacci, Historia di Bologna, Tom. I., p. 505.

and plausible explanations, including a petition for forgiveness to the municipal authorities. In the work cited the principal emissaries are designated doctores physiciæ,[83] or as written by Sarti, Fixice,[84] which at that period had begun to be the title of medical practitioners, excluding ultimately vernacular phraseology among the polite nations of Europe.[85]

Perhaps the most authentic writer upon whose judicious statements absolute reliance should be placed touching Mundino's birthplace, is Guy di Chauliac, nearly contemporaneous with this distinguished professor, whom he distinctly asserts to be Bolognese—Mundinus Bononiensis.[86] Soon after the event alluded to the uncle died, leaving the nephew to the full enjoyment of family grandeur and the performance of a duty to elevate to the decedent's memory a tablet on which was engraved the representation of a professor of medicine surrounded by a troop of eager disciples, before the professorial chair. The epitaph ingeniously compares his curative powers with the sublimest efforts of the Pergamic scientist, and accuses invidious fatality with suddenly severing the thread of so noble an existence.[87] Subsequent to his kinsman's decease, Mundino pursued his professorship of medicine at the Bolognese university, where he obtained the large compensation of a hundred liri annually for scientific lectures.[88]

The exact date of his death is unsettled. An annalist under the year 1326 fixes that period as the end of his earthly and valuable labors.[89] The chronist presumably in a summary form reproduces what appears to be the united accord of all, his great reputation as the most skillful surgeon of the universe, to whom the highest honors of Bologna were awarded.[90]

83 Ibid., p. 591.

84 Sarti, op. cit., Tom. I., Pars II., p. 227.

85 Rothii, Explicat. Vocab. Physic., § 13.

86 Chauliac, Tractat. I., Doctr. I., cap. 1, p. 3.

87 Tiraboschi, Storia della Litteratura, Tom. V., p. 278.

88 Ghirardacci, Historia di Bologna, Tom. II., pp. 18, 56.

89 Muratori, Scriptor. Rer. Ital., Tom. XVIII., p. 340.

90 "Che fu reputato uno de megliori Medici del Mundo." Ibid.

A conventual record earlier by one year, however, records the donation of certain gifts to a cloister, subject to the order of Saint Frances, for masses to the repose of Mundino's soul.[91] Guy di Chauliac, historian of surgical science down to his own time, narrates that during his studies in Bologna under the tutelage of this famed anatomist, Mundino was celebrated for the excellence of his lectures, and numerous treatises on dissection.[92] Some of these are still extant in manuscript among the libraries of Italy.

A writer of the period, describing one of Mundino's mechanical compositions used in illustrating the science of anatomy, declares him to have had exalted pre-eminence in synthetical demonstration of the art, and in the number and range of writings on medicine. The chronist, in the fervency of panegyricism, naively adds: "When he read them himself, his soul was filled with unlimited joy." He also urges as the specific source of Mundino's renown his dexterous preparation of human effigies designed to elucidate the literal portions of anatomical lectures. Upon this invention the annalist hesitates to express an opinion, "because the poverty of words must restrict a sounding eulogy."[93]

Faccioli affirms this Bolognese professor was the first to compose a full and complete treatise on dissection since the days of ancient surgeons; and so ponderous was the weight of his influence, that contemporary scientists cited a single paragraph from his works, as a guide for an entire reading before their disciples.[94] A statute of the Paduan university prescribed that medical licentiates matriculated there should follow literally and rigidly the comments and explanations of this distinguished anatomist in their studies on surgery—a regulation subsisting in full force until the sixteenth century.[95]

[91] Tiraboschi, op. cit., Tom. V., p. 279.

[92] Chauliac, Tractat. I., Doctr. I., De Anatomia, cap. 1, p. 3.

[93] Muratori, Scriptores Rer. Ital., Tom. XXI., p. 1162.

[94] Fasti Gymnas. Pat., Pars I., p. 48.

[95] "Ut Anatomici Paduani explicationem textualem ipsius Mundini sequantur." Portal, Histoire de l'Anatomie, Tom. I., p. 259.

It is admitted by medical historians, both in Italy and elsewhere, that Mundino is justly entitled to the honor of restoring anatomy to the proportions of an exact science, and in all respects, from the multiplicity of his writings explanatory of this art, passes as the precursor of the modern system.[96] At a time when deep and profound interest began to advance medicine swiftly along the plane of an accurate science, it was fortunate there were persons of erudition to translate, compendiously, the voluminous works of ancient and more recent sages into the professional Latinity of that age.

Many of these translators, doubtless deeply interested in the progress of the curative art, possessed, however, no further acquaintanceship with it than could be gleaned from versions carefully made of medical authorities, Greek or Arabic, for which they were abundantly compensated by municipal and university laws. When western scholars had acquired sufficient familiarity with oriental languages,[97] acting upon the example of Saracen predecessors in making translations of Syriac and Grecian writings,[98] they reproduced the literature of the Arabs into the learned idiom of mediæval Europe. Toward the end of the fourteenth century, when the European mind loosened slightly the crippling processes of irrational induction, Italian cities maintained their advance of scientific culture propagated from the Sicilian schools.

Padua and Venice vigorously upheld this rational distinction, and endeavored, especially the latter, by the repressive energy of legislative interdict, to retain their students within the educational limits of domestic colleges.[99] At this time the Paduan University possessed a register of eighteen thousand scholars attracted thither by diversified departments of science and art, which were remarkably endowed with the most com-

[96] Sarti, De Professoribus Bononiensis, Tom. I., Pars I., p. 463.

[97] Daru., Histoire de Venise, Tom. II., p. 308.

[98] Heeren, Sur l'Influence des Croisades, p. 51; and Leo African., De Viris Quibus Illust.; ap. Arab., cap. 1, p. 261.

[99] Daru., op. cit., Tom. II., p. 311.

plete collection of subjects illustrating natural history; a botanical garden, vast accumulations of manuscripts, a chemical laboratory, and a fully equipped amphitheatre exclusively devoted to anatomy.[100] Many cities of Italy during the century before us attained great celebrity on account of their aggregation of oriental books and numerous translations of the most important works.

Pisa, Milan, and Pavia, were distinguished for the ardent zeal with which they pursued such labors, while Venice appears to have been the first to furnish the best and purest version of Arabic authors, notably Avicenna—in the ensuing era.[101] Anterior to 1345, translations of nearly the entire writings of Galen were made by Nicholas de Reggio from the original Greek. To this literary pursuit he devoted his linguistic culture over a period of thirty years, during which he certainly produced the most authentic translation of this venerable authority on medicine.

Contemporaneous with Guy di Chauliac, he had early obtained favorable notice for such services, and although an unprofessional scholar, his versions were accepted as the purest and most perfect, so much so that upon production at the papal court in Avignon, they were commended by expert linguists to be of a style more elevated and lucid than those reproduced from Arabic sources.[102] Some years prior to Nicholas, a Montpelier professor of medicine by the name of Armengardus Blasius, translated the Canons of Avicenna directly from Arabic into the Vulgate. This version also included the commentaries of Averroes. Avicenna's treatise was entitled: "De partibus Medicinæ," and in its translated form was so arranged as to provide a means of ready use to physicians, both for memorizing and instruction.[103]

---

[100] Ibid.

[101] Daru., Histoire de Venise, Tom. II., p. 309 seq.

[102] Chauliac, Tractat., Prœm.

[103] Herman. Corneri, Chronicon, sub an. 1293 ap. Eccard.; II., p. 947.

CHAPTER XXVIII.

Status of Physicians in the Middle Ages—Their Practice—Clergy Eagerly Adopt this Profession—Its Lucrativeness—Interdicted the Monks—Decretals of Synods—Physicians Confined to the Laity—Pharmacists Sell Drugs and Confections—Gallic Disgust of Medicaments—Specimen of German Surgery of the Twelfth Century—Mediæval Surgical Practices—Barbers and Phlebotomy—Fame of Jewish Physicians—Unscrupulous Charlatans—High Ecclesiastics Disprove Medicine—Contempt of Scientific Treatment—Clerical Division of Medicine—Popular Respect for Practitioners—Often Satirized by Romancers—Fees According to Wealth or Indigence of Patients.

ALTHOUGH ecclesiastical society in its numerical majority naturally inclined to the study of theology, many clerics, influenced by secular gain, or impelled by innate taste, eagerly sought the important culture of medicine. For this reason priestly physicians incurred the censure of sensitive reformers, and among these, no less a personage than Saint Bernard himself, who bitterly complained, about the middle of the twelfth century, that monks, professedly under church discipline, preferred the rescripts of Justinian to the sacred laws of the Lord, and charged that it profited little to religion to seek corporeal medicines,[1] administered by worldly-minded recluses.[2]

Out of this general incrimination directed at clerical scholars of the Pandects, the writings of Galen and Hippocrates developed frequent decrees of Synods, whose uniform design was the extinction of the thirst for lucre, superinduced by the practice of medicine and civil law. As early, therefore, as the year 1130, a general council held at Rheims ordered that the

[1] "Propterea minime competit religioni medicinas quaere corporeales." Bernardi, Abbat. Clairæ V., Epistolæ, Ep. 345, Tom. V., p. 550.

[2] Ibid., Ep. 491, Tom. I., p. 706.

study of the Roman codes and physic should thenceforth be interdicted the monks.[3] The immediate causes leading to this canonical law, as previously stated, doubtless originated in the accusation that the acquisition of these sciences necessarily demanded the absence of monastic students from the cloisters, during prolonged and intolerable periods of time. This decree was frequently reiterated—nine years afterwards, and in the years 1163 and 1180, through a decretal of Pope Alexander III.[4]

At a provincial council, held in the city of Montpelier, where fifteen years previously a magnate of the province had established a school of medicine, subsequently so celebrated that in 1220 new statutes for better government were obtained from a pontifical legate, in the year 1195 the following canon was promulgated as a proper norm for the monasteries: "It is prohibited under strictest ecclesiastical penalties, for monks or regular canonicals to pursue the study of law or physic."[5] The statutes authorized by Alexander at Montpelier and Tours, regulating this infraction of church discipline, were formally reaffirmed, empowering diocesan bishops to punish the priestly offender. In order to accelerate the penalties prescribed, other regulations equally minute were enacted by the Narbonnese synod.[6] An important extension of this forbiddance emanated from the decretal of Honorius III., issued in the year 1219.

According to a fragment of this rescript still extant, this restriction was made to include all priests. It was found, however, by actual experience to be impossible to maintain the rigidity of the decree, and consequently curates of a rectorship

[3] "Leges temporales et medicinam gratia lucri temporalis," etc. Labbe, Concilia, sub an. 1130, Con. V., Tom. XXI. p. 438.

[4] Ibid., Con. IX., sub an. 1139.

[5] "Ne quis monachus vel canonicus regularis aut alius religiosus ad seculares leges vel physicam legendas accedat." Concil., Monspeliense, sub an. 1195, Can. XV.

[6] Concil., Monspeliense, sub an. 1195, Can. XX.; ap. Baluz., I., p. 35 seq.

were, in the interest of their patrons, exempted from its operation. The most significant means adopted at this period to hold in check these violations, were edicts of Innocent IV., who directed all pupils of law and medicine should largely draw on their foreign benefices.[7]

When at a later date in the papal metropolis, a celebrated professor of civil and canon law publicly read his lectures in 1285, this pontiff, evidently realizing the necessity of securing the attendance of suitable disciples upon these lectures, so far modified this regulation as to admit the presence of all clergy, excepting bishops, abbots and monks.[8] In the next century, the University of Bologna procured a similar dispensation permitting the matriculating of clerics as licentiates to both readings of law and medicine—a decretal subsequently re-affirmed in the year 1321 and 1419.[9] About the same period in 1344, the school of Pisa received like authorization for regular and uninterrupted attendance upon medical lectures. The principal object of such dispensations was the important privilege of clergy, absent from their prebendaries and churches, to receive and enjoy revenues arising from these distant and neglected rectorships.[10] For similar reasons a papal decretal, in the year 1220, directed that clerical students upon such readings in the University of Paris should be peremptorily placed under the ban, inasmuch as Roman law was not applied in the civil courts of that muncipality.[11]

On account of undisputed precedence given by this great school to theological studies, it has been fairly assumed that the foregoing decree was designed to definitely crush out by the weight of Vatican authority any attempt among scholars indiscriminately to perpetuate lectures on civil law.[12] Although

[7] Savigny, Geschichte des Römischen Rechts, Th. III., p. 365.

[8] Ibid., p. 366.

[9] Ghirardacci, Historia di Bologna, Tom. I., p. 539; and Tom. II,, pp. 7 and 626.

[10] Savigny, op. cit., Tom. III., p. 366.

[11] Ferriere, Histoire du Droit Romaine, cap. 29.

[12] Savigny, Geschichte des Rœmisch. Rechts, Th. III., p. 367.

the licentiates in the Italian Universities, during the twelfth and thirteenth centuries, were semi-clerical, and until the sweeping canon of church synods and papal rescripts, composed largely of enthusiastic ecclesiastical students of medicine, the evident determination of the sacerdoty to enforce their legislative decrees materially altered the character of scholastic frequenters of medical instruction, especially before the year 1190, and throughout the entire course of the ensning age.

Medical students were therefore from the first three decades of the twelfth century recruited in greater numbers from the laity, subject however to a partial sacerdotal discipline, which prevented their marriage until the fifteenth century,[13] and obliged them to assume a quasi-clerical costume. It was perhaps unfortunate for the development of this science upon the elevated plane of a rational system, that the most cultivated minds of the time were debarred by the repressive power of synodal and decretal interdict from that searching inquiry, which the scholastic intellect was competent alone to furnish. Naturally depressed by hierarchical hindrance and canonical rulings, the curative art too often was dwarfed into the stinted companionship of ignorance and charlatanism, until toward the close of the Middle Ages, when the standard of professional inquirers reacted favorably upon medical practitioners.

History may narrate the occasional prominence incidentally given the licentiate of medicine at infrequent intervals during the progressive expansion of the scholastic establishments of Southern Europe; and although the lack of medical and surgical skill may painfully surprise, it should be remembered that the critical rule of modern times must constitute the most illiberal accusation against the mediæval profession. Physicians in those remote periods seem to have prescribed certain rules by way of sanitative precaution in the ordinary details of domestic life, including the order of diet, food and drink at the table. Pharmacists sold drugs and conserves indifferently,

---

[13] Pasquier, Recherches Sur l'Histoire de France, Liv. III., p. 244.

as may be gathered from the following extract of the Guiot Bible:

Lors dient-il, ce m'est avis,
Qu'il ont gigimbret et pleris
Et diagragent et rosat,
Et penidium et violat.[14]

But these attractive medicines, eagerly sought by feminine invalids, recede before the necromancing preacher Monk, who seriously ordered his patients to eat snakes and frogs as a specific against all infirmities, particularly for the cure of eye diseases.[15]

The chronicler's charging this practitioner with abandoning urinal inspection in diagnosing for maladies,[16] is convincing proof of the survival of this adjunct of practice since the time of Cassiodorus.[17] It was adopted during the sickness of William the Norman[18] and the foundation of permitted practice under the Jerusalem code in the year 1090.[19] Deviation from this regulation entailed public scourging.[20]

In the place of such test, the Teutonic preacher-physician used small closed pouches, the contents of which no one was permitted to inspect, and as a remedy suspended them over the diseased at night. A Polish nobleman and his wife partook of the medicinal diet of snakes, lizards and frogs, and as the annalist avows, were completely cured.[21] As early as the year 1055, juniper berries, perhaps an extract, were found to

---

[14] Notices et Extraites des MSS. du Roi, Tom. V., p. 506.

[15] "Comedere serpentes, lacertas et ranas contra quamlibet infirmatatem, sive fuit dolor oculorum vel aliud." Annales Polonor., sub an. 1278.

[16] Ibid.

[17] Cassiodor, Formulæ, XIX.

[18] Flor. Wigior., Chronicon, Tom. II., p. 29. In 1195 sagacious prediction from such examination. Golscheri, Gestæ Archirpp. Trevierens, sub an. 1195, op. Ecc. II., p. 2205.

[19] Le Assisse et Bone Usauge del Reaume de Hyerusalem, cap. 218.

[20] Ibid.

[21] "Bursiculas clausas singulas super singulos infirmos per notem." Annales Polonorum, sub an. 1278.

be an excellent remedy for colic, and made a matter of permanent record by the conventual chronicles.[22]

In France especially, where the inhabitants, according to Villannova, evinced the utmost disgust at taking medicines,[23] attention was early directed to the adaptibility of edibles and their suitable admixture with potable liquids as a sanitary substitute for other means of preserving health. In order to aid the natural warmth of the stomach, ragoûts and sauces, strongly flavored with spices, were partaken for principal food, which should be followed with aromatic wines and flavored essences.[24] The use of fruits was either dispensed with entirely, or indulged in with defiance and grave apprehension. Many of the great mediæval professors of medicine regarded these productions rather for medicinal than dietary qualities,[25] and consequently ordered both robust and invalid to eat them invariably at the commencement of repasts, so that the seasoning of meats, combined with the fermenting heat of wines, might correct the pretended pernicious effect of their frigidity.

For this reason it was a standing prescription to the close ot the Middle Ages that fruits the most readily decomposing must be eaten before, while astringents, such as chestnuts, almonds, pears, and figs, should be reserved for dessert. Excepting perhaps the individual accomplishments of a few priestly medicists, the Jewish physicians were certainly honored with more frequent summons to attend Christian patients, on account of their famous medical skill.

Wherever the Israelites had domiciled in the provincial towns and cities of occidental Europe, many of them, as early as the tenth and eleventh centuries, had embraced the lucrative practice of law and medicine.[26] In this science they became distinguished at a period when their Christian rivals

---

[22] Annales Corbeienses, sub an. 1055.

[23] Villannova, Breviarii, Lib. IV., cap. 22, p. 1419.

[24] Legrand D'Aussy, Histoire de la Vie Privée des Français, Tom. III., p. 332.

[25] Villannova, Regimen Sanitatis ad Inclytum Regem Aragonum, cap. 11.

[26] Wm. Neubrigens, Historia Anglicana, Lib. IV., cap. 10.

were almost wholly given up to the suppositious material benefactions of superstitious devices,[27] but were frequently charged with administering poisons under the guise of medicines, as happened in their treatment of Hugo, a Gallic prince in the tenth century.[28]

Doubtless the most eminent and famous professor of medicine among this people was Moses Maimonides, to whose writings we have repeatedly referred, a native of Cordova, who died about the year 1208. In addition to this science, his knowledge swept the entire range of mediæval liberal arts, including astrology, philosophy, and mathematics.[29] In France, in 1009, great multitudes of this nationality, of whom many were accomplished surgeons, were remorselessly slain amid the operations of war provoked by Caliph Haken becoming possessed of the holy sepulchre.

Under Richard the First of England, whose celebrity made him an exemplar for the closing years of the next age, Jewish citizens were exposed first to the fiery zeal of the London Christians, which culminated in wholesale assassinations in the city of Lynn. Here, under the incitement of hatred surreptitiously evoked by foreign youth present for commercial traffic, the rage increased to such an extent that all Jews were murdered, including an Israelitish personage whose great medical skill, successful practice, and modest merit, had endeared him to Christian patrons.[30]

By a decretal of the Avignon Synod, held in the year 1327, Christians were forbidden to invoke the medical or surgical science of this people, unless in an emergency when it was impossible to procure other professional attendance. The decree recites that recourse was had by unscrupulous and ungodly persons to Jewish medicastres for noxious drugs and

[27] Sismondi, Histoire des Français, Tom. I., p. 191.

[28] Richerius, Historiarum, Lib. IV., c. 101.

[29] Leo Africanus, De Medicis et Philosophis Hæbraeis, cap. 20, p. 296; and Buddæus, Histor. Philosoph. Hæbrorum, p. 124.

[30] Neubrigensis, Historia Anglicana, Lib. IV., cap. 7.

potions.[31] These medications, objects of sacerdotal animadversion, were provided, it appears, equally by male and female physicians.[32] This law was repeated forty years later, a sufficient indication of the radical tenure which this illicit practice maintained in defiance of canon law.[33] In the year 1410, Henry IV., of England, issued letters of safe conduct to Elia Sabot, a Hebrew doctor of medicine, to travel withersoever he pleased throughout the realm.[34]

Leopold, Duke of Austria, whose heartless captivity of Richard the Lion-Hearted was the frequent subject of mediæval romances, was overtaken by a frightful calamity in the year 1195, which contemporary and later English annalists accepted as a just punishment of Deity, who had "placed the remorseless axe at the tree's root." While celebrating Christmas festivities with haughty pride, exhibiting his personal grandeur to admiring subjects amid martial pomp, Leopold was thrown from his horse, which fell violently upon the rider's foot, fracturing it so terribly that the bones protruded through the flesh.[35]

On the arrival of surgeons or medici, quickly summoned to attend the aggravated wound, they prescribed such remedies as might possibly heal the grievous fracture.[36] The following day the wound presented such a sombre appearance that the surgeons decided it to be absolutely essential to amputate the mutilated member.[37]

Wendover, who evidently transcribed official documents of later date than the annals cited, distinctly affirms when the medical advisers consulted upon the sinister presentment of

---

[31] "Pro medicamentis imò verius nocimentis indifferenter recurrunt." Concilium Aveniense, Can. LXXII.

[32] "Judaeis utriusque sexus ut in curandis." Ibid.

[33] Concilium Vaurense, cap. 114.

[34] Rymer, Fœdera, Tom. VIII., p. 667.

[35] Flor. Wigior., Cont. Chronic., Tom. II., p. 160.

[36] Neubrigensis, Historia Anglicana, Lib. V., cap. 8.

[37] Ibid.

the mortified limb, they announced to the ducal sufferer that the application of a searing iron, combined with the tumid aggregation around and above the broken bones, would cause excruciating agony,[38] and in such a deplorable conjuncture, it was futile to attempt a cataplasm.[39] The duke refusing to subject himself to tortures thus plainly stated, ordered imperatively the injured foot to be forthwith severed from the tibia. The most singular part of this strange narrative, which provides a significant specimen of mediæval surgery in the twelfth century, remains to be related. When the noble patient had directed amputation, there was no one sufficiently skilled in surgery to attempt this operation: regardless of his earnest adjurations to prolong life, surgeon, friend and son equally declined the risk.[40]

His chamberlain being called, under duress and minatory compulsion, while the duke himself held a battle-axe upon the diseased limb—a service refused by horror-struck bystanders with a heavy mallet or beatle, severed the foot in three blows.[41] The physicians thereupon applied their medicaments to the wound, and when, the next morning at dawn, they visited the sufferer, immediately recognized signs of approaching mortality,[42] which originated, as our chronicler says, in the brutal operation driving consuming fires nearer the vital parts of the body, instead of alleviating crucial pangs.[43] By their voice and countenance, the medical attendants announced to him: "Fix thy house, for thou shalt die and not live."[44]

Canonical rules, existing for more than a half century, inter-

---

[38] "Quin igne quem infernalem vacant, tumori admixto intolerabiliter cruciaretur." Flores Historiar., Tom. III., p. 88.

[39] "Nullo medicorum potuit cataplasmate sedari." Ibid.

[40] Neubrigensis, op. cit., Lib. V., c. 8.

[41] "Dum ipse dux dolabrum manu propria tibiæ apponeret, malleo vibrato, vix trina percussione pedem ejus abscidit." Ibid.; and Wendover, op. cit., Tom. III., p. 88.

[42] Hemingburg, Chronicon, sub an. 1194, Tom. I., p. 210.

[43] Wendover, Flor. Historiar., Tom. III., p. 88.

[44] Neubrigensis, Historia Anglicana, Lib. V., cap. 8.

dicting the practice of surgery and medicine to the clergy, might warrant the presumption that these physicians were not of monastic profession, notwithstanding the solemn and significant quotation of the Vulgate Bible.[45] It is needless to add, the Austrian ruler died as a sacrifice to ignorant surgery.[46]

Of the diversified filiations of medicine, to which the mediæval mind naturally turned with unremitting zeal, engaged in constant and cruel warfare, surgery, or the cure of wounds, was doubtless of transcendent attraction, although the science itself does not appear to have progressed beyond the simplest treatment known to remote antiquity,[47] which indeed recognized its utility.[48] It is barely possible the delicate surgical operation of trepanning may have been known at a distant epoch of the Middle Ages.

In the year 891, a monk afflicted with agonizing cephalic pains was directed "to saw into his head."[49] About the same epoch, an eminent Gallic ruler lost his life through surgical ignorance in amputating a wounded member. Richerius, the devoted student of a medical compilation in the tenth century, describing the results of this operation, is redolent with learned technical verbosity,[50] but his diagnosis of the march of the disease terminating Lothair's existence in 986 is a most admirable specimen of disease-sketching.[51] Mediæval surgeons were doubtless abundantly able to protect their personal interests in defiance of sacerdotal interdicts, by means of guilds;[52] although the apparent dishonor attaching to this curative art may be understood, when it is stated that the status of practitioners

45 Reg. II., c. 21.

46 Neubrigensis, op. cit., p. 139; and Hemingburg, Chronicon, Tom. I. p. 211.

47 Goujet, Origin des Arts et Metiers, Tom. I., p. 216.

48 Celsi, De Medicina, Lib. I., Præf.; and Lib. VII.

49 "Jussus est pro remedio in capite secari." Annalista Saxo, sub an. 981; ap. Eccard. I., p. 229.

50 Historiarum, Lib. I., c. 2.

51 Ibid., Lib. III., c. 109.

52 Ungewitter, Geschichte der Hændel, p. 234. Guilds of actors and acrobats in 1040. Otto Frising., Chronicon, Lib. VI., cap. 32.

was assimilated to the social degradation of barbers and blood-letters until the year 1406, at which time Wenclaus, emperor of Germany, by imperial rescript ordered that thenceforth this profession should be deemed honorable.[53]

Repulsive and barbarous methods, involving the terrible usage and frequent abuse of the searing-iron, preserved a vigorous existence beneath the pressure of canon law and ignorance, which abandoned such operations to ambulatory charlatans or rural empirics[54] and vagrant monks, wandering unlicensed along the public highways of Europe.[55] In the time of Tertullian, a red-hot iron was universally used to attest the presence of death in the human cadaver,[56] which, however, was not invariably satisfactory, since it was recognized the results were not uniform.[57] On account of surgery being subjected to the dishonoring censure of both civil and ecclesiastical society, and its consequent abandonment to barbers and perhaps Jews,[58] whenever history has preserved notice of their operations, until the resurrection of the science by Italian professors, they excite contempt and disgust.

In contemplation of mediæval statutes, surgeons united to their occupation that of pharmacy, and oftentimes prescribed medicines for patients, subjecting themselves to the discipline of excommunication in case of vending injurious drugs, whether for poison or unnatural uses.[59] Like penalty was placed upon the purchasers.[60] In the year 1337, by a synodal decree, it became mandatory for apothecaries to make oath

---

[53] Friedlander, Geschichte der Heilkunde, p. 231.

[54] Goujet, Origin des Arts et Metiers, Tom. I., p. 215.

[55] Chronicon Engelhusii, sub an. 1097.

[56] Apologetica, cap. 15.

[57] Celsi, De Medicina, Lib. II., c. 6; and Plinii, Histor. Natural., Lib. VII., cap. 52.

[58] Per contra, Abulfagus, Annales Moslem., Tom. III., p. 599. Christian surgeons 1164 to Chalif of Bagdad.

[59] Notices et Extraites des MSS. du Roi, Tom. V., p. 506.

[60] "Herbas mortiferas in mortem vel abortivam." Concilium Vaurense, an. 1368, Canon. 156.

before civil courts, to observe this law.[61] Count Richard, marshal of the English king, and his lieutenant in Ireland in 1234, by the unscrupulous infamy of a surgeon, terminated a short but brilliant life. After an engagement provoked by the treachery of his advisers, this warrior was captured. Although severely wounded, he was able to move about his chamber and at dice. Finally, the pain of his wounds caused him to summon a physician to relieve him. Whereupon Muricius, chief of the Irish justiciary, under whose custody the marshal was placed, ordered the attendance of a surgeon, the ability of whom, it is charged, "was greater for destruction than preservation."[62] The illustrious soldier seems to have felt an instinctive defiance of the surgical operator, and before submitting to carnal medication, received the viaticum and made a legal testament. The medicastre afterwards presented himself to perform the functions of the profession. With a long iron implement, used in this horrible ordeal, heated to a glowing red, he burned open and into the tumescent wounds of the moribund count so frequently and so profoundly, as started the vital fluids to flowing freely.[63] Immediately following this severe searing, the valiant warrior succumbed to a hasty fever a fortnight subsequently, and was interred in a sepulchre prepared for him by Minorite monks at Kilkenny, as an unusual example of modest erudition for the age.[64] It is evident the sneer of the annalist touching the surgeon's utter incompetency, produced by an enemy to attend the martial invalid, is justified by the unequivocal complaisance exhibited in assassinating a suffering patient under the indelicate exterior of professional skill.

Equally important and germane to this inquiry is the curious legend touching the legitimacy of Frederick the Hohenstauffen emperor of Germany, which illustrates the evident depravity

---

[61] Concilium Aveniense, cap. 23.

[62] Wendover, Flor. Historiar., sub an. 1234, Tom. IV., p. 307.

[63] "Medicus autem ad eum accedens cum ferro longo et ignito vulnera ejus aperuit, et tam sæpe et profunde ferrum demersit," etc. Ibid.

[64] Annales Waveliens, sub an. 1234, p. 314.

of medical practitioners in the thirteenth century. When in the year 1220, this enlightened ruler was crowned by the Roman pontiff, he was asserted to be of illegitimate birth, being the son of Henry, his putative father, only in name.[65]

The following statement is given touching this singular accusation. At the time of her marriage to the Emperor, Constantia was upwards of sixty years of age. By virtue of an ante-nuptial settlement, in case the imperial spouse should die childless, the royal provinces of Apulia, Sicily and Calabria reverted to certain heirs, and in consequence grave apprehension was expressed concerning the empress' possible sterility. At this important juncture the imperial physicians suggested a plan by which the domination of the countries designated could be retained within Teutonic lineage. Upon their responding for the success of the nefarious scheme, he sanctioned the proposition to provoke fecundity.

By the uterine introduction of energetic medicaments, which these crafty and unscrupulous professors themselves compounded, the noble lady began gradually to reveal the appearance of fully answering the necessity of providing an heir to the throne in question,[66] and the emperor himself, as the chronist ingenuously relates, "most vehemently asserted the imperial dame advanced in pregnancy."[67] Towards the maturity of gestation, the complaisant medical advisers arranged for the production of an infant from several women; and at the period of the consummation of this impudent plot a new-born child was transferred secretly within the regal bed-chamber of Constantine, which was ultimately recognized in public as the heir apparent—subsequently renowned as the illustrious Frederick II.

Notwithstanding the uniformity of the use of the searing-iron as a necessary remedy in the treatment of wounds, the cure of Edward king of England by different means is a not-

---

[65] Albert Stadensis, Chronicon, sub an. 1220; ap. Schilt. I., p. 302.

[66] "Fecerunt autem uterum ejus per medicinas paulatim intumescere." Ibid.

[67] "Ut Imperator eam vehementer crederet impraegnatem." Ibid.

able instance of contrary practice. The Soldan of Babylon, seeking a method of ridding his territory of the English monarch, dispatched a Saracen menial to assassinate him, and succeeded in wounding the King with a poisoned dagger. It is stated he was unexpectedly healed from the destructive effect of this blow by means of certain medicines,[68] which seems to imply an unusual knowledge and thorough familiarity of the attending physician with antidotes. When Jewish suitors at law were in mediæval courts formally complaining against Christian defendants, they were required to take the juridical oath by Sabaoth, Eloi, and Adonai, and the ten names of Jehovah; and as corporeal punishment for perjury against this imposing array of divinities, they were placed under the invocation of fevers, to which they agreed by responding Amen.[69] The remedy for a malady thus provoked, which appears to have possessed the attributes of infallibility, was suspending the patient between two dogs.

Bernard of Clairvaux advises the less summary curatives for these fevers—the Quartain remedied by manual labor, and the Tertian with cold or tepid water; if still obstinate, wine or warm potions should be administered.[70] Superstitious or saintly usages, in preference to terrestrial medicaments, maintained uninterrupted existence throughout the Middle Ages, and were invariably sought when the complications of disease surpassed the science of secular and clerical physicians, who, in defiance of canonical law, persisted in practicing medicine. In the year 1137, the celebrated Abbot of Clairvaux was called to Salerno in order to accomplish a celestial cure of a person whose bodily infirmity had exhausted the resources of medicists.[71] A dream having advised the invalid to drink the water with

---

[68] Steron., Annales Altahensis, sub an. 1270.

[69] "On annoncait la fièvre tierce, quatre, et quotidienne, s'ils se parjuraient." Voltaire, Essai Sur les Moeurs et Usages, Tom. III., p. 52.

[70] Apologia ad Guillelmum, cap. 4, § 7.

[71] Fleury, Histoire Ecclesiastique, Tom. XIV., p. 509.

which Saint Bernard washed his hands, the priestly physician proceeded thither and healed an incurable disease.[72]

Annalists oftentimes expressed contempt for scientific treatment of maladies. Thus, in the year 1100, when the monkish medicastres, or archiatri, attending the Dauphin of France, announced his approaching death, summoned a physician from Barbary—perhaps a Saracen country is generally to be understood—Odericus Vitalis, in recording the event, alludes slightingly to him as a "hairy person."[73] Hugo St. Victor illustrates in brief the medical theories of the mediæval profession, which are worthy of reproduction in their original form: "Medicina continet occasiones operationes. Occasiones sunt sex: aer circumdans nos, cibus et potus, somnus et vigiliæ, motus et quies, inanitio et repletio et accidentiæ animæ. Operationes siunt intus et foris. Intus ut ea, quæ intromittantur per os, per anum, adexcitandas sternutationes, vomitiones, purgationes. Foris, ut amplastra, incisio, ustio."[74]

In his treatise of Medicine of the Soul, St. Hugo lays down the rule that a physician should not only know the present but the past of a disease, so as to decide upon its future progress.[75] The doctrine of temperaments constituted a leading feature in Middle Age medical culture,[76] doubtless more extensively than in modern times. From the quotation above—accidentiæ animæ—as an integral element in the curing of diseases, it would seem that a pathology of the soul was regarded as essential to successful practice. Under the distinction ustio was included searing-iron, and operations necessitating abnormal heat. In the thirteenth century great diversity of systems was developed in detail by Italian professors of medicine,

---

[72] "De boire de l'eau dont il auroit lavé ses mains." Ibid.

[73] "Apodixem medicinalis peritiæ super desperatum, juvenem excere coepit—quidam hirsutus de Barbarie." Oderic Vital., Annales, Lib. XI., cap. 7.

[74] Tractat. de Origine et Divisione Artium, Lib. I., cap. 21; De Medicina, p. 201.

[75] De Medicina Animæ, cap. 9.

[76] "Quator humores corporis humani, sanguis, cholera rubra, cholera nigra, et phlegma." Ibid., cap. 2.

while the science itself advanced slightly through apparent indifference to experimental observations.

Some of these appear to have contemplated the use of immense quantities of medicines, which a monkish annalist of this age hesitated not to satirize, although his experience of such things was gleaned by professional visits during a prolonged illness.[77] The clergy continued to study the curative art as licentiates in the next age, and were oftentimes sufficiently distinguished for their skill to perform diplomatic missions to the papal court,[78] notwithstanding the decretals against priestly practice of medicine were rigidly maintained.[79] In England so universally were clericals preferred incumbents of secular offices that they were made secretaries of government, the privy seal, cabinet counsellors, treasurers of the crown, ambassadors, commissioners to open Parliament, presidents of king's council, supervisors of royal works, chancellors, and masters of the rolls.

Added to these, which would seem to exclude other offices, physicians to Henry VI. and his celebrated regent, Duke of Gloucester, were regularly recruited from the monastic professors.[80] In the fourteenth year of this monarch, a petition was received in council to grant the request of a Greek, styling himself a Master in Medicine, to become a citizen of England.[81] Surgeons in France under the unfortunate reign of Charles VI. were largely involved in the revolutionary troubles of the year 1355, when Jean de Troyes, regarded as the most skillful practitioner of his age, was an active element of revolt. Curiously enough, fifty-nine years later, called before the Dauphin for in-

77 "Die paratus nono elleborum,
Dolce non est ut mel aut zuccarum,
Quod Magistrorum propter ministerum,
Mihi confertur in refrigerium."

Rycardo San Germano, Chronica, sub fin an. +1239, p. 158 seq.

78 Chronica Comit. de Marka, sub an. 1357.

79 Jaffé, Regesta Pontific. Romanor., pp. 562, 585.

80 Turner, History of England, Vol. III., p. 217.

81 "Maistre en Medicine, natif. de Grece." Rymer, Fœdera, Tom. X., p. 35.

surrectionary conduct he concluded a rhetorical censure, by imposing upon the royal head a white cap as a distinctive symbol of liberty.[82] An English physician was prominent in 1333, according to the records of Durham, in aiding an adjustment of archiepiscopal troubles agitating this affluent See.[83]

Popular respect in general during the Middle Ages was accorded physicians unreservedly, although accused, with a unanimity quite significant, of avarice. A metrical romance charges them, in conjunction with jurists, of possessing only those principles of idolatrous reverence due to well filled purses. A versifier of the thirteenth century complains bitterly of excessive prices demanded for drugs by physicians:

"Triois cuillerètes de syrop,
Qui, à envis valent un œuf,
Nos vendent-ils, dix sols ou neuf."[84]

The Romance of the Rose thus inveighs against the disciples of law and medicine vending for filthy lucre their scientific knowledge:

"Advocatz et physiciens
Sont tous liéz de telz liens,
Ceulx pour deniers sciences vendent
Trestous à ceste harte se pendent
Tant ont le gaing et doulx et fade.
Que cil vouldroit pour ung malade,
Qu'il a qu'il en fust bien cinquante."[85]

The indignant romancer proceeds to inculpate them with disloyalty and covetousness:

"Tant les art, couvoitise et guille,[86]
Ceulx ne vivent pas loyaulement,"[87]

and that many of them in following these professions were

[82] Sismondi, Histoire des Français, Tom. II., p. 35 seq.

[83] Graystones, Hist. Dunelh., cap. 43.

[84] Mir. de Notre Dame; ap. Extraites des MSS. du Roi, Tom. V., p. 506.

[85] Roman de la Rose, vv. 5307–5312.

[86] Ibid., v. 5316.

[87] Ibid., v. 5321

influenced by vain glory to the damnation of their souls, concluding with this melancholy satire:

"Il est moult de telz deceveurs."[88]

It was a standing incrimination against mediæval physicians that they had neither friends nor relatives whom they desired to find robust and well, when going through the empty formality of a visit.

The Guiot Bible makes the sweeping inculpation of charlatanism as the principal attribute of Montpelier licentiates, whose skill was particularly displayed in imposing upon the credulity of patients in order to enhance the price of their drugs.[89] Raymund Lully asserted practitioners of medicine were more dexterous in killing invalids, under the weighty exterior of doctorates, than saving jeopardized lives by science.[90] Municipal authority was frequently invoked during the Middle Ages to readjust charges for medical services, upon more equitable and reduced rates[91]—an evident attestation of that same pecuniary avarice urged against Æsculapius himself.[92]

The Statutes of Nice forbid the association of medicists and apothecaries, in order to guard against extortions.[93] In the earlier ages the attendance of professors was recognized as a luxury so costly as to place ordinary citizens beyond the reach of medicines. Oftentimes chronicles turn upon excessive demands by physicians as an inducement for saintly remedies. Frequently, before recourse was had to these curatives, an entire patrimony was swallowed up in medical attendance.[94]

---

[88] Roman de la Rose, v. 5325.

[89] "S'il reviénent de Montpellier électuaire
Lor lectuaire sont moult chair."

Notices et Extraites des MSS. du Roi, Tom. V., p. 506.

[90] In Contemplatione Dei.

[91] Constitutiones Regni Siculi, Tit. XXXIV., Lex 3.

[92] Clemen. Alexand., Cohortat. ad Gentes, cc. 1 and 2.

[93] Monumenta Histor., Patr. Ital., Leg. Munic., Tom I., p. 80.

[94] Vita Godehardi, cap. 2.

Celestial cures were, notwithstanding, assumed to be worth terrestial compensation. In the year 1094, the Monastery of Corbey accepted three conditioned beeves for prayers so efficacious as to restore health.[95]

Many physicians regulated their schedule of charges according to the affluence or indigence of invalids. Consequently, influenced by an inflexible rule of diversified application to wealthy gentlemen and matrons, they prescribed specific and uncommon pharmaceutical compounds as necessary medicaments, or assigned double portion of drugs for remedies, while for impoverished or pauper patients the smallest allowance was ordered from apothecaries, upon the presumption that this quantity sufficed to cure the indigent, which for the rich was utterly inadequate.[96]

The illustrious medical practitioner, Johannes Gaddesden, in the opening years of the thirteenth century, especially distinguished as author of the Anglican Rose—Anglicanæ Rosæ—invented a graduated system of medicines to be used in treating the varied classes of society: the refined, the noble and affluent. He urged most diligently upon his disciples, both by example and voluminous treatises, to peremptorily decline transmitting these graded drugs to the diseased and infirm without receiving in advance the compensation fixed for professional services and pharmaceutical compounds.[97] This writer, against whom the charge of necromancy was freely made, did not hesitate to declare that man's credulity was the most successful element of medical practice[98]—a reproduction of Constans Afer's solemn argumentation.[99]

Another surgeon of Great Britain, in the same age, exhorts

---

[95] "Tres boves saginatos misit conventui pro reconvalescentia filii sui, precibus Fratrum nostrum impetrata." Annales Corbeienses, sub an. 1094.

[96] Rothii, Disquisit. Nomin. Loch., etc., cap. 2, § 5.

[97] "Quod tamen medicamentum dari non debeat, nisi acceptis prius salaris." Freind, Historia Medicinæ, p. 553.

[98] Ibid., p. 551.

[99] De Incantat. et Adjurat., Epistol., p, 318.

the profession to proportion salaries and perquisites in exact accord with unreasonable demands of patients. Gaddesden himself invariably advised his disciples to exact double fees from the affluent.[100] It is evident eminent English practitioners of the ensuing era were enabled to demand and obtained enormous compensation for their services. In 1333, the professsional skill of Pontius de Coutrone, was so gratefully appreciated by Edward II., that his successor endowed him with an annual pension of a hundred pounds sterling.[101]

Thirty years later, Joannes Paladyn was paid twenty pounds as a fee for medical attendance upon Edward III.[102] His queen caused a Florentine physician named Petrus de Florentia to be enrolled as a pensioner for twice that amount annually.[103] In referring to exemplary rules established by Johannes de Saliceto touching medical ethics, the renowned English scientist, Gaddesden, recommends members of the profession to tolerate no familiarity from the laity, "because too great familiarity breeds contempt,"[104] and what was more deplorable, rendered the demand for increased compensation of increased difficulty. But the paragraph of this statute regulating the profession ethically, which must provoke admiration from the members of all learned avocations, is the significant suggestion that large fees for attendance rendered a physician more estimable to the invalid, and conferred on him proportionate authority and respect.[105]

Guildic co-operation of surgeons doubtless aided in maintaining this pleasing rule in full practice, although some Italian municipalities forbid conjurations of every kind.[106] In

---

[100] "Duplum ejus quod pauperibus detur; pro divitibus imperat." Freind, op. cit., p. 551.

[101] Rymer, Fœdera, Tom. IV., p. 560.

[102] Ibid., Tom. VI., p. 417.

[103] Ibid., p. 587.

[104] Freind, Historia Medicinæ, p. 551 seqq; and Rothii, Disquisit. Nomin. Lach., etc., p. 93.

[105] Freind, op. cit., p. 551.

[106] Monument, Patr. Ital., Leges., Tom. I., p. 724.

France, under Louis IX., it is possible these unions may have suggested incorporations—the actual precursors of the modern societies.[107] An ordinance of Philip IV., issued 1311, promoted the substantial interests of surgery by directing that thereafter no surgeon, whether male or female, should pursue this profession unless first submitting to an approved examination into their abilities before a sworn syndicate—per magistros Chirurgicos—and receive a formal license in the nature of a diploma.[108] A guild of physicians was in existence at the metropolis of Lombardy as early as the year 1228.[109] In the hospital infirmary of the Order of Saint John at Jerusalem, four surgeons and an equal number of practitioners of medicine were assigned to the proper treatment of the sick and disabled.[110]

Whether or not the allegation of Eichhorn[111] be chargeable with exaggeration, that the thirteenth century in its manifestations of advancing culture is inferior to the ages succeeding and preceding, strict justice should admit that so far as medical science is concerned, the sweeping inculpation cannot apply to the profession so successfully pursued in the Universities of Italy. An important change of significant character occurred at this era, which energetically contributed to modify ecclesiastical dogmas, and largely aided in reducing the operations of the mind to the basis of sounder ratiocination. Up to this period, the teaching of Augustine had been in general an exclusive rule of guidance in argumentative inquiries touching matters profoundly agitating the mediæval reason.

From the thirteenth century, and with surprising velocity, they were wholly excluded by translations of Aristotle, pro-

---

107 Cuvier, Histoire des Sciences Naturelles, Tom. I., p. 408 seq.

108 Ordonnances des Rois de France, Tom. I., p. 491 seq.

109 "Collegio nobile di Medici Milanese prendendo principio dal 1228." Bettinelli, Risorgimento d'Italia, Tom. I., p. 116.

110 "Concedit ut in domo hospitalis semper quator medici totidem sint chirurgici." Jaffé, Regesta Pontificor. Romanor., N. 9766.

111 Geschichte der Beredsamkeit, Tom. II., p. 94 seq.

cured from the Arabs in part as hitherto stated, through the munificent patronage of Frederick II.,[112] whose legitimacy his papal enemies sought to question. Some of these Saracen manuscripts discovered by the Crusaders at Antioch were brought to Southern Europe and translated.[113] Anterior to the introduction of the Greek philosopher's writings into Germany by Otto Frisingen,[114] the illustrious Norman prelate, Lanfranc, appears to have had a profound acquaintanceship with the Dialectics of Aristotle in the eleventh century.[115]

These versions, when conjoined with the commentaries of Averroes and Avicenna, great scientists in philosophy and medicine, when publicly lectured upon in the Parisian University, seemed of so sinister presage to the fundamental dogmas of the Romish church, that a decretal was issued forbidding further readings of the Stagyrite, and directing his works burned by secular authority.[116] The spirit of searching investigation, however, arose uninjured from the ashes smouldering with the charred writings of the Hellenistic sage, and directed with subtle energy awakening minds to the splendor of exact sciences.

Scholasticism doubtless quickened a desire for more rational explanations of natural relations between causes and effective results, upon which system of investigation reposed the future of medicine, and while such tendencies progressed in graded value towards the solution of numberless problems glittering with undiminished but meretricious pomp, ages of superstition and painfully slow advances of intellectual culture were necessary to vindicate for the Æsculapian art the classi-

---

[112] Fabricius, Biblioth. Græca, Tom. III., p. 305.

[113] Muratori, Antiquitat. Ital., Tom. III., p. 993.

[114] Gesta Frederici Imperator, Lib. IV., cap. 11, sub an. 1158.

[115] Oderic, Vital. Histor. Ecclesiastic., sub an. 1090.

[116] Launoy, De Varia Aristotl. Fortuna, p. 139. Philip Augustus was present at the conflagration. Ibid., p. 138. Etabili, publishing a work of Aristotle in the year 1327, was burned alive. Maffei, Storia della Litteratura Italiana, Tom. I., p. 75.

fication of an exact science. That impress which medicine and its system of cures had received subsequent to Galen's time unfortunately preserved with vigor the undaunted miraculous remedies and astrological preventatives throughout the Middle Ages to Paracelsus, who sought in the fifteenth century to introduce a novel scheme of medicinal curatives.[117]

[117] Hallam, Introduction to the Literature of Europe, Vol. I., p. 363.

APPENDIX A.

Legum Wisigothorum, Liber XI., Titulus I., De Medicis et Ægrotis. Circa A. D. 504.

Lex 1. Ne absentibus propinquis mulierem medicus flebotomare præsumat. Nullus medicus sine præsentia patris, matris, fratris, filii, aut avunculi, vel cujuscunque propinqui, mulierem ingenuam flebotomare præsumat: excepta si necessitas emerserit ægritudinis, ubi etiam contuigat supradictas personas minime adesse, tunc aut coram vicinis honestis, aut coram servis aut ancillis idoneis, secundem qualitatem ægritudinis, quæ novit pendat. Quod si aliter præsumpserit X., solidos propinquinis aut marito coactus exsolvat: quia difficillimum non est, ut sub tali occasione ludibrium interdum adhærescat.

Lex 2. Ne medicus custodia retentos visitare præsumat. Nullus medicorum ubi comites, tribuni aut judices, aut villici in custodiam retruduntur, introire præsumat sine custode carceris: ne illi per metum culpæ suæ mortem sibi ab eadem explorent. Nam si aliquid mortiferum his ab ipsis medicis datum vel indultum fuerit, multum publicis rationibus deperit. Si quis hoc medicorum præsumpserit, sententiam cum ultione præcipiet.

Lex 3. Si medicus pro ægritidine ad placitum expectetur. Si quis medicum ad placitum pro infirmis visitando, aut vulnero curando poposcerit: ut viderit vulnus medicus, aut dolores agnoverit, statim sub certo placito cautione emissa infirmum suscepiat.

Lex 4. Antiqua. Si ad placitum susceptus moriatu, infirmus. Si quid medicus infirmum ad placitum susceperit, cautionis emisso vinculo infirmum restitutat sanitati. Ceste si periculum contigerit mortis, mercedem placiti penitus non requirat, nec ulla inde utrique parti calumnia moveatur.

Lex 5. Si de oculis medicus ypocismata tollat. Si quis ypocisma abstulerit, et ad pristinam sanitatem perduxerit infirmum V. solidos pro suo beneficio consequatur.

Lex 6. Si per flebotomum ingenuus vel servus mortem incurrat. Si quis medicus dum flebotomum exercet, ingenuum debilitaverit, C. solidos coactus exsolvat. Si vero mortuus fuerit, continuo propinquis tradenduus est, quod de eo facere voluerint, habeant potestatem. Si vero servum debilitaverit aut occiderit, hujusmodi servum restituat.

Lex 7. Antiqua. De Mercede discipuli. Si quis medicus famulum in doctrina susciperit, pro beneficio suo duodecim solidos consequatur.

Lex 8. Antiqua. Ne indiscussus medicus custodiæ deputatur. Nullus medicus inauditum, excepta homicidii causa, in custodiam retrudat. Pro debito tamen sub fidejussore debet consistere.

APPENDIX B.

Le Assisse, et Bone Usauge del Reame de Hyerusalem, A. D. 1090.

Caput 218. De li fisici che medicano li amalati, dandoli medicine, siropi et altre cose li quali morino per la mala cura.

1. Sel avien che un schiavo ò schiava sià amalata, e un medico vien al suo patron, ò patrona, e li dice volerlo guarire, accordandosi con esso per nominato precio, et accade poi che quel medico li dà cose calde, e molificative, e egli li doveva dar cose frede, e restretive, e nol fece, per il che more; la rason commanda, e judica, che liu sia obligato restituir un servo simile al suo patrono, ò il precio che li costò fina quel giorno che morite de jure.

2. Similimente sel avien che uno servo sia amalato da caldo che ha di dentro grande, e il medico li fa trar sanguine avanti el termine conveniente, e li traze troppo sangue, si che per la grau debilità il calore li dà sopra la testa, e more, la rason vole che quel medico debe refar al patrona del servo il valor di quello, civè quanto valeva il di che morite, overo quanto l'haverà comprato de prima comprita de jure.

3. Parimente sel avien che uno mio servo sia amalato da fredo, e un medico me vien a dire di volerlo guarire, e s'accorda meco, e tuol la cura guarirlo, e li fa trazer sangue sopra quel fredo, il che fa per la sua poca cognition de urina, e però secca l'orina, e perde la favella per causa del sangue trattoli, e con questo more, la rason vole che mi debbe far restoro di tanto quanto mi costava quel mio servo de jure.

4. Similiter s'io ho un servo, ò serva dropica, e un medico si mette a guarirlo, e li taglia il ventre là dove è il male, e poi non fa trarge li humori di dentro con rasone, anzi lassa insio la prima, ò la seconda volta, che se indebilisse, e perde il fiato, e more, la rason vole che mi deba pagar el mio servo. Similimente se un servo, ò serva è amalato con la febre quotidana, e un medico prende di guarirlo con purge de medicine, e li dà poi la medicina a strashora, e tanta schamonea in quella medicine, e la farà si forte, che more il servo bevendola, overo andarà del corpo tanta che suddi il ventre, el figito, e il pulmone, e more, overamente non tempera il medico la medicina bene, si che non lo menarà, e per questo more, la rason vole chel medico sia tenuto de pagar al patron del servo il valor di quello.

5. Cosi se un servo ha male al fondamento, e un medico tuol in si de guarirlo, e piglia un ferro ben calde e li vol curare, del qual vene quel male, el lui non saverà farlo, e brusa el budello talimente che si retira, e non potra pui andare del corpo, e more, la rason judica, che il medico dia tenuto pagar del servo il precio che l'ha comprato, ò quanto valeva.

6. Parimente se un schiavo ò schiava ha mal di san Lazaro ò rogna secha, ò alcun' altra malatia, e un medico s'accorda de guarirlo con condition che la mità del precio che sarà venduto sia del medico, e l'altra mità del patron del schiavo, e il medico li fa quanto sa, ma non lo giova, e more, la rason judica che in questo caso el medico non è obligato de restorar el schiavo, ò schiava, per che lui perde prima le sue fatiche, e poi quanto doveva haver; e questo è de jure per l'assisa.

7. Similiter se un medico medicarà à questo modo alcun homo libero, ò donna libera, le rason judica che esso medico debba esser impicato, e tutta la sua facultà dove esser del signor de la terra, e avanti chel sia impicato, deve esser menato frustrandolo per la terra, con uno urinal in man, per spaviar li altri da simel caso de jure.

8. Ben dovete sapere ch'è di rason che vi siano do testimonii, avanti chel medico sia convinto, sel denega d'haver medicato nel sopra ditto caso, e deveno jurar li testimonii, come in presentia loro ha medicato con tal medicine, e siropi, per li quali morite quello amalato, e come intesono dir à l'amalato che per le cose datali ha sentito dentro al cor suo ch'era per morire; e con questo deve esser convinto el medico de jure, per quello homicidio del servo che diè restrorar, ò del Christian, per el qual deve esser impicato, e non altramente.

9. Silimente nessun medico extraneno, che venisse d'oltra mar, ò da li infideli non deve medicar de urina nessun, fin che non sia provato da li miglior medici de la terra, in presentia del Vessovo de la terra; e cognoscendolo sufficiente à medicar li deve esser data licentia de medicar per urina, e questo è di rason per l'assisa de Hierusalem. Et se non sara bon medico, el Vescovo, et la corte deveno commandarlo che debba suddar la città ò stando a la città chel non debba medicar alcuno.

10. Et sel avien che alcun medico medicarà in la città senza licentia de la corte, et del Vescovo, la corte deve prenderlo, et farlo frustrar per la terra, de jure, et per l'assisa del Reame de Hierusalem.

APPENDIX C.

Constitutiones Regni Siculi, Titulus XXXIV., De Probabili Experentia Medicorum.

Lex 1. Rex Rogerius. Quisquis amodo mederi voluerit, officialibus nostris, et judicibus se præsentet, eorum discutiendum judicis; quod si sua temeritate præsumpserit, carceri constringatur, bonis suis omnibus publicatis. Hoc enim prospectum est, ne in regno nostro subjecti periclitentur ex imperitia medicorum.

Lex 2. Imperator Fredericus. Utilitati speciali prospicimus, cum communi saluti fidelium providemus. Attendentes igitur grave dispendium, et irrecupababile damnum, quod posset contingere ex imperitia medicorum, jubemus in posterum nullum medici titulum prætendentum audere practicari aliter, vel mederi, nisi Salerni primitus, et in conventu publico magistrorum judicio comprobatus, cum testimonialibus litteris de fide, et sufficienti scientia, tam magistrorum, quam ordinatorum nostrorum, ad præsentiam nostram, vel nobis a regno absentibus, ad illius præsentiam, qui vice nostra in regno remanserit, ordinatus accedat, et a nobis, vel ab eo medendi licentiam consequatur: poena publicationis bonorum, et annalis carceris imminente his, qui contra hujusmodi nostræ serenitatis edictum in posterum ausi fuerint practicare.

Lex 3. Idem. Quia nunquam scire potest scientia medicinæ, nisi de scientia logicali præscribatur, statuimus, quod nullus studeat in medicinali scientia, nisi prius studeat ad minus triennia in scientia logicali: post triennium, si voluerit, ad studium medicinæ procedat: it quod chirurgiam, quæ est medicinæ, infra prædictum tempus addiscat. Post quod, et non ante, concedatur sibi licentia practicandi, examinatione juxta curiæ formam præhabita, et nihilominus recepto pro eo de prædicto tempore studii testimonio magistrali. Iste medicus jurabit servare formam curiæ hoctenus observatam, eo adjecto, quod si pervenerit ad notitiam suam, quod aliquis confectionarius minus bene conficiat, curiæ denuntiabat; et quod pauperibus consilium gratis dabit. Iste medicus visitabit ægrotos suos ad minus bis in die, ad requisitionem infirmi semul nocte: a quo non recipiet per diem, si pro eo non egrediatur civitatem vel castrum, ultra dimidium tarrenum auri. Ab infirmo autem, quem extra civitatem visitat, non recipiet per diem ultra tres tarrenos cum expensis infirmi; vel ultra quator tarrenos, cum expensis suis.

Non contrahat societatem cum confectionariis, nec recipiat aliquem sub cura sua ad suas expensas pro certa pretii quantitate; nec ipse etiam habebit propriam stationem.

Confectionarii vero facient confectionem expensis suis, cum testimoniis medicorum, juxta formam constitutionis: nec admittentur ad hoc, ut teneant confectiones, nisi præstito juramento, quod omnes confectiones suas secundem prædictam formam facient sine fraude. Lucrabitur autem stationarius de confectionibus suis secundem istum modum: de confectionibus et simplicibus medicinis, quæ non consueverint teneri in apothecis ultra annum, a tempore emptionis, pro qualibet uncia poterit et licebit tres tarrenos lucrari. De aliis vero, quæ ex natura medicaminum, vel ex alia causa, ultra annum in apotheca tenentur, pro qualibet uncia licebit lucrari tres (sex?) tarrenos.

Nec stationes hujusmodi erunt ubique, sed in certis civitatibus per regnum, ut inferius describitur. Nec tamen post completum quinquennium practicabit, nisi per annum integrum cum consilio experti medici practicetur.

Magistri vero infra istud quinquennium libros authenticos, tam Hippocraticos quam Galeni, in scholis doceant tam in theorica quam in practica medicinæ. Salubri etiam constitutiones sancimus, ut nullus chirurgicus ad practicam admittatur, nisi testimoniales literas offerat magistrorum, in medicinali facultate legentium, quod per annum saltem in ea parte medicinæ studerit, quæ chirurgiæ instruit facultatem; et præsertim anatomiam humanorum corporum in scholis didicerit, et sit in ea parte medicinæ perfectus; sine qua nec incisiones salubriter fieri patuerent, nec factæ curari.

Lex 4. Idem. In terra qualibet regni nostri nostræ jurisdictioni subjecta, duos viros circumspectus et fide dignos volumnus ordinari et corporali per eos præstito sacramento teneri, quorum nomina ad curiam nostram mittentur, sub quorum testificatione, electuaria, et sirupi, ac aliæ medicinæ legaliter fiant, et sic factæ vendantur.

Salerni maxime per magistros in physica hoc volumus approbari. Præsentia etiam lege statuimus, ut nullus in medicina vel chirurgia, nisi apud Salernum vel Neapolim legat in regno, nec magistri nomen assumat, nisi diligenter examinatus in præsentia nostrorum officilalium, et magistrorum artis ejusdem.

Conficientes etiam medicinas sacramento corporaliter præstito volumus obligari, ut ipsas fideliter juxta artes et hominium qualitates, in præsentia juratorum conficiant; quod si contra fecerint, publicatione bonorum suorum mobilium sententialiter comdemnentur. Ordinati vero, quorum fidei prædicta sunt commissa, si fraudem in credito ipsis officio commisisse probentur, ultimo suplicio feriendos esse censimus.

APPENDIX D.

Ordonnances des Rois de France, Sub Philippe IV., dit le Bel, A. D., 1311.

Edicto presenti statuimus, ut in Villa et Vicecomitatu Parisiensi, nullus chirurgicus, nulla chirurgica, seu opus quomodolibet exercere præsumat, seu se immiscere eidem publice, vel occulte, in quacumque jurisdictione, seu terra, nisi per magistros chirurgicos juratos, morantes Parisius vocatus per dilectus magistrum Joannem Pitardi chirurgicum nostrum juratum Castelleti nostri Parisius tempore suo, ac per ejus successores in officio, qui ex juramenti sui vinculo, chirurgicos alios prædictos juratos vocare pro hujusmodi casu, quoties fuerit tenebuntur, et prius examinati fuerint diligenter, et approbati in ipsâ arte, ac ab ipso, vel ejus successoribus in officio, ut est dictum, juxta approbationem aliorum chirurgicorum, vel majoris partis eorum, ipsius vocantis voce inter alias numeratâ, licentiam operandi in arte prædicta meruerint obtinere: ad quem ratione sui officii, quod a nobis obtinet, et ad ejus successores in hujusmodi officio habebit licentiæ concessionem, non ad alium volumus pertinere.

Qui quidem per eum et ejus successores, modo præmisso examinati et approbati, antequam officii sui ad ministrationem attingant, juramentum prestare teneantur coram Preposito Parisiensi nostro, de hujusmodi officio fideliter exercendo, quod insuper vulneratum quemcunque non visitabant, seu parabant, in locis sacris, seu privilegiatis, nisi solum in prima vice, et quod statim factâ illâ primâ visitatione, sen paratione, vulnerationem illam Præposito nostro Parisiensi, vel ejus locum tenenti, seu Auditoribus Castelleti prædicti revelabunt, vel etiam intimabunt.

Damus itaque Præposito nostro Parisiensi moderno, et aliis pro tempore fuerint, præsentibus in mandatis, quatenus sub virtute juramenti quo administrationis suæ ratione tenentur, hujusmodi presens nostrum statutum faciant nunc et alias, cum expediens fuerit in villa et vicecomitatu prædictis publicari et firmiter observari, banneriasque omnium chirurgicorum et chirurgicarum prædictorum, non approbatorum et juratorum, ut permittur, post publicationem hujus Edicti domibus eorum appositas, coram domibus ipsorum publice comburi, personas capi, et in Castellum nostrum Parisiensi conducti, et tamdiu tenere quosque nobis fuerit legitime emendatum, eisdem districte et firmiter inhibendo, ne de cætero in arte prædicto practicare præsumant, nisi prius per dictum magistrum Joannem Pitardi, vel successores suos in officio dicto ut præmissum est, examinati et approbati fuerint, et juramenta præstiterint antedicta.

Si quis vero ipsorum ipsa præstare recusaverit. Nos eidem dictæ artis opus et exercitium penitus interdicere volumus. Et si contra interdictum et prohibitionem nostram dictæ artis practicæ se immiscere præsumpserint, ipsos per Præpositum nostrum prædictum, prout facti, qualitas poposcerit, et ad ipsum pertinuerit, volumus prima ratione puniri.

Quod ut ratum et stabile permanent, in futurum præsentes litteras sigilli nostri fecimus appositione muniri.

INDEX.

B.

C.

M.

N.

O.

P.

Q.

R.

S.

T.

X.

Y.

Z.